Improving Medical Outcome - Zero Tolerance

Anthony G. Gallagher • Gerald C. O'Sullivan

Petra Apell
Series Editor

Fundamentals of Surgical Simulation

Principles and Practices

Springer

Authors
Anthony G. Gallagher, PhD
School of Medicine
Brookfield Health Sciences Complex
College Road
University College Cork
Cork
Ireland

Gerald C. O'Sullivan, FRCSI, FACS
Consultant Surgeon
Mercy University Hospital
& Director in Chief
Cork Cancer Research Centre
University College Cork
Cork
Ireland

Series Editor
Petra Apell, M.Sc
Gothenburg, Sweden

ISBN 978-1-4471-2699-7 ISBN 978-0-85729-763-1 (eBook)
DOI 10.1007/978-0-85729-763-1
Springer London Dordrecht Heidelberg New York

British Library Cataloguing in Publication Data
A catalogue record for this book is available from the British Library

Cover design: eStudioCalamar, Figueres/Berlin

Printed on acid-free paper

Springer is part of Springer Science+Business Media (www.springer.com)

The art of progress is to preserve order amid change and to preserve change amid order.

—Alfred North Whitehead
(15 February 1861–30 December 1947)

Foreword and Introduction of Authors

From a health care administrative perspective, poor quality is primarily associated with higher cost. From a medical staff perspective, poor quality is a cause of disappointment and frustration for individuals and teams wanting to provide best possible care. For a patient, poor quality may result in a medical error drastically changing their quality of life.

With 20 years of experience in life sciences, primarily in medical skills training and business development, I have met powerful and insightful individuals with groundbreaking ideas whose research has contributed directly or indirectly to patient safety. What often strikes me, however, is that despite evidence of more people dying due to medical errors than from motor vehicle accidents, AIDS, and breast cancer; and despite recent improvement initiatives with proven clinical effect, such as the WHO Surgical Checklist, few practical solutions have been implemented and our society still puts very limited resources into issues concerning patient safety. To increase awareness and perhaps catalyze change, the book series "Improving Medical Outcome – Zero Tolerance" has been created. Each book will tackle a specific area of quality and patient safety; and leading experts will share their expertise and personal views on quality improvement strategies.

In this book, Prof. Anthony Gallagher and Prof. Gerald O'Sullivan have combined and integrated their unique perspectives on surgical training to produce a scholarly volume on training, learning, and practice of modern surgery. Prof. Gallagher is an experimental psychologist of international renown and a highly cited researcher in the field of human factors, objective assessment, and simulation. Prof. O'Sullivan is internationally renowned for his work as a practicing surgeon, cancer researcher, and professional leader within Irish, European, and World surgery. Using their expertise to analyze why modern image guided surgery is difficult to learn and practice, they have concluded that the difficulties faced are not just related to human factors, but arise from fundamental problems associated with a century old way of training in surgery. Gallagher and O'Sullivan propose the current Halstedian apprenticeship approach to training surgeons should be supplanted with a systematic, evidence-based, quality-assured approach based on simulation and not on clinical exposure and experience alone. They propose using a metric-based, deliberate practice curriculum requiring trainees to objectively demonstrate a pre-defined level of skills before being allowed to implement and consolidate their skills in the clinical environment. The authors give a detailed account of the principles and practices of how this approach to training works, i.e., Proficiency Based Progression (PBP), including insights into a number of clinical trials utilizing this approach. Prospective, randomized, and blinded clinical trials have shown that proficiency-based progression trained surgeons perform significantly better than their traditionally trained counterparts.

The implications of this proficiency-based approach to the training of surgeons are profound. Appropriately trained surgeons and fellow medical staff team members can be expected to more reliably and uniformly provide the best possible care to patients. Improved care and less medical errors will lead to reduced costs. Most importantly, the ramifications of the proposed training approach will have a real impact on the quality of care and safety at individual level.

It is my wish that this book will become a true companion for individuals working with medical skills training and assessment. A companion, giving valuable advice or perhaps just make you think and act differently.

Petra Apell, M.Sc.

Disclosure: Mrs. Apell has held senior positions at Orzone AB, Mentice AB and Johnson & Johnson. Mrs. Apell is owner of Aproficio AB, holds shares in Orzone AB, and ensures she has not influenced the authors of this book to favor any of the companies in which she has financial interests.

Preface

The spectacular developments in surgery and procedure based treatments brought to the agenda concerns about the training and development of skills by young doctors and the acquisition of modern techniques by experienced surgeons. There is a widespread recognition that the traditional system of skill development in the operating room is no longer adequate. Many of the operations that were commonly performed and were used in whole or in part for basic training experiences are no longer in common usage. Forty years ago a third-year general surgical resident could expect, each week, under supervision to perform or significantly participate in several open abdominal "set piece" operations such as vagotomy and drainage, open cholecystectomy, and hernia repair. The cure of ulcers by medical treatment replaced vagotomy and the widespread adoption of minimally invasive surgery for cholecystectomy and hernia repair removed large and important educational opportunities fundamental to the basic training programs of most of the surgical specialties. In addition, the introduction of working time directives and the requirement to train more surgeons without commensurate expansion of services restricted the clinical experience of the individual trainee.

The introduction of minimally invasive surgery, particularly laparoscopic cholecystectomy, was accompanied by an increased frequency of complications, many life-threatening, particularly during the early experiences. That these problems could occur when experienced surgeons, well versed in open procedures and with knowledge of anatomy and pitfalls embraced new procedural practices heightened concerns about the training of novices who lacked such a background in open surgery. But the agenda was now set, surgery needed to develop new methods for training the novice in surgical approaches in general and for training experienced surgeons in the newer techniques. A series of high profile adverse medical events drew the attention of the general public to issues of clinical training. The societal response was best epitomized by The Bristol Inquiry – "there can be no more learning curve on patients." Surgery was forced to confront realities and to consider new approaches to surgical training – particularly the development and use of simulation to train and develop new techniques and procedures "off site." Surgeon Trainers were forced to engage with psychologists and computer engineers to develop new simulation technologies and to validate simulation based transfer of training to the clinic and operating room.

In *Fundamentals of Surgical Simulation* we attempt to provide a resource for program directors, surgical trainers, surgical trainees, psychologists, simulation engineers, and researchers. For trainers, this book gives explicit theoretical and applied information on how this new training paradigm works thus allowing them to tailor the application of simulation training to their program, no matter where in the world they work. For the trainee, it allows them to see and understand the rules of this new training paradigm thus allowing them to optimize their approach to training and reaching proficiency in as efficient a manner as possible. For the simulation researcher, engineer, and medical profession *Fundamentals of Surgical Simulation* poses some difficult questions that require urgent unambiguous and agreed answers.

This book is the product of a friendship and mutual respect between an experimental psychologist and a practicing surgeon/surgeon trainer. This friendship permits forthright exchanges of views and endures many agreements and disagreements particularly on the science and philosophy of surgical simulation, training, assessment, and validation. The outcome has been consensus, fellowship, friendship, and an abundance of (Irish) *craic*.

AGG
GCO'S

Acknowledgments

We wish to acknowledge the following for their contributions not only to this book but also for their many generous discussions which shaped our thinking:

Mrs. Lorna Doherty (Jordanstown, NI) for her diligence, patient proof-reading, and helpful comments on the first complete draft of each chapter.

Dr. Kieran McGlade (Medicine, Queens' University Belfast), Prof. Brendan Bunting (Psychology, University of Ulster, Derry), and Prof. Lars Lonn (Radiology, Rigshospitalet, Copenhagen) for reading and commenting on specific chapters.

Paul Coulter (Queen's University, Belfast) for invaluable computer and technical support during the writing.

Dr. Dwight Meglan for technical advice and discussion about haptics, full-physics simulation, and open surgical simulation.

Prof. Peter Hamilton (Pathology, Queen's University, Belfast) for discussions about imaging and image compression.

Prof. Rick Satava (University of Washington, Seattle) who suggested the title for the book, for his friendship and fellowship over the years.

Prof. Sir Alfred Cuschieri who (along with Rick Satava) is one of the most original scientific thinkers in modern surgery.

Prof. Dana K. Anderson who as Chief of Surgery at Yale University (during AGG's time as Fulbright Distinguished Scholar there) made the first prospective, randomized, blinded clinical trial on proficiency-based virtual reality training possible.

Prof. Neal Seymour (Surgery, Tufts University, Springfield) who was the surgeon PI on the Yale clinical trial.

Prof. Randy Haluck (Surgery, Penn. State, Hershey) for numerous enjoyable and insightful conversations and discussions about the practicalities and detail of surgical simulation.

Outstanding surgeons who got the whole "metrics thing" so quickly and helped to clarify and expand our understanding: Mr. Sean Carroll (Plastic Surgery, St. Vincent's Hospital, Dublin), Mr. Paul Neary (Colorectal Surgery, Tallaght Hospital, Dublin), Mr. Tom Diamond (Hepatobiliary Surgery, The Mater Hospital, Belfast), Mr. Jim McGuigan (Thoracic Surgery, Royal Victoria Hospital, Belfast), Prof. Howard Champion (Trauma Surgery, USUHS, Bethesda, Maryland), Prof. Sean Tierney (Vascular Surgery, Tallaght Hospital and RCSI), Prof. Lorraine

Cassidy (Ophthalmic Surgery, Trinity College, Dublin), Prof. Gerry Leonard, (Otolaryngology, Hartford, Connecticut), Dr. Pat Cregan (Nepean Hospital, NSW), Prof. John Collins (Breast Surgery, RACS).

Also, colleagues in medicine who helped to shape our thinking beyond surgery: Dr. Christopher U Cates (Cardiology, Emory University, Atlanta) and Dr. Peter Kearney (Cardiology, University College Hospital, Cork), Dr. Steve Dawson (Radiology, Brigham and Women's Hospital, Boston) and Prof. Dave Gaba (Anaesthetics/Simulation, Stanford, Palo Alto).

Prof. George Shorten (Anaesthetics/Dean of Medicine, University College Cork): A new breed of medical leadership that understands the opportunities and threats offered by simulation based training.

We specifically want to acknowledge the leadership given and the contributions by Prof. Gerry Healy (Children's Hospital, Boston) and Prof. Carlos Pellegrini (University of Washington, Seattle) for championing simulation in the American College of Surgeons, the American Board of Surgery, and the American Surgical Association.

We are particularly grateful to the surgical colleagues, Fellows, and trainees at the Mercy University Hospital, Cork Cancer Research Centre, Yale University, Emory University, School of Psychology, Queen's University Belfast, Royal Victoria Hospital Belfast, and the Royal College of Surgeons in Ireland for their friendship, support, and patience.

This work could not have been possible without the enormous support of our families – Liz, Conor, and Cullen; Breda, Orla, Gearoid, and Eoghan.

Anthony G. Gallagher
Gerald C. O'Sullivan

Contents

Chapter 1
Agents of Change

Halsted: The Beginning of the Modern Surgical Training Program

In August 1922, Dr. William Stewart Halsted returned to Baltimore from his summer retreat (High Hampton, North Carolina) with symptoms of choledocholithiasis. He had had his gallbladder successfully removed at Johns Hopkins Hospital in August 1919 and had remained symptom free until this occasion. However, despite a successful reoperation and attentive care by his colleagues he developed pneumonia and pleurisy of which he died on Thursday, 7 September 1922. Even at the start of the twenty-first century the stature of Halsted's contribution to medicine remains undiminished despite revelations about his private life. He was educated at Yale University (where there is no record of him ever borrowing a book from the library) and the University College of Physicians and Surgeons in New York, after which he took up a position as a house physician at the New York Hospital. One of his earliest contributions to patient care that still exists to this day is the introduction of the temperature, pulse, and respiration recordings to the patients chart. In 1884, Halsted commenced a series of experiments on himself and his colleagues investigating the anesthetic powers of cocaine. Unfortunately, during the process of these experiments Halsted and several of his colleagues became addicted to cocaine. Although hospitalized and treated for his addiction on at least two occasions it emerged after his death that his addiction had been treated by switching from cocaine to morphine, to which he remained addicted throughout his life. Most of his peers and colleagues assumed that his addiction to cocaine had been cured during his hospitalization in Rhode Island. However, private diary notes by Sir William Osler (the first chief of medicine at the Johns Hopkins Hospital), who was also Halsted's physician, clearly indicated that Halsted was never able to eliminate his daily use of morphine. Osler noted that Halsted could work comfortably and maintain his "excellent physical vigor" on three grains of morphine per day (about 180 mg). In later years (i.e., 1912), Osler noted that Halsted had reduced his consumption to about 1½ grains/day.

A.G. Gallagher and G.C. O'Sullivan, *Fundamentals of Surgical Simulation*, Improving Medical Outcome - Zero Tolerance,
DOI 10.1007/978-0-85729-763-1_1,

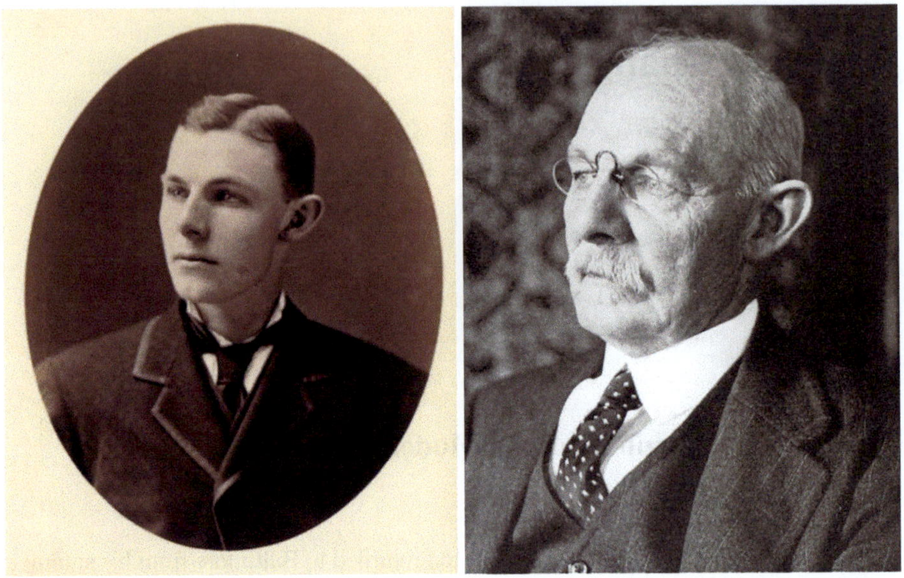

Fig. 1.1 Dr. William Stewart Halsted (1852–1922). Portrait of William Stewart Halsted, Yale College class of 1874 (Photograph courtesy of the Yale University Manuscripts & Archives Digital Images Database, Yale University, New Haven, CT)

During his time living and working in New York, Halsted was outgoing, gregarious, sociable, energetic, and vigorous. However, when he moved to Baltimore he led a quiet and scholarly life which bordered on reclusive. He appeared to be a solitary figure with few friends or close acquaintances at Hopkins throughout his career. Dr. John Cameron (1997) a subsequent Chairman of Surgery at Johns Hopkins speculated that this marked change in Halsted's demeanor probably resulted from his humiliation by his addiction. Despite this burden Halsted's contributions to surgery included recognizing the importance of submucosal suturing for intestinal anastomosis, development of radical mastectomy for cancer of the breast, and development of a surgical procedure for inguinal hernia repair. He was also the first surgeon to promulgate the philosophy of safe surgery by introducing rubber gloves into the operating room and advocating that the gentle handling of tissues, careful hemostasis, and the use of meticulous surgical technique. Even though general anesthesia had been introduced in the early nineteenth century, during Halsted's time most surgeons still operated rapidly with little concern for hemostasis (as though the patient was still awake during the procedure). By the time of his death the American surgical community had accepted his philosophy of safe surgery and took full advantage of the operative benefits anesthesia afforded for technical skills application during surgery. However, Halsted's (Fig. 1.1) single greatest contribution to modern healthcare was the development and implementation of the first system to train young surgeons.

Surgical Training

In the latter part of the nineteenth century there were no formal training programs in surgery. Individuals who were qualified or experienced in the practice of surgery were not particularly interested in training other surgeons who might then become competitors in private practice. Halsted devised a surgical training program at Johns Hopkins Hospital based on what he had learned from a number of well-known European surgeons. He established a surgical training program that was based on strict dedication to the bedside study of disease and graded responsibility with a clinical teacher. He also established that surgery was best learned by hands on experience and education within a hierarchical training program. His training program consisted of a 1-year internship, followed by 6 years as an assistant resident. If successfully navigated, this period culminated in 2 years as a house surgeon. The term (surgical) "resident" comes from Halsted's training program. His trainee surgeons were discouraged from marrying, lived in the hospital where room, board, and training were provided in exchange for service to the hospital 24 h a day, 7 days a week. This pattern of long work hours and service commitment was wedded (and indeed probably still is in some quarters) to the persona of becoming a surgeon.

The training system developed by Halsted at John Hopkins Hospital was based on the German system, and as such, it was autocratic and pyramidal in structure. Although eight residents entered training in first year, four of these positions were for only 1 year and of the remaining four, only one became a surgeon and the other three spent long periods of time with no guarantee of becoming staff surgeons. The system aimed at producing one outstanding surgeon that then went on to become a Professor (Grillo 2004). In this sense, the Johns Hopkins training model worked very well as graduating surgeons went on to establish training programs at other distinguished institutions such as Yale, Duke, and Brigham Hospital based on the Halsted training model.

One of the first major changes to this training system was introduced by Dr. Edward Delos Churchill (1895–1972) at Massachusetts General Hospital (MGH). Churchill was critical of the Halstedian training model for two reasons. The first was that the training model developed at Johns Hopkins unintendedly produced a number of poorly trained surgeons because they left training after completion of 1 year or shortly afterward. The second reason was that the training system was somewhat authoritarian in that it depended on the formation of a relationship between the dominant master surgeon and the docile trainee. Churchill believed that this was anti-intellectual (Pellegrini 2006). Churchill proposed a new training structure at MGH which intellectually and philosophically departed considerably from the traditional Halstedian approach to training. In the traditional MGH training structure there were eight residents, six of which were trained for 2 years with two being advanced to the 4th year level. The first change that Churchill advocated was that the total number of residents entering the training system in any given year should be decreased to six, with four of them obtaining a 4-year training (which meant they were fully trained) and two would remain in the hospital and might be destined to become master surgeons at MGH or go on to take up leading academic positions at other institutions. However, he also proposed that the residents should be trained by a group of master surgeons rather than a single dominant personality. One of his intentions in implementing this training structure appears to have been to minimize or obviate the self-aggrandizing and authoritarian relationship which was such an integral part of the apprenticeship model of training (Grillo 2004). The rectangular system proposed by Churchill would remain, with minor modifications, the core structure of the residency training systems in the USA until the end of the twentieth century. As Pellegrini (2006) points out, Churchill believed that the residency training structure should be implemented in such a way that it allowed for flexibility which enabled individual residents to follow up any specific interests they had and it also allowed the acquisition and development of proficiency. This idea of proficiency and flexibility in progression will be discussed further in Chap. 8.

The enactment of the servicemen's readjustment act of 1944 (or the GI BILL) was a defining moment for surgical training. It was created to train medical officers returning from World War II and marked the first time that surgical trainees in the USA received payment (Sheldon 2007). Although surgical trainees received some payment, the life of surgical trainees remained austere up until the 1970s. Just as in Halsted's era, they rarely left the hospital which provided them with meals, white uniforms, laundry, and somewhere to sleep. The next major change in surgical trainees' lifestyle was initiated by the Medicare and Medicaid Act of 1965 which provided a mechanism for surgical trainees to receive financial compensation for care that they had previously given for free (Sheldon 2007). Surgical trainees observed huge increases in their salaries as a result of this landmark health care legislation. Possibly as a result of these changes and changes in attitudes to work during the 1960s and 1970s, the restrictive lifestyle of the Halstedian training paradigm began to lessen. Trainees began to marry and move out of the hospital and were no longer available for service delivery 24 h a day (Wallack and Chao 2001). Despite these changes, surgical training remained arduous with the trainees working long hours, frequently on call every other night and going home only after the work was completed. Indeed, this work ethic and culture persisted in surgical training until the late twentieth century when the death of a young woman in a New York hospital brought into question the safety of having trainee doctors who had been on duty for long hours take care of sick patients.

Agents of Change

The Halstedian approach to training in surgery existed for the best part of a century, and despite its critics was effective. Indeed, it was so effective that the rest of medicine, more or less imitated the training program that had been pioneered at the Johns Hopkins and refined at MGH in Boston. However, all that was to change in the latter part of the twentieth century. Surgical training was about to undergo a paradigm shift in the way surgeons were trained and this revolution would impact on how *all* doctors were trained. Thomas Kuhn (1962) argued that science does not progress via a linear accumulation of new knowledge but undergoes periodic revolutions or so-called *paradigm shifts* in which the nature of scientific enquiry within a particular field is abruptly transformed. He also argued that paradigm shifts do not occur by accident, but instead are driven by agents of change. An agent of change can be something as simple as a growing body of evidence that demonstrates significant anomalies against an accepted paradigm or approach (such as the Halstedian approach to training). At some point in the accrual of this evidence the discipline is thrown into a state of crisis. During this crisis, new ideas, perhaps ones previously discarded are tried. Eventually, a new paradigm is formed which gains its own new followers and an intellectual battle takes place between the followers of the new paradigm and those who held on to the old paradigm. However, Kuhn (1962) argues that this is not simply an evolution of ideas, but a revolution. Furthermore, the new paradigm is *always* better and not just different. Paradigm shifts have occurred most frequently in the natural sciences and have always been dramatic, particularly in what appeared to be a stable and mature area of research and study. For example, Lord Kelvin in an address to an assemblage of physicists at the British Association for the Advancement of Science in 1900 famously stated that "there is nothing new to be discovered in physics now. All that remains is more and more precise measurement" (Smith and Wise 1989). Five years later, Albert Einstein published his paper on special theory of relativity which fundamentally challenged the bases of Newtonian mechanics (Pais 2005). In this chapter we will argue that the agents of change impinging on the discipline of surgery were worldwide, varied, pervasive and persuasive and cried out for a different and better way to prepare surgeons for operating on patients. The outcome of this revolution has been precisely that. In the coming pages, we will describe what we believe have been the agents of change.

The Libby Zion Case, USA

Libby Zion was an 18-year-old woman admitted to the New York Hospital, Cornell Medical Center, with fever, agitation, delirium, and strange jerking movements of her body on March 4, 1984 (Asch and Parker 1988). Within 8 h of admission, she was dead. The exact cause of her death was never conclusively demonstrated although it is widely suspected that she died because of serotonin syndrome. Her father, a lawyer and New York Times columnist, believed that she had died as a result of inadequate care from overworked and inadequately supervised medical residents. Her father conducted a very public and emotional campaign against the hospital and doctors and claimed that the death of his daughter was tantamount to murder. In 1987, the intern and resident who cared for Libby Zion were charged with 38 counts of gross negligence and/or gross incompetence. The grand jury considered evidence that a series of mistakes contributed to Libby Zion's death including the improper prescription drugs and the failure to perform adequate diagnostic tests. Under New York law, the investigative body for these charges was the Hearing Committee of the State Board for Professional Medical Conduct. The hearing committee unanimously decided that none of the 38 charges against the two residents were supported by evidence (Spritz 1991). However, the final deliberations on this case rested with another body, the Board of Regents. In a surprise decision the Board of Regents voted to censure and reprimand the resident physicians for acts of gross negligence. Although the decision did not affect their right to practice as doctors and was overturned in the appeal Court in 1991, the decision of the Board of Regents caused considerable concern among practicing physicians in New York City and nationally.

As a result of a grand jury indictment of the two residents, the New York State Health Commissioner (David Axelrod) established a blue ribbon panel of experts headed by Dr. Bertrand M. Bell from Albert Einstein College of Medicine to address the problems in residency training. The Bell Commission put forward a series of recommendations that addressed several patient care issues one of which was resident work hours (Asch and Parker 1988). In particular, they recommended that residents could not work more than 80 h a week or more than 24 consecutive hours. In 2003 the Accreditation Council for Graduate Medical Education (ACGME) adopted similar regulations for all accredited medical training institutions in the USA (Philibert et al. 2002). These changes in training practices shook the medical establishment to its very roots and continue to reverberate. In general, both residents in training and attending surgeons thought that the quality of care given to patients had been negatively affected by the introduction of an 80 h work week (Whang et al. 2003) despite objective evidence that found no differences in the quality of care received by patients or quality of education experience received by trainees pre-and post the introduction of the ACGME work hour limit (Hutter et al. 2006).

European Working Time Directive

In the USA, pressures to reduce the number of hours worked by doctors in training emanated from an incident that occurred in medicine. However, pressures to reduce the number of hours worked by junior doctors in training in the UK and Europe derived from an entirely different source. The European Union Working Time Directive (EWTD) was first drafted in 1993 and was introduced to improve the living and employment conditions of workers within the European Economic Community. The most commonly known clause within the directive is that which is associated with a 48-h working week and the opt-out associated with it (Adnett and Hardy 2001). The directive, adopted in 1993 and amended in 2003 has been incrementally introduced in European nations with the final stage introduced on August 1, 2009. When first adopted in November 1993 the working time directive excluded the air, rail, road, sea, inland waterway and lake transport, sea fishing, offshore work, and the activities of doctors in training, as it was decided that these sectors required individual specific legislation to accommodate working time measures. A further directive covering these sectors, known as Horizontal Amending Directive was adopted on August 1, 2000. The entitlements in this legislation include:

- A limit of an average of 48 h work a week, up to maximum of 60 in any one week
- A limit of an average of 8 h work in 24, but no more than 10
- A right for night workers to receive free health assessments
- A right to 11 h rest a day
- A right to a day off each week
- A right to an in-work rest break if the working day is longer than 6 h
- A right to 4 weeks paid leave per year

It is fair to say that few issues have generated as much controversy or legal challenges as this directive, particularly within the medical profession. Doctors' leaders argued that if their American colleagues found it challenging to train doctors in the ACGME mandated 80 h/week, they would find it impossible within a 48-h time frame. When the legislation was first introduced there was some compromise with its implementation. However, in 2008 the European Parliament voted to end the right of individual doctors in member states to opt out of the directive. There is little doubt that the EWTD posed considerable organizational difficulties for its implementation in medicine. It was also widely believed that the directive compromised the training of future surgeons (Lowry and Cripps 2005) and as such was unpopular with UK trainee and trainer surgeons. In the UK, the implementation of the EWTD meant that doctors had to move to a shift pattern of working. This type of work practice allows important information loss about clinical care during the increased number of handovers. However, it should be remembered why this legislation was introduced in the first place.

The practice of working at night was made possible by Edison's commercialization of electric light in 1882. This extended the working day to 24 h a day, 7 days a week; fatigue caused by working longer hours and round-the-clock became a major social issue. The emerging labor movement in the early 1900s eventually influenced work hour regulations and laws and the concept of hours of service regulation emerged. As a result, the issue of workplace fatigue became intertwined with labor pay and rights issues and led to regulatory limits on work duration and minimums of off-duty time duration in all transportation modes by the middle of the twentieth century (Moore-Ede 1993). Research conducted in the late 1970s demonstrated that the brain's circadian clock exerted strong control over time, duration, and stages of sleep. Because of this circadian regulation of sleep, there was an important difference between sleep opportunity and the amount of sleep it was possible to obtain during that opportunity. For example, even under ideal sleeping conditions, individuals who slept 8 h when they went to bed at 11 p.m. would only sleep 6 h if they went to bed at 3 a.m., and only 4 h if they went to bed at 11 a.m. even though they had been kept awake all night (Åkerstedt and Gillberg 1986; Daan et al. 1984).

Around about the same time studies reporting on the link between sleep pattern, fatigue, and accidents started to appear in the scientific literature (Dembe et al. 2005; Samkoff and Jacques 1991; Schuster and Rhodes 1985; Wojtczak-Jaroszowa and Jarosz 1987). Furthermore, a series of major industrial accidents occurred between 1970 and 1990 where human operating errors related to fatigue were linked. These included:

- The Chernobyl nuclear reactor explosion in the Ukraine, where 237 people suffered from acute radiation sickness of whom 31 died within the first 3 months, 135,000 people were evacuated from the area (Hallenbeck 1994).
- Flixborough, where a chemical plant explosion destroyed an English Village on 1 June 1974, killing 28 people and seriously injuring 36.
- Piper Alpha North Sea oil platform which exploded and killed 167 people in 1988.
- In the city of Bhopal, India, December 3, 1984 a poisonous gas cloud escaped from the Union Carbide India Limited (UCIL) pesticide factory. The cloud contained 15 metric tons of methyl isocyanate (MIC) covering an area of more than 30 square miles. The gas leak killed at least 4,000 local residents instantly and caused health problems for at least 50,000 others.

These types of incidents led to in-depth analyses of how they occurred and precipitated the evolution of a systematic understanding of the relationship between human operative error and fatigue. These efforts have been greatly informed by the work of Prof. James Reason (1990) who had been an advisor to the Royal Air Force and NASA on human error. Reason pointed out that most major accidents are the result of multiple latent system errors and not just by the immediately obvious act of error by the human controller (Reason 1990). He suggested that many accidents were in fact not accidents but a series of events that set the occasion for an adverse event to happen. All that it took for these "accidents" to occur was the right set of environmental circumstances which invariably revolved around a person or persons. Avoidable human factors such as fatigue due to sleep deprivation which are known to be associated with increased probability of errors should not be allowed to happen, should be specifically anticipated and dealt with at a senior organizational level.

The relationship between errors in medicine and sleep deprivation was established in the 1970s (Friedman et al. 1971). Friedman et al., reported that interns made almost twice as many errors reading electrocardiograms after an extended workshift (i.e., 24 h or more) than after a night's sleep. More recent studies have shown that surgical residents make up to twice as many errors in the performance of a simulated laparoscopic surgical task after working overnight than after a night of sleep (Grantcharov et al. 2001). Although the literature as a whole suggests that sleep deprivation causes substantial decrements in physicians' performance (Gaba and Howard 2002; Weinger and Ancoli-Israel 2002) this is not accepted by some in the medical community. For example, Dr. Malcolm Lewis, Director of Postgraduate Education for General Practice at the School of Postgraduate Medical and Dental Education in Cardiff University (Wales) and chairman of the Committee of General Practice Education Directors, (a UK-based forum) has questioned the relationship between fatigue, work hours, and medical errors. In an interview for a Canadian medical Journal, he stated that "the perceived advantages [of the EWTD] are of less tired workforce and of improved patient safety as a result. This is of course theoretical and I am not aware of a body of evidence to support the perception" (Villaneuva 2010). It is of course possible that Dr. Lewis is unaware of the large volume of well-controlled, quantitative research that directly links decrements in performance to fatigue and sleep deprivation. However, what is less believable is that he is unaware of the results from studies in medicine, published in leading medical journals that have directly established a relationship between medical error, sleep deprivation, and fatigue. For example, Landrigan et al. (2004) investigated the effects of reducing intern work hours on serious medical errors in intensive care units, using a prospective, randomized study design. They compared performance of interns working according to a traditional schedule with extended (i.e., 24 h or more) work shifts every other shift (i.e., and every third night call schedule) and a schedule that eliminated extended work shifts and reduced the number of hours worked per week to 63 h. They found that interns made significantly more serious medical errors when they worked frequent shifts of 24 h than when they worked shorter shifts. Interns made approximately 21% more serious medication errors during the traditional schedule and they were also five times more likely to make a serious diagnostic error. Furthermore, the data for this study was from direct observation of the intern's performance rather than self-reported.

From the wealth of published data on the effects of fatigue on performance in a variety of industrial and occupational settings, the results are unambiguous, i.e., it significantly degrades human performance and considerably increases the probability that an error will be enacted. However, fatigue poses a particular and very real problem on a daily basis for particular types of surgical specialties such as neurosurgery, ophthalmic surgery, otolaryngology surgery, plastic surgery, or any type of surgery requiring a microsurgical techniques (e.g., tendon repair, vascular anastomosis, etc.). Physiological tremor arises from mechanical and neuromuscular sources and is made worse by a number of factors such as dehydration, caffeine, cigarettes, anger, fear, stress, and fatigue (Patkin 1977). Unfortunately for surgeons using this particular technique, increased hand tremor is a natural result of normal operating procedures and is a simple fact of the job resulting from muscle fatigue (Slack and Ma 2007). Surgeons who employ microsurgical techniques on a regular basis go to great lengths in an effort to control their hand tremor. These include biofeedback training, maintenance of a healthy lifestyle, ensuring they are well hydrated before operating, abstaining from coffee and nicotine, and sometimes resorting to taking beta-blockers (Elman et al. 1998; Ferguson and Jobe 2004; Harwell and Ferguson 1983). However, within these operators, fatigue is recognized as the most tremor producing factor and situations which induce fatigue prior to operating should be, where possible, avoided. Unfortunately, injuries which require the application of these types of surgical skills occur irregularly but commonly at inconvenient times such as during the night, in a patient admitted to accident and emergency as a result of a road traffic accident. The only safe approach to this type of scenario is for the surgeons to maintain a state of readiness, and that means minimizing surgical interventions by fatigued surgeons.

Other factors that need to be kept in mind are the findings from the 1960s, relating performance to levels of arousal and the presence of others, who would appear to have important implications for the practice of surgery. Scientific investigation of the effects of an audience dates back over a century. In 1904, a German researcher conducted experiments concerned with muscular effort and fatigue. He noted that the subjects were able to exert far more muscle effort on days that he watched as compared to the days on which they were not watched (Meumann 1904). However, Zajonc (1965) suggested that the situation was not that simple, and that the presence of others energized individuals and increased their drive level. An increase in drive strengthens the dominant response of the organism, i.e., the response most likely to occur. At the same time, an increase in drive weakens responses that already are weak. What this means is that under stressful conditions individuals will respond in a way that is very familiar or is easier for them. For example, in a simple or well-learned task, familiarity with what is required exists or the task has been practiced several times, thus the strongest and most likely response is the one that is appropriate and correct. In a complex and difficult task on the other hand, the strongest response is likely to be the wrong one. Complicating matters further is the Yerkes–Dodson law (Yerkes and Dodson 1908) which establishes an empirical relationship between arousal and performance. The law dictates that performance increases with physiological or mental arousal, but only up to a point. When levels of arousal become too high, performance decreases. The process is often illustrated graphically as a curvilinear, inverted U-shaped curve which increases and then decreases with higher levels of arousal. What this means for the practicing surgeon is that the skills which are very familiar and or well trained are more likely to be performed well in situations of stress whereas surgical skills which are unfamiliar and or novel to them will not be performed well. These predictions have profound implications for trainee surgeons, particularly in stress provoking situations such as in accident and emergency or in the operating room when unanticipated complications occur. This type of response is most likely to occur for surgical trainees (of *any* level of seniority) if the skills they are required to practice are novel, unpredictable, not under the control of the individual, and required to be practiced in the presence of an experienced evaluator (e.g., a more senior surgeon part of whose job is to appraise their performance). Lupien et al. (2007) have reviewed the evidence of the psychophysiological effects of stress hormones (glucocorticoids) on the process of forming long-term memory. They concluded that mildly elevated levels of glucocorticoids enhanced long-term memory formation. In contrast, long-term memory formation is impaired after adrenalectomy (which causes chronic low glucocorticoid levels) or after exogenous glucocorticoids administration (e.g., subcutaneous injection) thus demonstrating an inverted U-shaped performance reminiscent of the Yerkes–Dodson effect.

The Bristol Case, UK

In 1989 Dr. Stephen Bolsin moved from the Brompton Hospital in London to take up position as a consultant cardiac anesthetist at the Bristol Royal Infirmary. He very quickly formed the opinion that the Bristol Royal infirmary had significantly higher complication and mortality rates than what he was accustomed to, and probably higher than the national average complication rate. He identified that too many babies were dying during heart surgery and although he raised his concerns with senior hospital administrators, they refused to investigate. He eventually took his concerns to the media and the ensuing investigation became known as *The Bristol Case* (Smith 1998). The Bristol case centered around three doctors: Mr. James Wisheart, a former medical director of the United Bristol Healthcare trust; Mr. Janardan Dhasmana, a pediatric and adult cardiac surgeon; and Dr. John Roylance, a former radiologist and Chief Executive of the Trust. The central allegations against these individuals were that they knowingly allowed to be carried out or carried out operations on children, knowing that the mortality rates for these operations in the hands of the surgeons were higher than the national average. Furthermore, the operating surgeons were accused of not communicating to the parents the correct risk of death for these operations in *their* hands.

One of the earliest concerns raised by Dr. Bolsin was that Mr. Wisheart's operations took up to three times as long as those at the Brompton Hospital and were associated with more complications. By 1993, he had concluded a formal audit that showed that while national average mortality rate for repair of tetralogy of Fallot was 7%, Mr. Wisheart's was 33% and Mr. Dhasmana's was 25%. The audit also showed that while national average mortality rate for atrioventricular canal surgery was 10%, Mr. Wisheart's was 60% and Mr. Dhasmana's was 17%. By the time Mr. Wisheart had retired in 1995, seven of the last eight children that he operated on died. At about the same time Mr. Dhasmana began performing arterial switch procedures on neonates. Although he stopped after performing the procedure on 13 patients, 9 of them died and 1 of them had sustained serious brain damage. A team in Birmingham (87 miles north-east from Bristol) who were performing the same procedure had only 1 death in 200 patients. Mr. Dhasmana's results in older children were also cause for concern with a mortality of 30% compared to about 1% in centers of excellence.

Although Dr. Bolsin contacted the Department of Health in 1993, it was not until 1995 that a new consultant cardiac surgeon was appointed. The Bristol Royal Infirmary Inquiry was chaired by Professor Sir Ian Kennedy and was a landmark case in that it changed how medicine was learned and practiced in the UK (Bristol Royal Infirmary Inquiry 2001). Mr. Wisheart and Dr. Roylance were struck off the medical register and Mr. Dhasmana was disqualified from practicing pediatric cardiac surgery for 3 years. The enquiry concluded that a substantially and statistically significant number of excess deaths (between 30 and 35) occurred in children between 1991 and 1995. The mortality rate over the period was probably double the rate in England at the time for children under one and was even higher in children under 30 days (Bristol Royal Infirmary Inquiry 2001).

Dr. Richard Smith (1998) in his editorial in the British Medical Journal (BMJ) seemed to summarize very well the impact that the Bristol Case would have on medicine in the UK and the international reverberations from it when he said that medicine would be transformed by the case. It had thrown up a long list of important issues that British medical practitioners would take years to address which has proved correct. These included:

- The need for clearly understood clinical standards
- How clinical competence and technical expertise are assessed and evaluated
- The training of doctors in advanced procedures
- How to approach the so-called learning curve of doctors undertaking established procedures
- The reliability and validity of data used to monitor doctors' personal performance

There were many other issues raised, which included an appreciation of factors other than purely clinical ones that affect clinical judgment performance and outcome, team leadership, and responsibility and communicating with patients and families. One of the more uncomfortable issues that The Bristol Case raised was the need for doctors to take prompt action at an early stage when a colleague was in difficulty in order to offer the best chance of avoiding damage to patients and a colleague to put things right.

Just like the Libby Zion case in New York, the problems that were encountered in Bristol met with intense and sustained political, media, and public interest both in the UK and internationally (Walshe and Offen 2001). It also brought into sharp focus issues relating to professional regulation, clinical competence, and health care quality improvement in medicine. Furthermore, much of this debate was conducted on the front page of national newspapers and television chat shows. One of the aspects of this case that was very striking to the UK general public was the fact that senior hospital managers (some of whom were doctors themselves) knew that some of their surgeons were underperforming and despite frequent, often public, protestations from clinical colleagues they did not act. The trust between doctors and patients had been compromised by this case and the general public was unambiguously aware of this fact. It was a very public failure of doctors and the health care system.

The Neary Case, Ireland

Our Lady of Lourdes Hospital is a 340-bed public hospital located in Drogheda, County Louth, Ireland. It provides acute-care hospital services, including a 24-hour emergency department for the population of County Louth and the North East of the Irish Republic. In serves a population of about 110,000 out-patients, and more than 20,000 in-patients. It is also a very busy maternity hospital with more than 4,000 births a year. It had previously been owned by the Medical Missionaries of Mary who were founded in 1939 by Mother Mary Martin. It was the first hospital founded by the order. The order set up the hospital, then called the "International Missionary Training Hospital," in Drogheda. It served the people of Drogheda and the surrounding regions, and it also served to train personnel for hospitals in Africa. Nurses and patients for the most part refer to the hospital as "The Lourdes," a shortened version of its full title Our Lady of Lourdes Hospital. Many of the older consultants referred and still refer to the hospital as the IMTH (International Missionary Training Hospital). The hospital provided services that accorded with the ethos of the Roman Catholic Church – including its teachings on human reproduction (Harding Clark 2006). In sum, the hospital had a strong Irish Catholic history.

In 1998 Dr. Michael Neary was asked by his employer to take administrative leave for 2 weeks from his post as a consultant gynecologist at the hospital after concerns about his clinical practice were expressed by two experienced midwives. In 1998 three senior consultant obstetricians from major teaching hospitals in Dublin were asked to review the practices of Dr. Neary between the years 1996 and 1998. Seventeen caesarean hysterectomies identified from the maternity theater register were to be reviewed. The three obstetricians met with Dr. Neary and considered each case in turn. However, of the 17 cases they were asked to review, 8 were excluded on the bases that Dr. Neary had informed them that these were consented hysterectomies necessitated because of the prohibition in the hospital of tubal ligation. Their reports exonerated Dr. Neary's clinical practice. The health board was uncomfortable with this report and asked for a fourth opinion. They requested a review from a very senior practicing obstetrician consultant at St Mary's Hospital in Manchester where he was lead clinician in the labor ward which had more than 6,000 births each year. The Manchester obstetrician reviewed the same nine cases previously reviewed by the three obstetricians acting for Dr. Neary. His report stated that he had major concerns about Dr. Neary continuing to practice as a consultant obstetrician. Unfortunately this report was leaked to the press and it made national headlines throughout the subsequent investigation into the case.

The Medical Council of Ireland received complaints from 15 patients who had procedures carried out by Dr. Neary during the years 1986–1990, including ten complaints alleging unwarranted peripartum hysterectomies. The Medical Council commenced its enquiry on 6 June 2000 and continued taking evidence over the next 2 years. These ten complaints included the nine cases reviewed by Dr. Neary's review group and the English obstetrician from Manchester. On 29 June 2003 the Medical Council's Fitness to Practice Committee found that the facts in relation to the ten complaints alleging unwarranted peripartum hysterectomies were proved and that Dr. Neary was found guilty of professional misconduct. The Medical Council determined that his name should be erased from the General Register of Registered Medical Practitioners.

The Inquiry into peripartum hysterectomy at Our Lady of Lourdes Hospital, Drogheda, chaired by Judge Maureen Harding Clarke S.C. was established by the Government in 2004 following the decision of the Medical Council to remove Dr. Neary from the Register of Medical Practitioners. They found that a total of 188 peripartum hysterectomies were carried out in the 25-year period between 1974 and 1998. Of the 188 cases, 129 cases were attributed to Dr. Neary. An average consultant obstetrician would perform about five or six operations in an entire career. The rate of Caesarean hysterectomies at the hospital for the period was 1 in every 37 Caesarean sections. In contrast, the rate at other hospitals of similar ethos ranged from 1/300 to 1/254 Caesarean sections. Although concerns were raised in 1978/1979 by the then matron her concerns were not heeded. Indeed, no issues were raised about Dr. Neary's practice until 1998 when the two midwives raised the issue with the Health Board solicitor. Furthermore, the unit was passed for training by the Royal College of Obstetricians and Gynaecologists in 1987 and again in 1992. The unit was also passed by the Royal College of Surgeons in Ireland (RCSI) for undergraduate training and by Bord Altranais for midwifery training. The inquiry also found that 23.4% of obstetric hysterectomy records (44 cases) for the period 1974–1998 were missing and were intentionally and unlawfully removed from the hospital with the object of protecting those involved in hysterectomies or protecting the reputation of the hospital. In 40 of the 44 cases the birth registers were also missing (Harding Clark 2006).

This case is important because, just like the Bristol Case in the UK, it changed the public's perception of doctors in an otherwise very conservative country where doctors were held in very high esteem. Indeed, when Dr. Neary was suspended there was enormous support for him and outrage by many of his patients and colleagues at his treatment. However, as the facts of the case emerged sympathy turned to anger. In particular, there was considerable anger at what the public perceived as the medical profession's attempts to cover up its own mistakes. The three consultant obstetricians who conducted the original review were perceived as trying to protect their own and this was specifically commented on in the inquiry (Harding Clark 2006).

This was the worst case of medical misconduct ever to have occurred in Ireland. It resulted in significant modifications to the Medical Practitioners Bill in the country which made continuing professional development and education compulsory for all medical practitioners. It also established in law for the first time a statutory obligation for competence assurance for medical practitioners. More than a decade after questions first started to be asked about this case, medical practitioners are still dealing with the impact of the changes initiated by it.

The Bundaberg Hospital Scandal, Australia

In 2003 Dr. Jayant Patel, who trained in India and the USA, was appointed surgical medical officer and later promoted to the post of Director of Surgery at Bundaberg Base Hospital, Bundaberg, in central Queensland. Over the following 2 years he operated on about 1,000 patients of whom 88 died and 14 suffered from serious complications (Burton 2005). However, all this may not have happened had the 2003 registration of Dr. Patel by the Queensland Medical Board been more rigorously scrutinized (Van Der Weyden 2005).

Although Dr. Patel obtained his preliminary medical education in India, and was awarded a Masters Degree in Surgery, he completed his intern year and residency training at the University of Rochester School of Medicine in Upstate New York. While working at a hospital in the city of Buffalo (New York) in 1984, Dr Patel was cited by New York health officials for failing to examine patients before surgery and placed on 3 years clinical probation. In 1989, he moved to Portland, Oregon, to work at the Kaiser Permanente Hospital system. Staff reported that his practices (including hygiene) were unusual and bizarrely he would frequently turn up to perform surgery on patients, some of whom were not even his responsibility. In some cases, the surgery was not required and in other instances he caused serious injuries and death to patients. After a review in 1998 the Kaiser Permanente Hospital system in Portland restricted his practice and banned him from doing liver and pancreatic surgeries and required him to seek second opinions before performing surgeries. After a further review, the Oregon Board of Medical Examiners made the practice restrictions statewide in September 2000 and in relation to a separate (previous) case, New York State health officials required him to surrender his license to practice in April 2001.

After this Dr. Patel moved to work for the Queensland Health Department in Australia. Unfortunately, they employed him without conducting due diligence regarding his qualifications and experience. Had this review been conducted by the Queensland Medical Board they would have discovered his placement on probation in 1983 by Rochester Hospital, New York, for "gross negligence"; they would have discovered the Oregon Board of Medical Examiners placing restrictions on his surgical practice; and they would also have discovered the threat by New York state to have his license to practice revoked before he voluntarily surrendered it. None of this information was disclosed by Dr. Patel at the time of his appointment. Also, just like the Neary case in Ireland and the Bristol Case in the UK, the concerns about Dr. Patel's performance at Bundaberg Hospital did not emerge from clinical governance systems but from concerns expressed by individual doctors and nurses about his surgical performance and prowess. Once again it was a communication from a member of the nursing staff about this matter which led to a question being tabled at the Queensland Parliament, which eventually resulted in the establishment of a Commission of Inquiry (Van Der Weyden 2005).

After the issues pertaining to Dr. Patel were raised in the Queensland Parliament, an award-winning Australian journalist succeeded in uncovering Patel's past which resulted in a media frenzy surrounding the case. Dr. Patel left Australia shortly after this and returned to his home in Portland, Oregon. A warrant was issued for his extradition from the USA on three charges of manslaughter, five charges of causing grievous bodily harm, four of negligent acts causing harm, and eight charges of fraud. He was extradited to Australia on 21 July 2008. He was tried in the Queensland Supreme Court for the unlawful killing of three patients and grievous bodily harm to a fourth. On 29 June 2010, Dr Patel was found guilty of four charges and on 1 July 2010 he was sentenced to 7 years in prison. Even after his sentencing there was considerable public anger as many believed his sentence was too lenient considering the gravity of the charges and the lack of remorse that Dr. Patel showed during the trial.

Just like the UK and Irish cases outlined here, a similar pattern appears to be emerging. At the center of this pattern is a doctor who is underperforming but fails to recognize that he is or fails to do anything about. In fact, Dr. Patel went to great lengths to cover up and deny his failures. Deficits in his clinical performance were not brought to light by clinical governance systems but by concerned members of staff who had to go outside the health care system to raise their concerns. Once the case reached the public scrutiny brought about by the media, the facts of the situation exploded on to the front pages of the Australian and world press. Similar to the Bristol and Neary cases, the Queensland Health Care system came under considerable criticism. It was depicted as a gigantic dysfunctional conglomerate with a corporate center that was more concerned with performance indicators, revenue generation, and cost control than people. Furthermore, of the 64,000 employees of Queensland Health, fewer than one in five were clinicians (Forster 2005).

The Medical Board of Queensland has since introduced extensive measures for the registration of overseas doctors, including receiving a certificate of good standing on each and every jurisdiction in which a doctor has practiced and getting the primary degree, registration, and transcripts of applicants verified by the Educational Commission for Foreign Medical Graduates International Credentialing Service. Just like the UK and Ireland, corporate and professional medicine moved to put structures in place that would ensure that this type of incident did not occur again. However, by the stage that this had happened the good standing of medicine and doctors had once again been significantly undermined by a doctor who had behaved less than honorably but also by a medical system that was patently seen to fail to regulate itself.

The Institute of Medicine Report, USA

The Institute of Medicine (IOM) is an independent, nonprofit organization that works outside of government in the USA to provide unbiased and authoritative advice to decision makers and the public. Established in 1970, the IOM is the health arm of the National Academy of Sciences, which was chartered under President Abraham Lincoln in 1863. Nearly 150 years later, the National Academy of Sciences has expanded into what is collectively known as the National Academies, which comprises the National Academy of Sciences, the National Academy of Engineering, the National Research Council and the IOM.

In 1999, the IOM published the report, "To Err is Human; Building a Safer Health System," (Kohn et al. 2000) which made the astonishing claim that between 44,000 and 98,000 people die in USA hospitals each year as a result of medical errors that could have been prevented. This report very quickly became a citation classic and was the focus of discussion in almost every major health care journal across the world. The content of the report shocked USA citizens and health care workers by the starkness of the message. In a single publication they had brought the issue of medical errors and patient safety to the forefront of discussions about health care. Ironically, the data that the IOM used to make these claims had been published in two papers in the *New England Journal of Medicine* almost a decade earlier (Brennan et al. 1991; Leape et al. 1991). In these two reports, the researchers reviewed 30,121 randomly selected records from 51 randomly selected acute care, nonpsychiatric hospitals in New York State in 1984. From these records, the researchers developed population estimates of injuries and computed rates according to age

Table 1.1 Rates of adverse events and negligence among clinical specialty group

Specialty	Rate of adverse events		Rate of negligence	
	Percent	Population estimate	Percent	Population estimate
Orthopedics	4.1±0.6	6,746	22.4+4.7	1,514
Urology	4.9±0.8	4,819	19.4±-6.5	933
Neurosurgery	9.9±2.1	2,987	35.6±8.6	1,063
Thoracic and cardiac surgery	10.8±2.4	3,588	23.0±9.3	826
Vascular surgery	16.1±3.0	3,187	18.0±8.1	575
Obstetrics	1.5±0.2	5,5013	38.3±7.0	1,920
Neonatology	0.6±0.1	1,713	25.8±6.9	442
General surgery	7.0±0.5	22,324	28.0±3.4	6,247
General medicine	3.6±0.3	37,135	30.9±4.4	11,475
Other	3.0±0.4	11,097	19.7±4.9	2,183

Plus–minus values are means±SE. Values differ from the sums of those reported above because of rounding

and gender of the patients as well as error rates for the specialties of the physicians. The study was the largest and most comprehensive ever to investigate the incidents of adverse events that occurred to patients, while they were being cared for in hospital. In general, the medical profession and the general public had some awareness that hospitals were associated with an increased risk of bad things happening to patients while they were hospitalized. However, their estimates were on nothing like the same scale of adverse events reported by these two studies and discussed in detail by the IOM report. It is fair to say that the data shocked citizens and healthcare workers in the USA and around the world.

Adverse events occurred in 3.7% (95% confidence interval; 3.2–4.2%) of hospital admissions, and of these 27.6% (95% confidence interval; 22.5–32.6%) were due to negligence (i.e., 1%).

It should be noted that error and negligence may be correlated but they are not the same. Medical negligence is defined as failure to meet the standard of practice of an average physician practicing in the specialty in question (Oxford English Dictionary 2004). Negligence occurs, not merely when there is error, but when the degree of error exceeds an accepted norm. The presence of error is a necessary but not sufficient condition for the determination of negligence. Sometimes the evidence of negligence appears clear cut as when a physician fails to evaluate a patient with rectal bleeding. Other cases are less obvious.

Using weighted averages they estimated that in the 2,671,863 patients discharged from New York hospitals in 1984 there were 98,609 adverse events of which 27,179 were due to negligence. Rates of adverse events rose with age with more adverse events due to negligence occurring in the elderly group. There were also marked differences between the rates of adverse events among the different physician groups and these are shown in Table 1.1.

Table 1.1 shows that the highest percentage of adverse events observed in the study was for vascular surgery (16.1%), followed by the thoracic and cardiac surgery (10.8%), neurosurgery (9.9%) and then general surgery (7%). The actual

Table 1.2 Incidence of specific types of performance errors ($n = 697$)

Type of error	No.	%
Inadequate preparation of patient before procedure	59	9
Technical error	559	76
Inadequate monitoring of patient after procedure	61	10
Use of inappropriate or outmoded form of therapy	24	3
Avoidable delay in treatment	41	7
Physician or other professional practicing outside area of expertise	13	2
Other	75	14

population estimates that these percentages represent was 22,324 adverse events in general surgery and an even higher incidence of 37,135 in general medicine. Despite the difference in observed incidence of adverse events between the different medical specialties the percentage of adverse events judged to have occurred as a result of negligence was fairly similar across the different specialties (range 35.6–18%). Obstetrics had the highest incidence of negligence (38.3%) followed by neurosurgery (35.6%). The incidence of adverse events as a result of negligence was 28% in general surgery (which represents 6,247 incidents) and 30.9% in general medicine (which represented 11,475 incidents). The data from this study are probably more accurate than the estimates from the only other large-scale study to have been conducted. The California Medical Association's Medical Insurance Feasibility Study (Mills 1978) was carried out in the 1970s to estimate the incidence of iatrogenic injury and substandard care. In this study, adverse events were estimated as occurring in 4.6% of the cases examined, with a negligence rate of 0.8% which was 20% lower than the Brennan et al. (1991) study. Of the 98,609 adverse events studied by Leape et al. (1991) 56,042 (56.8%) of them led to minimal disability with complete recovery in 1-month. In 13,521 (13.7%) incidents, the adverse events led to minimal disability with complete recovery in 6 months. However, 2,550 (2.6%) of them produced permanent total disability and in 13,451 (13.6%) led to death.

The researchers expressed surprise at the number of adverse events caused by negligence. In the New York study in 1984 they estimated that 27,179 injuries, including 6,895 deaths and 877 cases of permanent and total disability resulted from negligent care. Furthermore, the researchers (Brennan et al. 1991; Leape et al. 1991) point out that they did not measure all negligent acts, but only those that led to injury. Thus, their figures only reflected a consequence of negligence and not the actual true rate and as such probably represented a significant underestimation of the true rate of negligence in clinical care in the 30,121 randomly selected records that they studied.

The researchers also categorized the different types of errors as to their perceived cause. There were 397 events that were attributable to prevention errors, 265 events that were attributable to diagnostic errors; 153 that were due to drug treatment errors; and 68 that were due to system errors. However, the greatest single category was performance errors (697) and these are summarized in Table 1.2. More than three quarters of this type of error were due to technical performance. Nearly half of all adverse events (48%) resulted from operations and the location of the largest

Table 1.3 Number of adverse events by medical specialty

Specialty	No. (%) of records reviewed	No. of patients with adverse events DETECTED All (%) of records	Preventable (% of events)
General medicine	273 (27)	24 (8.8)	18 (75)
General surgery	290 (29)	41 (14.1)	17 (41)
Obstetrics	174 (17)	7 (4)	5 (71)
Orthopedics	277 (27)	38 (13.7)	12 (32)
Total	1014	110 (10.8)	52 (47)

percentage of adverse events was the operating room (41%) followed by the patient's own hospital room (25%). The emergency room, intensive care units, labor and delivery rooms sites accounts for approximately 3% of the adverse events.

In a similar but less extensive study Vincent et al. (2001) assessed the incidence of adverse events in 1,014 hospital case notes randomly selected from two acute hospitals in London between July and September 1999 in one hospital and December 1999 and February 2000 in the second hospital. Table 1.3 shows the number and percentage of records reviewed by medical specialty which they were drawn from. The highest number of adverse events occurred in general surgery ($n=41$), followed by orthopedics ($n=38$) and then general medicine ($n=24$). The greatest number of preventable adverse events occurred in medicine ($n=18$), surgery ($n=17$) and orthopedics ($n=12$). They found that 10.8% of patients admitted to hospital experienced adverse events and an overall 11.7% rate of adverse events when multiple adverse events are included. About half of these events were judged preventable. A third of adverse events led to moderate or greater disability or death.

The Rhetoric and the Reality of Follow-Up to the IOM Report

The Institute of Medicine (IOM) report had a profound effect on the health care community in the USA and across the world. It is not clear why the report made such an impact given it was based on data that was more than 10 years old (Brennan et al. 1991; Leape et al. 1991). Possibly it was the unambiguous and sheer number of adverse events and deaths as a consequence of health care that shocked and emboldened the healthcare community to do something about it. Within days of the Institute of Medicine's report, the Clinton administration asked a federal task force to examine the recommendations made in it. The task force quickly agreed with the majority of the recommendations that were made in the report (Quality Interagency Coordination Task Force (QuIC) 2000). In spite of the initial flurry of activity that the report stimulated, activity and progress slowed once the media moved on to the next crisis. When the IOM published a follow-up report in March 2001 the release barely registered with the media and the public (Millenson 2002). Indeed, one of the architects of the IOM report and scientific lead of the study on which the report was based concluded that movement toward systematic change to the healthcare system remains frustratingly slow (Leape and Berwick 2005). More than a decade after the release of the IOM report, efforts to reduce the harm caused by medical care systems have been few and fragmented.

The IOM report included recommendations to prevent medication errors, create accountability within the healthcare system through transparency and to establish a national focus by actually measuring the extent of the problem. The IOM report identified medication errors as a substantial source of preventable error in hospital. They recommended stronger oversight by the Food and Drug Administration to address safety issues connected with drug packaging and labeling, similar name drugs and post marketing surveillance of doctors and pharmacists(Kohn et al. 2000). Many medication errors are caused by the confusion of medicines with similar names and labels. Despite the fact that the FDA has had procedures in place since 1999 for assessing the potential of name confusion and monitoring of the market for instances of medication confusion, few existing names have been changed. Available evidence suggests that prescribing and administration problems associated with look-alike/sound-alike drugs has not been adequately dealt with by the FDA. Furthermore, the use of technology to minimize prescription or administration errors has been inadequately adopted by healthcare institutions and so patients continue to receive the wrong drug or the wrong dosage because of a doctor's poor handwriting. A federal law passed in 2008 offers bonus Medicare payments to physicians who use e-prescribing and physicians not using this facility will face reductions in Medicare payments starting in 2012. These relatively simple changes in physician behavior have failed to happen despite the existence of evidence that shows physician e-prescribing reduces medication errors by 81% (Bates et al. 1999) and the inclusion of the pharmacists with the team when doing rounds results in 66–78% reduction of preventable adverse drug reactions (Kucukarslan et al. 2003; Leape et al. 1999).

One of the primary recommendations made by the IOM report was for better data collection, particularly on adverse events to more reliably quantify the extent of the problem but also so that doctors and other members of the healthcare community could learn from mistakes. However, even this simple goal has met with only very variable success. For example, the National Quality Forum is a private membership group that works to set national priorities and goals for performance improvement. It publishes a list of voluntary consensus standards related to patient safety and includes a list of medical events that should never occur. The list of serious reportable events (sometimes known as the "never event" list) includes:

- Surgery performed on the wrong body part
- Surgery performed on the wrong patient
- Wrong surgical procedure performed on a patient
- Intra-operative or immediately post-operative death in an ASA Class I patient
- Patient death or serious disability associated with the use or function of a device in patient care, in which the device is used for functions other than as intended (Leape 2002; Wachter 2004)

Despite apparent widespread consensus on these types of efforts only 17 states had established a confidential reporting system by the time a federal framework was created in the Patient Safety and Quality Improvement Act of 2005 (which was not implemented until 2008 (Fassett 2006)). Progress has been almost entirely focused on voluntarily, confidential or aggregate reporting systems which although offer some benefits it hinders efforts to identify specific hazards, their antecedents (which are extremely valuable in helping to identify solutions) and the outcome of interventions put in place as a result of this analysis.

Knowing the incidence and potential origins of adverse events is a very valuable starting point in the development of a strategy to reduce these adverse events. One study which clearly showed the effectiveness of this approach targeted catheter-associated infections in the Michigan-affiliated Intensive Care Units. They found that they had an incidence of 7.7 bloodstream infections for every 1,000 days catheter used. In response to this problem they initiated a state-wide safety initiative called "Michigan Health and Hospital Association" Keystone: ICU and set a goal of reducing catheter-associated bloodstream infections. They instituted a short checklist of best practices related to catheter use and empowered nurses to ensure that doctors were following best practices. They tracked catheter associated bloodstream infection rates in 103 participating ICUs. Bloodstream infections across the participating ICUs dropped from 7.7 to 1.4/1,000 days catheter use during the study (Pronovost et al. 2006). The results also showed that 18 months after the study began the Michigan Health and Hospital Association reported that at least 50% of the participating ICUs had completely eradicated catheter-associated bloodstream infections.

These efforts represent a rare success story. The Agency for Health Research Quality (AHRQ) is the closest federal agency to the IOM's vision of a center for patient safety and coordinated national resources on patient safety. It was established as a direct result of initiatives that stemmed from the IOM report and funds numerous research projects on quality and safety. It also publishes the National Healthcare Quality Report (NHQR), which is the vehicle for discussion and reporting on progress on patient safety which includes collecting evidence on the prevalence adverse events. The agencies patient safety indicators focus mainly on surgical errors and does not use data contained in forms such as patients case-notes. As an indicator of how little progress has been made towards accounting for preventable medical harm the 2009 NHQR (Agency for Healthcare Research and Quality (AHRQ) 2009) used data from the IOM work (Kohn et al. 2000) as the best estimate of the magnitude of medical errors!

One of the reasons for the limited impact of the IOM report may have to do with how well the AHRQ has been funded. The AHRQ was established around 1999 with a funding stream from Congress starting in the same year and it was tasked with dealing with issues pertaining to patient safety. Table 1.4 shows the amount of funding received by AHRQ in the years 1999, 2000, 2005, and 2010. It also shows the amount of funding received by different National Institutes of Health. AHRQ received $28 million in 1999 which has increased to $55 million by 2010. In contrast, the National Library of Medicine received $35 million in 1999 but had

Table 1.4 The amount of research dollars (in $000,000) available from the Agency for Healthcare Research Quality for funding research from 1999 through to 2010 in comparison to the amount of funding available to a number of organizations within the National Institutes of Health (NIH)

	1999	2000	2005	2010
AHRQ	28	36	55	55
National Library of Medicine (NLM)	35	43	67	70
National Institute of Mental Health (NIMH)	860	973	1,400	1,500
National Cancer Institute (NCI)	3,000	3,300	4,800	5,100
National Centre for Complimentary and Alternative Medicine (NCCAM)	NA	68	122	129
Office of the Director (OD)	306	282	358	1,200
Total NIH Budget	15,000	17,800	28,500	31,000

increased to $70 million in 2010. The amount of research monies received by AHRQ pales into insignificance when compared with the amount of research money received by the National Cancer Institute which received $3 billion in 1999 and had increased to $5.1 billion by 2010. Even the National Institute of Mental Health (which globally is notoriously underfunded), received significantly more funding than AHRQ. In fact, even the Office of the Director of National Institutes of Health (NIH) was significantly better funded than AHRQ. In 1999, the Office of the Director received 11 times the funding of AHRQ and by 2010 this had increased to 22 times more funding. Even the National Centre for Complimentary and Alternative Medicine (NCCAM) received more funding than AHRQ, despite not being established until the year after (NIH 2010). Lack of funding for this laudable enterprise is surprising, particularly given the furore that the IOM report created when it was published in 1999. However, with hindsight, perhaps the lack of funding is understandable, given that the majority of the first decade of the twenty-first century was under a Bush and Republican administration and all efforts took second place after the horrendous events of the World Trade Center in 2001. However, the problem of medical errors and adverse events is not going to go away on its own, in the USA or in any other country around the world. The issue will require a concerted and systematic approach to understand the problems and then develop evidence based solutions.

Patients as Consumers

Unfortunately for medicine and surgery, all of these events occurred at a particular time in the historical development of public health care delivery when governments sought to empower patients. The clearest example of this occurred in the UK where the Conservative government led by Margaret Thatcher introduced the internal market to the National Health Service (NHS). This was outlined in the 1989 White Paper, Working for Patients (Health Committee 1989) which passed into law as the NHS Community Care Act 1990. The bill had been designed to increase the responsiveness of the service to the consumer, to foster innovation, and to challenge the monopolistic influence of the hospitals on health-care in which community-based services were increasingly important. After the establishment of the internal market and the purchaser–provider split (purchasers' were health authorities and some family doctors and providers were acute hospitals, organizations providing care for the mentally ill, people with learning disabilities, and ambulance services), purchasers were given budgets to buy health care from providers. One of the goals of this major NHS reorganization was to reduce waiting lists and to make health-care more efficient and responsive to patients. However, one of the unexpected consequences was precisely how much the general public would take the concept of "consumer" to heart. Around about this same time the consumer society was taking off and the general public had more and more access to better information and communication technologies such as satellite TV and the Internet. Under Prime Minister John Major, the Patient's Charter reflected the idea of an "empowered client" as seen in the Citizen's Charter, which was enacted in 1991. Although this charter did not have the force of law, it encouraged patients to complain and assert their health care rights (Harpwood 2001). It set out details of what patients could expect from the NHS, thereby establishing a standard by which doctors could be judged. In this respect, it significantly raised public awareness of rights and standards and encouraged the health care providers to focus on the gap between perceived and actual levels of care. The result was that the general public expected more from the health services and was better informed by the media about whether they were or were not getting better health care. Scandals such as the Bristol Royal Infirmary case could not have occurred at a worse time. Furthermore, although Bristol and many other scandals originated in the 1980s and early 1990s, responsibility for dealing with many of them came under the watch of a Labour government led by Tony Blair, who had publicly committed to the expansion of the NHS and ensuring better quality of patient care.

During this time also, there was a process of demystification of the medical profession. In the past, the public generally regarded physicians highly for three main reasons: (1) physicians' control of knowledge, (2) the public's perception that physicians worked in the patient's best interest, and (3) physicians control of the decision-making process with regard to health care. The cause and effect of this relationship is not clear, but doctors have gradually lost their status as keepers and infallible source of medical knowledge (Haug 1973). In part this may be due to the fact that the average length of formal education among the general public has increased. This, combined with growing access to information, especially through Internet websites like WebMD (www.webmd.com), have decreased the knowledge gap between the patient and physician. What is clear is a greater level of information has empowered patients to question the decisions about their diagnosis and treatment (McKee and Healy 2002). In general, during the 1980s, people started to question these assumptions. There was a growing awareness standards of care and decisions about the single best treatment based on past effectiveness did not exist for many illnesses. Furthermore, as treatments became more technical it was difficult to know with certainty that one treatment option was better than another. In addition, the general public became more aware of small variations and different treatments for similar conditions, based not on clinical determinants but on other factors, including physician preferences, in a particular region (Charles et al. 1999). Patients also began to realize since they had to live with the consequences of the doctor's medical decisions they should participate in the evaluation of the trade-offs.

There was also growing concern about whether the doctor really was acting in the patient's best interest. The medical profession to a greater extent throughout the twentieth century was almost entirely self-regulated. The profession chose to establish the General Medical Council (GMC) which is financed by the profession but accountable to Parliament as a form of self-regulation (Salter 1998). Originally, the GMC was charged with establishing a register of medical practitioners who were qualified to treat patients (Davies 2007). As part of discharging this duty, the GMC has the authority to discipline members whose actions are of poor quality and if necessary to revoke medical licenses. In theory, the GMC concerns itself with claims of serious professional misconduct, which according to the GMC means no more than serious misconduct judged according to the rules, written or non-written, governing the profession. One therefore might expect the GMC to review a wide range and large number of claims. However, it interprets this mandate narrowly. For example, from 1970 to 1984, no doctor was struck from the register for failing to attend a patient, but four were struck off for sexual misconduct with patients. Brazier (1992) summarizes the appearance of this situation particularly well when she asks, "has the GMC got its priorities right in punishing the adulterer with greater vigor than the uncaring doctor"? The answer, she explains, is that serious professional misconduct is interpreted to consist not of negligence or failure to attend to patients, but rather of actions that disgraced the profession. The general public and parliamentarians had access to this information and the ensuing discussions. The consequence for medicine was that doctors were not held in the same esteem that they had been when the NHS was first established. Overall, the relationship between a patient and their physician has changed considerably over the past few decades. The power of doctors associated with their professional autonomy and dominance has gradually weakened. The image of an idealized, infallible medical professional has undergone significant changes.

"Keyhole Surgery": The Tipping Point

The tipping point for the belief that surgery, and perhaps medicine needed to consider a radical change in the way that doctors were trained came with the widespread introduction of minimally invasive surgery (MIS) in the 1990s. "The Tipping Point" (Gladwell 2000) was a very influential book by a staff writer from the *New Yorker* magazine (Malcolm Gladwell). He argued that certain exceptional people can initiate change. These individuals can be characterized (individually or simultaneously) as "Connectors," "Maverns," and "Salesmen." Connectors are individuals who know lots of people and establish large social networks which means they have the capacity to spread information on ideas or products which they are particularly taken with. Maverns are individuals who enjoy collecting information and then sharing that information with others. The third characteristic which Gladwell described was Salesmen, who are characterized by charm, enthusiasm, and likeability, i.e., the personality elements required to win others to a particular way of thinking. Gladwell suggested these characteristics Connectors (as the social glue), Maverns (as databank or informationists) and salesmen (selling the idea, concept or product) brought to a project interacted to create a very powerful endorsement. The surgeons who were learning and practicing minimally invasive surgery at the outset were probably best typified by all of these three characteristics. They were (youngish) enthusiastic adopters of a new advanced technology which allowed for the performance of traditional surgery in a very novel way. Furthermore, the surgical Establishment was not particularly in favor of this new approach to performing surgery and so the proponents seemed like rebels in an otherwise very conservative profession. This small group of surgeons traveled the world giving lectures and seminars at international surgical meetings describing their experience of this new approach to performing surgery. However, Gladwell also suggests that for a message or idea to take hold, it has to be somehow memorable. The media supplied this last ingredient when they referred to minimally invasive surgery as "keyhole surgery". This term captured the world's attention and news of it spread like wildfire around the globe.

The surgery proponents of MIS did not actively discourage the use of the term "keyhole surgery" and this new approach to the performance of surgery quickly captured the public imagination. Surgeons were regular guests on news programs and documentaries promoting this approach to the performance of surgery for certain surgical procedures. The approach seemed to resonate with a consumer minded general public because it meant less scarring due to smaller incisions; incisions that were made were much easier to disguise (e.g., around the umbilicus); there was less pain associated with the procedure and patients returned to normal activities faster than they would after recovering from the same procedure performed with a traditional open surgical incision. It was also popular with cost-conscious hospital administrators because patients could have major surgical procedures performed minimally invasively with a much shorter hospital stay than they would with a traditional surgical incision. This approach to surgery was also very popular within industry as new types of surgical instruments, laparoscopes, cameras, monitors, etc. (some of them in the developmental stages) were required for the performance of surgery and the majority of the surgical instruments were disposable (and not inexpensive). This created a new large volume market from an existing customer base (surgeons) who traditionally, rarely replaced operating room instruments. In many respects, the development and evolution of MIS equipment manufacturers morphed into something resembling the pharmaceutical industry. However, nothing in life is that simple!

It soon became clear this new approach to performing surgery was associated with a higher complication rate than the traditional approach to performing the same procedure by the open technique, particularly for establishing procedures such as laparoscopic cholecystectomy (Davidoff et al. 1992; Peters et al. 1991; The Southern Surgeons Club 1991). The minimally invasive approach to diagnostic procedures was not particularly new and had been used throughout the 1980s. Fiber-optic technology, closed-circuit television, and electocoagulation equipment led to widespread introduction of laparoscopic techniques by gynecologists throughout the 1970s. General surgeons incorporated diagnostic laparoscopy into their practice during the 1980s for laparoscopic liver biopsy and cancer staging (Litynski 1999). The first laparoscopic cholecystectomies were in fact performed by European gynecologists in the late 1980s. Kurt Semm, a German gynecologist, performed the first laparoscopic appendectomy in 1983; the first documented laparoscopic cholecystectomy was performed by Eric Műhe in Germany in 1985, but Phillipe Mouret has been credited with performing the first laparoscopic cholecystectomy in Lyon, France, using video technique in 1987. This is important because it was the laparoscopic cholecystectomy operation which proved to be the precise tipping point for a revolutionary change in the way some surgical procedures were performed and as a consequence how surgeons were trained to perform them safely. Despite this period of exposure to the technique and the technology surgery was unprepared for the changes in training that were required for the safe adoption of this procedure.

By the time surgery had accepted there were "difficulties" in learning to perform surgery laparoscopically the approach had already achieved widespread acceptance by the general public, hospital administrators, and the health care establishment. What surprised many in the surgical and medical community was the degree of the difficulties associated with acquiring the surgical skills to practice this technique safely. After all, medical courses around the world attracted the brightest and best, and in general, surgery recruited the cream of them. However, surgery had made a fundamental and important miscalculation about the human factor difficulties associated with the practice of minimally invasive surgery. These will be discussed in detail in Chaps. 3 and 4. The trainee has to overcome considerable psychomotor and perceptual problems before even learning to perform MIS surgery safely and these problems arc considerable and multiple. Firstly, the surgeon has to learn to coordinate 18 in. long surgical instruments that pass through trocars in the patients abdominal wall. Thus, they had lost important tactile and haptic information that they would normally receive through their fingers and the palms of their hands. They also had to perform surgery while looking at a pixelated image on a monitor. It may be a high quality image but it is still a pixelated image which required the brain to work harder than if it was processing information captured by the eye while viewing under natural seeing conditions. Images displayed on the monitor are captured from a single camera which means that many of the binocular cues that were associated with the judgment of depth of field are also lost. Lastly, perhaps the most significant obstacle to the learning and practice of safe laparoscopic surgery was the apparent counterintuitive movement of surgical instruments. For example, when the surgeon moved his or her hand (holding the handle of a surgical instrument) to the right inside the patient's abdomen, the working end of the instrument moves to the left on the monitor. This causes a fundamental proprioceptive-visual conflict for the operator.

Their proprioceptive system tells the brain that the instrument is moving to the right while their visual system simultaneously informs the brain that the working end of the instrument is moving to left. Compounding these problems are the reduced degrees of freedom (in comparison to the hand and fingers) afforded by these new surgical instruments. These complexities make learning the psychomotor coordination necessary to perform laparoscopic surgery difficult and protracted. Furthermore, the reduced degrees of freedom afforded by the surgical instruments also meant that new techniques had to be developed for relatively straightforward surgical maneuvers such as suturing. In traditional open surgery, suturing is a precise but a very straightforward technique to learn. The widespread acceptance of MIS changed all that and it quickly became apparent that the traditional apprenticeship model (of learning on-the-job while practicing on patients) which had served surgery well for more than a century was not a viable training model, particularly for the early stages of the learning curve.

"More" Training

In September 1992 the American NIH convened a consensus development conference on Gallstones and Laparoscopic Cholecystectomy (NIH 1993). They brought together surgeons, endoscopists, hepatologists, gastroenterologists, radiologists, and epidemiologists as well as other health care professionals and the public. They came to a number of conclusions one of which was that most patients who experienced symptoms of gallstones should be treated and that laparoscopic cholecystectomy provided a safe and effective alternative treatment to open cholecystectomy, for most patients. They also concluded that every effort should be made to ensure that surgeons performing laparoscopic cholecystectomy were properly trained and credentialed (and proctored for their first 15 procedures). As a result, there was a rapid expansion of training courses in laparoscopic surgical technique each expounding the ethos of the course organizer. It also led to the establishment of national and regional training centers around the world. However, a fundamental and detailed understanding of the specific human factor aspects of this surgical technique which made it difficult to learn eluded the majority of the surgical community except for leaders such as Prof Sir Alfred Cuschieri at Ninewells Hospital in Dundee and Dr Michael Patkin in Australia. The precise explanation as to why laparoscopic surgery is difficult to learn will be discussed in detail in Chaps. 3 and 4 but it is fair to say that it was not until the late 1990s that the extent and magnitude of these difficulties were documented and quantified (Berguer 1999; Crothers et al. 1999; Cuschieri 1995; Gallagher et al. 1998; Patkin and Isabel 1993). However, in the interim surgeons who wanted to learn to practice MIS needed more training.

These early courses were primarily led by industry. In the early 1990s, device manufacturers such as Ethicon Endo Surgery, Auto Suture (later to morph into US Surgical), Karl Storz, to name but a few, arranged courses for consultant surgeons who wanted to learn to perform surgery using the new laparoscopic technique.

These were very well run courses, staffed with well known national and international surgical faculty and they were also exceptionally well resourced. However, it is generally acknowledged that industry ran these courses in their efforts to increase sales of their product. Nevertheless, this should not detract from the quality of the courses offered by these organizations when at that time, academic surgery departments around the world were completely unprepared and had nothing to offer. These courses taught surgeons what they could and could not do with the devices they were going to use to perform the surgery. In reality, this meant that the surgeon was not going to have to work out what they were going to do with an instrument the first time they opened the packaging in the operating room, just prior to operating on a real patient. In this sense, industry provided the first human-factor safety training for devices in surgery. These same industrial organizations and a great many more continue to organize courses to this day. However, academic departments of surgery have become much more proactive in the establishment and running of a wide variety of courses as have professional organizations such as SAGES and EEES.

In general, these courses (industry and academic) lasted 1 or 2 days, usually over a weekend. Although the didactic and knowledge aspect of the course was well developed and reasonably standardized, there was a complete absence of standardization for the skills training component. Surgeons were familiarized with the imaging equipment, endoscopes, electrocautery, surgical instruments, and had some opportunities to acquire the psychomotor skills necessary for instrument handling. The training models used varied from course to course (and are discussed in more detail in Chap. 2) and included anything from an anesthetized pig in a fully equipped operating room through to inanimate bench top animal parts (e.g., chicken leg) or silicon models. Training simply consisted of exposure and, time permitting, some repeated practice. Performance metrics were subjective appraisal of task performance and possibly task completion time. There were no benchmarks for trainees to reach before applying their "skills" on a real patient and there was an implicit assumption that these types of course would be more than sufficient to familiarize and prepare the surgeon for this new type of surgical practice.

What is probably most surprising about this whole state of affairs is that the problems encountered by the surgeon in their efforts to acquire the skills for the safe practice of laparoscopic surgery were entirely predictable and understandable from human factors perspective (Gallagher and Smith 2003) and had been for at least half a century. What is also hard to believe is the fact that surgeons leading the vast majority of these training courses were blissfully unaware of this fact. However, this ignorance was not malicious and slowly but surely, detailed quantitative analysis of the human factor difficulties associated with the acquisition of the skills necessary for the practice of MIS started to appear in mainstream surgical journals. Furthermore, there was increasing awareness by the leaders in the MIS community that human factors, ergonomics, education, training, and validation were assuming an increasing importance in surgery. The endoscopic surgical movement grasped this reality first and started to populate their mainstream journals such as Endoscopy and Surgical Endoscopy with studies that validated the basic laparoscopic surgical approach by comparing minimally invasive surgery to the traditional open approach for the same procedure. They also started to publish studies on the learning curve for a particular surgical procedure and the different approaches to training. Although at this time the understanding of "metrics" was crude e.g., using completion time as surrogate measure of performance, surgeons appeared to grasp the basic premise that subjective appraisal of trainee and intra-operative performance was inadequate for quality assurance purposes.

Virtual Reality Simulation

For a period the surgical community offered training courses for a diverse and wide variety of laparoscopic procedures (even before their clinical efficacy over open procedures had been demonstrated). However, after the initial novelty of these offerings, which were very popular, widely covered in the media, well attended and well sponsored by industry, the actual costs of running courses became clear, i.e., they were relatively expensive to run in terms of faculty and course materials, such as instrumentation, consumables (e.g., suture material), and surgical training tasks. The most expensive training models were live animals that were fully anesthetized and operated on in a very high spec operating theater. Of course, training courses that offered operating experience on a live animal were the most popular with the surgical community, probably because they had the greatest face validity to the attending surgeons. As well as the expense of these courses, there was also the issue of animal rights which meant that running these types of courses was a sensitive issue. The surgical community argued that to train them to operate safely on patients they needed the highest fidelity training model possible. The irony is that although the porcine model offers some similar features to operating on a patient there is minimal direct anatomical equivalency.

Dr. Richard Martin Satava was a general surgeon in the U.S. Army who had been seconded to work for the Defence Advanced Research Projects Agency (DARPA) at the start of the 1990s. Thus, he was very well-informed about the difficulties which learning MIS posed for surgeons. He was also aware of the risk that taking a traditional Halstedian approach to training MIS skills would pose for the patient. In the military, whenever something is too dangerous, expensive, or distant in time or place or imagination, physically experience, there have been attempts to simulate the experience (Satava 1993). This is the approach the military and NASA had taken over the training of aviation and space flight skills. Some years after that, he wrote that simulation is a fundamental activity of virtually all species; it is the replacement of one dangerous activity by the enactment of a similar activity in a non-dangerous environment. It is the primary way in which children are taught to deal safely with the real world, and frequently includes the setting of play, theater, practice or sports. Surrogates (simulators) are used as replacements for real objects; they include dolls and puppets, props, and games among other substitutes (Satava 2008). During his first secondment to DARPA, Satava began to envision a simulation approach to solving the problem of training minimally invasive surgical skills. Although anesthetists had been using mannequin simulation for team training for a number of years (Gaba and DeAnda 1988), no virtual reality simulator existed for training surgical skills. Asmund Laerdal, a successful plastic toys manufacturer had produced Resusci-Anne in the 1960s, which made possible the training of ABC (airway, breathing, circulation) for cardiopulmonary resuscitating (Safar et al. 1961). Cooper and Taqueti (2004) have reviewed the development of mannequin simulators and concluded that despite more than two decades of development the acceptance and market penetration of this type of simulation for clinical education and training was small. They also concluded that the acceptance of simulation and training would not occur until there was substantial validation evidence showing efficacy and cost-effectiveness for improving learning and producing better patient outcomes. Indeed, at the time of writing, this type of validation is was still not forthcoming for mannequin type simulations.

Validation

Dr. Dave Gaba one of the pioneers of mannequin type simulations believes that there are many obstacles to obtaining definitive proof of the impact simulation on clinical care. He also pointed out that “no industry in which human lives depend on skilled performance or responsible operator has unequivocal proof of the benefits of simulation before embracing it” (Gaba 1992). One of the major obstacles that Gaba alluded to was the development of reliable and valid measurement instruments and methodologies necessary for the assessment of performance and behavior change as a result of simulation training. We believe that these were very perceptive insights by Dr. Gaba. Furthermore, we believe that the lack of widespread acceptance and penetration of simulation into education and training in medicine is primarily linked to the dearth of validation evidence. Furthermore, we also believe that there is a lack of validation evidence relating to simulation in medicine because it is fundamentally misunderstood. These issues will be addressed directly in Chaps. 10 and 11.

There is some clinical validation of the utility of simulation training in surgery (Seymour et al. 2002), however this evidence is still scant. There is a growing body of evidence in relation to the psychometric properties of simulation devices but there needs to be an expansion in the volume and quality of studies examining the value of simulation training for clinical performance. Like Gaba, we believe that these studies shouldn’t really be necessary to convince the medical community that there is a better way to train clinical skills. However, all the indicators are that they are indeed required. The methodology which led up to and was used by the Seymour et al., study is probably the most robust clinical validation study that has been conducted on surgical simulation to date. The methodology used in the metric validation of the simulator used in this clinical trial was not new, and was derived from extensive knowledge of validation studies in the behavioral sciences. Likewise, the clinical validation methodology (i.e., proficiency-based progression training and objective assessment of intra-operative performance) used, were also drawn from the behavioral sciences. These methods will be covered in detail in Chap. 5 (where we will detail how to identify, define, and measure performance); Chap. 6 integrates metrics into simulation training; Chap. 7 validates the metrics that have been developed and Chap. 8 harnesses the simulation for metric-based training to proficiency for improved intra-operative performance.

Understanding and Implementing an Alternative Training Strategy

What we have tried to do in this book is draw together the knowledge and quantitative findings that help to explain why certain types of surgical procedures are difficult to learn. It is only from an extensive and thorough knowledge of these factors and how they relate to normal cognitive and information processing that methodology for more efficient and effective skill acquisition in surgery can be developed (Chaps. 3 and 4). This knowledge is necessary to help us understand precisely what we want to simulate and why we want to simulate it. Unfortunately, in the past simulations that have been developed for training medical skills have concentrated on what the simulator looks like. Most physicians mistakenly believe that a simulator that looks like real patient anatomy is a good simulator. As the reader will become aware in the chapters ahead, this is not a belief we hold to. Physicians tend to accept the validity and utility of this type of simulator purely on how it looks, in other words, how *pretty* it is. While this feature of a simulator is nice to have, there are a lot more important functional features which are higher up the priority list when making an effective and efficient simulation training device. One of these is the capacity to emulate the device and procedure to be learned and give detailed, reliable, and valid quantitative measures of performance, i.e., metrics. We will make the point time and time again; a simulator without these metric attributes is nothing more than a fancy video game, no matter how pretty it is. In Chaps. 5 and 6 we shall outline in detail how metrics are developed from first principles in a variety of contexts. We will give a number of examples to demonstrate that the principles are always the same and can be applied to any procedure to be simulated, learned, and assessed. Much of this methodology will be new to readers from a medical (and possibly engineering) background however; they have been well tried and tested for about half century in psychology. These are probably two of most important chapters in the book and this can be applied to any area of medicine and any medical procedure (if the principles are fully understood).

While it is all well and good knowing how to develop simulation and the metrics necessary for making it an efficient and effective training device there is still the "small" matter of convincing the medical community that the simulation and metrics that have been developed actually work. There are two steps to this process. The first is the validation of the psychometric properties of the metrics you have developed. This is an extremely important part of the validation of simulation, particularly as the metric-based simulation and assessments are likely to be used for high-stakes purposes, such as determining training progression. Shoddy validation studies will not do! In Chap. 7, we will discuss the different types a psychometric validation required in the process of validating a simulator and its metrics. Again, this knowledge and expertise has been drawn from the psychology and educational testing sectors where this issue has been debated at length and international gold standard methodologies agreed standards (American Psychological Association, APA 1999). However, the nuances for their application in procedural medical simulation and clinical validation are somewhat novel. But, the rules of validation for these efforts are clear, if not completely understood as evidenced by some of the validation efforts in objective assessment of procedural skills and the development of metrics (see Chap. 7 for a full discussion of this issue). We will give explicit examples of what is acceptable and what is not acceptable, particularly regarding the assessment of inter-rater reliability.

Armed with validated metrics it is then necessary to demonstrate that metric based simulation training improves clinical performance in comparison to traditional training. In Chaps. 8, 9, and 10 we will describe how a complete education (e.g., e-learning) and training package should be put together, how it should be implemented and evaluated. We will also discuss lessons learned from training programs that have already been developed and implemented. The novelty of this approach to training means that mistakes (e.g., inefficiencies) are inevitable. However, mistakes are very valuable learning opportunities (for those who wish to learn). That is precisely the point that is made in Chap. 11 when we discuss the issue of feedback and deliberate practice in determining how education and training should be optimally configured.

The Paradigm Shifts

The combined impact of all of these events on surgery was profound and disruptive. Just as Kuhn (1962) had predicted, it created a crisis within surgery in particular and medicine in general. Medicine and surgery have been subjected to high profile medical error and negligence cases in the past. However, the cases that we have outlined here had an enormous impact on the medical community, but they also impacted on the general publics' perception of doctors and how they treated their patients. Furthermore, these cases occupied the headlines in the popular press for years, with the graphic lurid details of each case being discussed in detail in front of a shell-shocked general public. There is little doubt that in the aftermath of these cases the general publics' perception and possibly confidence in their doctors had been significantly shaken. Furthermore, these cases also brought about a fundamental and radical reconfiguration of how doctors were trained. There was a move away from the perception that doctors were competent once they "knew how" to do something. In the new configuration of training doctors had to "demonstrate" that they knew how (see Chap. 8).

Compounding these considerable problems was a demand by health care providers for greater productivity in medical care which meant targets for operations, targets for waiting lists etc. Although the development of MIS may have helped on this front it was a tipping point for the change in how surgeons were trained. The widespread introduction of MIS into clinical practice meant two things for surgeons in training. The first was that the introduction of MIS eliminated many potential training opportunities for the junior surgeon. For example, hernia repair and open cholecystectomy were relatively straightforward surgical procedures that provided frequent opportunities for the vast majority of surgeons to acquire their basic technical surgical skills in a relatively low-risk environment. The second was that not only were these training opportunities removed from the basic surgical training opportunities, but they had now become more advanced procedures, which required advanced training. Even when they did get an opportunity to perform them, this was probably as a result of a patient being too ill to perform the procedure laparoscopically or an MIS procedure that was converted to an open procedure; neither of these scenarios could be described as straightforward! Making this situation even worse was the reduced work hours that surgeons had available to them during which to learn their craft. Moreover, the rate of change through the introduction of new approaches and new technologies to the performance of surgery had increased exponentially. Although this was not just a problem for surgery, but all of medicine, it impacted worst on surgery and other procedural specialties because the acquisition of their skills could only occur (traditionally that is) in a relatively specialized environment, i.e., the operating room. To make matters worse, surgeons were also being required to achieve certain standards or levels of competence. Furthermore, although the assessment of the skills that had traditionally been left to the prerogative of the supervising consultant surgeon, new standardized assessment methodologies had been introduced and were a mandatory part of training and career progression.

There can be little doubt that all of these factors combined to create a sense of crisis among the surgical establishment. There can also be little doubt that surgery was confronted with an unanticipated training crisis of global proportions. Kuhn (1962) also predicted that during transitions and periods of crisis a wide range of potential solutions are examined and sometimes existing solutions are re-examined. This is precisely what happened with simulation. As we have described earlier, anesthetists had been using simulation since the 1960s in their educational and training curriculum, but this had not registered with the surgical community as a technology they were particularly interested in. However, the development of one of the first surgical simulators by Satava (1993) started a process which would move surgical simulation from a proof of concept, through to clinical validation (Seymour et al. 2002) to widespread acceptance as a primary training modality for the new training paradigm in surgery (Pellegrini et al. 2006). We will argue here that simulation based training was accepted and implemented before it was fully understood by the surgical and medical establishment. Although widely believed to offer the opportunity for repeated practice that had been lost in the operating room, simulation in fact provides the opportunity for deliberate practice. Deliberate practice differs from repeated practice in the use of metric-based formative feedback to hone the skills of the trainee. This means that the optimal development and application of metrics lies at the very core of effective and efficient simulation training. One of the goals of this book is to explain how these factors work together and should be optimally configured for an efficient and effective approach to training.

Lastly, we will also argue that although simulation based training technology affords the opportunity for more efficient and effective training in disciplines such as surgery, it also offers the opportunity to quality assure the skill levels of graduating trainees. Traditionally, surgeons have acquired their skills in an apprenticeship model, where they practiced on patients. This meant that individual surgeons had a considerably varied experience, i.e., it depended on what hospital they were working in during training, on what consultant they worked with, and what patients they got to operate on, which meant they graduated with variable skills levels. In the past, *in all probability* their skills would have been trained to at least a safe level of operating simply by the sheer volume of operating they had performed during their training. In a twenty-first-century health care this guarantee of case volume no longer exists during training. Furthermore, the number of cases performed and the amount of time in training are very poor predictors of the skill level of the surgeon (which we will discuss in detail in Chap. 8). The approach that has been taken in most developed medicine training programs around the world is to require trainees to reach a level of competency. Unfortunately, this is a basic level of competency about which there is widespread unease among very experienced practicing surgeons. To be frank, we share this unease, not least because of the lack of transparency of these levels of competency, their lack of unambiguous operational definitions (see Chap. 5), and the impact that this has on the reliability of the assessment process (see Chap. 7). What we have proposed here is that trainees should train until they reach a performance criterion level, i.e., a level of proficiency. Furthermore, this level of proficiency should be quantitatively defined using validated metrics implemented in simulation technology and based on the *in vivo* performance of experienced and practicing surgeons. This strategy achieves two things: First, it establishes an unambiguous, objective, transparent, and fair training goal for a trainee, which is based on the performance of practicing surgeons in the real world and not some abstract concept of "a just passing performance" (i.e., competence). Second, it ensures a considerably less variable level of skills of graduates. Both of these factors would go some way to reassuring the surgical establishment that this new approach to training surgical skills stands a better than average chance of producing surgeons who can become as good if not better as they are.

Conclusions

Whether by design or by accident, Halsted developed a training program which has served medicine well for a century. However, considerably more is known today about the cluster of human factors which are essential for the education and training of advanced skills such as surgery. The process of education and skill acquisition is not some unknown black box. Surgery has a unique opportunity to develop a training program that will serve medicine well for many years. However, this program should be built on an explicit and detailed understanding of human sensation, perception, cognition, kinesthetics, psychomotor learning, and performance. Considerably more is known about the performance characteristics and parameters of these human factors and on how they impinge on human learning and the practice of skilled performance. Equipped with this knowledge, surgery will be better able to build simulations which are optimally configured for the training and assessment of advanced procedural skills in surgery. This approach is important because other procedural disciplines in medicine are confronting the same problems as surgery. However, surgery has reached this point first, and is duty bound to ask and address the important questions that will shape the future of procedural training in medicine. This approach will also inform surgery of the deficits in simulations that currently exist for training surgical skills and ensure that these are not repeated in the next generation of simulations. We also believe that this revolution which started in surgery, probably one of the most conservative disciplines within medicine, will change all of medicine.

References

Adnett N, Hardy S. Reviewing the working time directive: rationale, implementation and case law. *Ind Relat J*. 2001;32(2):114-125.

Agency for Healthcare Research and Quality (AHRQ). National healthcare quality report. *Journal*. From: http://www.ahrq.gov/qual/qrdr09.htm. 2009 (accessed 19th September 2010).

Åkerstedt T, Gillberg M. A dose-response study of sleep loss and spontaneous sleep termination. *Psychophysiology*. 1986;23(3):293-297.

APA. NCME (American Educational Research Association, American Psychological Association, & National Council on Measurement in Education). *Standards for educational and psychological tests*; Washington DC: AERA Publications Sales; 1999.

Asch DA, Parker RM. The Libby Zion case. One step forward or two steps backward? *N Engl J Med*. 1988;318(12):771.

Bates DW, Teich JM, Lee J, et al. The impact of computerized physician order entry on medication error prevention. *J Am Med Inform Assoc*. 1999;6(4):313-321.

Berguer R. Surgery and ergonomics. *Arch Surg*. 1999;134(9):1011-1016.

Brazier M. *Medicine, Patients and the Law*. Harmondsworth: Penguin-Printed Resource; 1992.

Brennan TA, Hebert LE, Laird NM, et al. Hospital characteristics associated with adverse events and substandard care. *JAMA*. 1991;265(24):3265-3269.

Bristol Royal Infirmary Inquiry. *Learning from Bristol: The Report of the Public Inquiry into Children's Heart Surgery at the Bristol Royal Infirmary 1984–1995*. London: Stationery Office; 2001.

Burton B. Court ruling ends Patel inquiry. *BMJ*. 2005;331(7516):536.

Cameron JL. William Stewart Halsted: our surgical heritage. *Ann Surg*. 1997;225(5):445-458.

Charles C, Gafni A, Whelan T. Decision-making in the physician-patient encounter: revisiting the shared treatment decision-making model. *Soc Sci Med*. 1999;49(5):651-661.

Cooper JB, Taqueti VR. A brief history of the development of mannequin simulators for clinical education and training. *Br Med J*. 2004;13(suppl 1):i11-i18.

Crothers IR, Gallagher AG, McClure N, James DT, McGuigan J. Experienced laparoscopic surgeons are automated to the "fulcrum effect": an ergonomic demonstration. *Endoscopy*. 1999;31(5):365-369.

Cuschieri A. Whither minimal access surgery: tribulations and expectations. *Am J Surg*. 1995; 169(1):9-19.

Daan S, Beersma DG, Borbely AA. Timing of human sleep: recovery process gated by a circadian pacemaker. *Am J Physiol Regul Integr Comp Physiol*. 1984;246(2):R161-R183.

Davidoff AM, Pappas TN, Murray EA, et al. Mechanisms of major biliary injury during laparoscopic cholecystectomy. *Ann Surg*. 1992;215(3):196-202.

Davies M. *Medical Self-Regulation: Crisis and Change*. Hampshire: Ashgate Publishing Company; 2007.

Dembe AE, Erickson JB, Delbos RG, Banks SM. The impact of overtime and long work hours on occupational injuries and illnesses: new evidence from the United States. *Br Med J*. 2005;62(9):588-597.

Elman MJ, Sugar J, Fiscella R, et al. The effect of propranolol versus placebo on resident surgical performance. *Trans Am Ophthalmol Soc*. 1998;96:283-294.

Fassett WE. Patient safety and quality improvement act of 2005. *The Annals of pharmacotherapy* 2006;40(5):917-924.

Ferguson RL, Jobe K. A quiet hand for microneurosurgery: twiddle your thumb. *J Neurosurg*. 2004;101(3):541-544.

Forster P. *Queensland Health Systems Review Final Report*. Queensland: Queensland Department of Health; 2005 http://www.health.qld.gov.au/health_sys_review/final/qhsr_final_report.pdf (accessed 5th July 2011).

Friedman RC, Bigger JT, Kornfeld DS. The intern and sleep loss. *N Engl J Med*. 1971;285(4): 201-203.

Gaba DM. Dynamic decision-making in anesthesiology: cognitive models and training approaches. In: Evans DA, Patel VL, eds. *Advanced Models of Cognition for Medical Training and Practice*. Berlin: Springer; 1992:123-147.

Gaba DM, DeAnda A. A comprehensive anesthesia simulation environment: re-creating the operating room for research and training. *Anesthesiology*. 1988;69(3):387-394.

Gaba DM, Howard SK. Patient safety: fatigue among clinicians and the safety of patients. *N Engl J Med*. 2002;347(16):1249-1255.

Gallagher AG, Smith CD. From the operating room of the present to the operating room of the future. Human-factors lessons learned from the minimally invasive surgery revolution. *Semin Laparosc Surg*. 2003;10(3):127-139.

Gallagher AG, McClure N, McGuigan J, Ritchie K, Sheehy NP. An ergonomic analysis of the fulcrum effect in the acquisition of endoscopic skills. *Endoscopy*. 1998;30(7):617-620.

Gladwell M. *The Tipping Point: How Little Things Can Make a Big Difference*. Boston: Little, Brown & Company; 2000.

Grantcharov TP, Bardram L, Peter FJ, Rosenberg J. Laparoscopic performance after one night on call in a surgical department: prospective study. *BMJ*. 2001;323(7323):1222-1223.

Grillo HC. Edward D. Churchill and the "rectangular" surgical residency. *Surgery*. 2004;136(5): 947-952.

Hallenbeck WH. *Radiation Protection*. Boca Raton: CRC Press; 1994.

Harding Clark M. The Lourdes Hospital Inquiry–An Inquiry into peripartum hysterectomy at Our Lady of Lourdes Hospital, Drogheda. *Report of Judge Maureen Harding Clark SC. The Stationery Office, Dublin*; 2006.

Harpwood V. *Negligence in Healthcare: Clinical Claims and Risk in Context*. London: Informa; 2001.

Harwell RC, Ferguson RL. Physiologic tremor and microsurgery. *Microsurgery*. 1983;4(3):187-192.

Haug M. Deprofessionalization: an alternative hypothesis for the future. *Sociol Rev Monogr*. 1973;20:195-211.

Health Committee. Working for patients. Vol. 159 cc556-9W. 1989. From: http://hansard.millbanksystems.com/written_answers/1989/nov/07/working-for-patients. Retrieved October 21, 2010.

Hutter MM, Kellogg KC, Ferguson CM, Abbott WM, Warshaw AL. The impact of the 80-hour resident workweek on surgical residents and attending surgeons. *Ann Surg*. 2006;243(6):864-871.

Kohn LT, Corrigan JM, Donaldson MS. *To Err Is Human: Building a Safer Health System*. Washington DC: National Academy Press; 2000:196-197.

Kucukarslan SN, Peters M, Mlynarek M, Nafziger DA. Pharmacists on rounding teams reduce preventable adverse drug events in hospital general medicine units. *Arch Intern Med*. 2003;163(17):2014-2018.

Kuhn TS. *The Structure of Scientific Revolutions. International Encyclopaedia of United Science*. Chicago: University of Chicago Press; 1962.

Landrigan CP, Rothschild JM, Cronin JW, et al. Effect of reducing interns' work hours on serious medical errors in intensive care units. *N Engl J Med*. 2004;351(18):1838-1848.

Leape LL. Reporting of adverse events. *N Engl J Med*. 2002;347(20):1633-1638.

Leape LL, Berwick DM. Five years after to err is human: what have we learned? *JAMA*. 2005;293(19):2384-2390.

Leape LL, Brennan TA, Laird N, et al. The nature of adverse events in hospitalized patients. Results of the Harvard medical practice study II. *N Engl J Med*. 1991;324(6):377-384.

Leape LL, Cullen DJ, Clapp MD, et al. Pharmacist participation on physician rounds and adverse drug events in the intensive care unit. *JAMA*. 1999;282(3):267-270.

Litynski GS. Endoscopic surgery: the history, the pioneers. *World J Surg*. 1999;23(8):745-753.

Lowry J, Cripps J. Results of the online EWTD trainee survey. *Bull R Coll Surg Engl*. 2005;87(3): 86-87.

Lupien SJ, Maheu F, Tu M, Fiocco A, Schramek TE. The effects of stress and stress hormones on human cognition: implications for the field of brain and cognition. *Brain Cogn*. 2007;65(3): 209-237.

McKee M, Healy J. *Hospitals in a Changing Europe*. Buckingham: Open University Press; 2002.

Meumann E. Haus-und Schularbeit: Experimente an Kindern der Volkschule. [Home and school-work: experiments on children in school]. *Die Deutsche Schule*. 1904;8:278-303; 337-359; 416-431.

Millenson ML. Pushing the profession: how the news media turned patient safety into a priority. *Qual Saf Health Care*. 2002;11(1):57-63.

Mills DH. Medical insurance feasibility study: a technical summary. *West J Med*. 1978;128(4): 360-365.

Moore-Ede M. *Twenty-Four-Hour Society: Understanding Human Limits in a World That Never Stops*. Reading: Addison Wesley Publishing Company; 1993.

NIH. Consensus development panel. Gallstones and laparoscopic cholecystectomy. (National Institutes of Health Consensus Development Panel on Gallstone and Laparoscopic Cholecystetomy). *JAMA*. 1993;269(8):1018-1024.

NIH. The NIH almanac – appropriations. May 14, 2010. From: http://www.nih.gov/about/almanac/appropriations/index.htm. Retrieved September 19, 2010.

Oxford English Dictionary (ed) (Vol. 24) Oxford: Oxford University Press; 2004.

Pais A. *Subtle Is the Lord: The Science and the Life of Albert Einstein*. Oxford: Oxford University Press; 2005.

Patkin M. Ergonomics applied to the practice of microsurgery. *Aust N Z J Surg*. 1977;47(3): 320-329.

Patkin M, Isabel L. *Ergonomics and Laparoscopic General Surgery. Laparoscopic Abdominal Surgery*. New York: McGraw-Hill; 1993.

Pellegrini CA. Surgical education in the United States: navigating the white waters. *Ann Surg*. 2006;244(3):335-342.

Pellegrini CA, Sachdeva AK, Johnson KA. Accreditation of education institutes by the American College of Surgeons: a new program following an old tradition. *Bull Am Coll Surg*. 2006;91(3):8-12.

Peters JH, Ellison EC, Innes JT, et al. Safety and efficacy of laparoscopic cholecystectomy. A prospective analysis of 100 initial patients. *Ann Surg*. 1991;213(1):3-12.

Philibert I, Friedmann P, Williams WT. New requirements for resident duty hours. *JAMA*. 2002;288(9):1112-1114.

Pronovost P, Needham D, Berenholtz S, et al. An intervention to decrease catheter-related bloodstream infections in the ICU. *N Engl J Med.* 2006;355(26):2725-2732

Quality Interagency Coordination Task Force (QuIC). Doing what counts for patient safety: federal actions to reduce medical errors and their impact. *Journal.* From: http://www.quic.gov/report/mederr2.htm. 2000 (accessed 19th September 2010).

Reason J. *Human Error*. Cambridge: Cambridge University Press; 1990.

Safar P, Brown TC, Holtey WJ, Wilder RJ. Ventilation and circulation with closed-chest cardiac massage in man. *JAMA*. 1961;176(7):574-576.

Salter B. *The Politics of Change in the Health Service*. Basingstoke: Macmillan; 1998.

Samkoff JS, Jacques CH. A review of studies concerning effects of sleep deprivation and fatigue on residents' performance. *Acad Med.* 1991;66(11):687-693.

Satava RM. Virtual reality surgical simulator. The first steps. *Surg Endosc.* 1993;7(3):203-205.

Satava RM. Historical review of surgical simulation – a personal perspective. *World J Surg.* 2008;32(2):141-148.

Schuster M, Rhodes S. The impact of overtime work on industrial accident rates. *Ind Relat J Economy Soc.* 1985;24(2):234-246.

Seymour NE, Gallagher AG, Roman SA, et al. Virtual reality training improves operating room performance: results of a randomized, double-blinded study. *Ann Surg*. 2002;236(4):458-463; discussion 463-454.

Sheldon GF. Surgical workforce since the 1975 study of surgical services in the United States: an update. *Ann Surg*. 2007;246(4):541-545.

Slack PS, Ma X. Time dependency assessment of muscular fatigue index and hand tremor under operating conditions. *IEEE*. 2007:4822-4825.

Smith R. All changed, changed utterly. *Br Med J*. 1998;316(7149):1917-1918.

Smith C, Wise MN. *Energy and Empire: A Biographical Study of Lord Kelvin*. Cambridge: Cambridge University Press; 1989.

Spritz N. Oversight of physicians' conduct by state licensing agencies. *Ann Intern Med.* 1991;115(3):219-222.

The Southern Surgeons Club. A prospective analysis of 1518 laparoscopic cholecystectomies. *N Engl J Med.* 1991;324(16):1073-1078.

Van Der Weyden MB. The Bundaberg Hospital scandal: the need for reform in Queensland and beyond. *Med J Aust.* 2005;183(6):284-285.

Villaneuva T. European working time directive faces challenges. *Can Med Assoc J*. 2010;182(1): E39-E40.

Vincent C, Neale G, Woloshynowych M. Adverse events in British hospitals: preliminary retrospective record review. *BMJ*. 2001;322(7285):517-519.

Wachter RM. The end of the beginning: patient safety five years after'to err is human'. *Journal*, W4-534-545. From: http://content.healthaffairs.org/cgi/reprint/hlthaff.w4.534v1. 2004.

Wallack MK, Chao L. Resident work hours: the evolution of a revolution. *Arch Surg*. 2001;136(12):1426-1431.

Walshe K, Offen N. A very public failure: lessons for quality improvement in healthcare organisations from the Bristol Royal Infirmary. *Qual Health Care*. 2001;10(4):250-256.

Weinger MB, Ancoli-Israel S. Sleep deprivation and clinical performance. *JAMA*. 2002;287(8): 955-957.

Whang EE, Mello MM, Ashley SW, Zinner MJ. Implementing resident work hour limitations: lessons from the New York State experience. *Ann Surg*. 2003;237(4):449-455.

Wojtczak-Jaroszowa J, Jarosz D. Time-related distribution of occupational accidents* 1. *J Safety Res*. 1987;18(1):33-41.

Yerkes RM, Dodson JD. The relationship of stimulus to rapidity of habit formation. *J Comp Neurol Psychol*. 1908;18:459-482.

Zajonc RB. Social facilitation. *Science*. 1965;149(3681):269-274.

Chapter 2
Simulations for Procedural Training

While the art of simulation has been known for many centuries the science of simulation has only come to the fore in the late twentieth and early twenty-first century. Simulation is the imitation of some real thing, state of affairs, or process. The act of simulating something generally entails representing certain key characteristics or behaviors of a selected physical or abstract system. Simulation is used in many contexts, including the *modeling* of natural systems or human systems in order to gain insight into their function. Other contexts include simulation of *technology* for performance optimization (automobile engine design, *safety engineering*, *testing*, *training*, and *education*). Simulation can be used to demonstrate the eventual real effects of alternative conditions and courses of action. For example, what might happen to the flight path or handling ability of an airplane under certain wind conditions or at certain speeds? Key issues in simulation include acquisition of valid source information about the relevant selection of key characteristics and behaviors, the use of simplifying approximations and assumptions within the simulation, the fidelity of the simulation (i.e., how "realistic" it is) and the validity of the simulation outcomes (i.e., how likely are the outcomes portrayed in the simulation likely to happen in real life). The first medical simulators were simple models of human patients (Lanier and Biocca 1992). Since antiquity, these representations in clay and stone were used to demonstrate clinical features of disease states and their effects on humans. Models have been found from many cultures and continents. These models have been used in some cultures (e.g., Chinese culture) as a "*diagnostic*" instrument, allowing women to consult male physicians while maintaining social laws of modesty (Rosen 2008). A model is a simplified version of something complex. It is used in analyzing and solving problems or making predictions and are typically used when it is either impossible or impractical to create the original conditions. For example models are used to help students learn the *anatomy* of the *musculoskeletal, vascular, and organ systems*. A simulation is the implementation of a model over time. It brings a model to life and shows how a particular object or phenomenon will behave under certain conditions. It is useful for testing, analysis, and training on real-world systems or concepts that can be represented by a model. The models

A.G. Gallagher and G.C. O'Sullivan, *Fundamentals of Surgical Simulation*, Improving Medical Outcome - Zero Tolerance,
DOI 10.1007/978-0-85729-763-1_2,

Table 2.1 Simulator category options list Penn. State minimally invasive surgical skills laboratory*

	Model driven	Instructor driven	VR/haptic	Computer programs	Task specific model
Physical body	Yes	Yes	Some	No	Some
Automatic responses	Yes	No	Some	Yes	No
Performance feedback	No	No	Yes	Yes	No
Independent learning	No	No	Yes	Yes	Yes
Start-up cost	Medium to high, depending on model	Medium	High	Low	Low

*With permission from Prof. Randy Haluck

can be dynamic such as full physics computer generated virtual reality simulation of the human vascular and cardiovascular system that responds to real-time vessel–instrument interaction or a synthetic pad in which a trainee can excise a sebaceous cyst or practice suturing. Both model some aspect of human anatomy which facilitates a learning activity through simulation of characteristics of that anatomy. On the VR simulator it is possible to learn how not to behave dangerously with interventional devices such as catheters and wires and on the synthetic pad it is possible to learn how to suture while minimizing trauma to the sutured tissue and while closing the incision as neatly as possible.

Professor Randy Haluck (Hershey School of Medicine, Penn State.), one of the early adopters and pioneers of simulation, has compiled a comprehensive list which included descriptions of medical simulation technology. A complete list of the names of owners and description of these simulators can be found on the Minimally Invasive Surgical Training Unit, Hershey School of Medicine website (Halluck, accessed April 2010). A summary table is included which attempts to categorize the simulators by type and how they think each simulator works and what type of start-up costs might be associated with each type of simulator. This information is given below in Table 2.1. Please note that simulation nomenclature is not as yet standardized and the use of these terms may differ from site to site, and between manufacturers.

Physical body – Is the user interacting with a physical object (manikin body or part of a body) representing relevant patient anatomy?

- *Automatic responses* – Does the simulator autonomously respond (give immediate feedback) to interventions performed by the user with no instructor input?
- *Performance feedback* – Can the simulator itself evaluate performance and give feedback to the user after the session without an instructor being present?
- *Independent learning* – Can a user work through a module without instructor presence?
- *Start-up cost* – What is the average relative start-up cost for a system?

This list is based on the majority of simulations in a given category. There are exceptions in each category. Professor Haluck and his team have provided a very useful summary and information source on available simulators but do not make any critical appraisal. In order to supplement this information for the novice on medical simulation additional comments are provided below. Specific criticisms associated with a particular simulation/educational product are not provided unless, of course, we are commenting on data which has been published, which bears direct relevance to the point being made or it is something that has to be discussed openly at scientific or clinical meetings. To facilitate our discussion of available simulators we have organized our comments around the different types of available simulations (Table 2.2).

The different types of simulation have been divided into bench-top models, computer-generated experiences such as online simulations and different virtual realities experienced from part task trainers or emulators through to high fidelity full physics simulators. The use of animal models, cadavers and real patients as simulation models for the training and acquisition of skills are discussed. An extensive list of all the simulators available is not the function of this chapter. What we have done is given an outline of some of the more common types of simulators which are currently used in the training of residents and consultants in surgical skills. Throughout this book it is emphasized that the simulator one uses is probably not that important because there are numerous others which will probably do a similar job. What is important is that the right simulator is chosen for the job (taking account the costs). What is probably of paramount importance for trainers is that a simulator is simply a tool for delivering the curriculum, and for trainees the curriculum is king. When assessing the functionality of a potential simulation task there are two important questions: (1) Will this simulation task allow you to teach and train the required skills? and (2) will the simulation task allow you to assess the skills you wish the trainee to acquire? If one understands the purpose of these two questions and one (genuinely) knows how to go about answering them one truly understands the science of simulation. The different types of simulation (not an exhaustive list) to be discussed are shown in Fig. 2.1. They have been chosen as exemplars of the main categories or type of simulation because they are widely available and because the authors have direct personal experience with them.

Bench-Top Models

Animal Tissue

One of the most basic types of simulation task that has been around for decades and has been successfully used to help train medical students and junior doctors the skill of surgery, is the use of animal tissue such as pieces of chicken, pork, liver, or bowel. These models can be used for training a wide range of surgical skills

Table 2.2 A summary of the strengths and weaknesses of different types of simulations

Simulation examples	Strengths	Weaknesses
Bench-top models e.g., Limbs & Things, animal parts etc.,	Ready to use today, inexpensive, good face validity, no hygiene/health and safety issues, hygienic (for some)	Cost, reusability, assess ability, cost of real instruments, hygiene/health and safety issues, messy, ethics
Computer simulators		
Online simulation e.g., School for Surgeons (RCSI), ESSQ (RCSE), FLS (SAGES), CASES (SCAI) etc.,	Flexible, easily configurable, easily delivered, huge (as yet untapped) potential Most have no automatically generated metrics	
Part task trainers/VR emulators e.g., MISTVR, PROMIS, surgical science	Ready to use today, configurability (easy to hard), poor face validity, extremely well validated, costs, can be set up anywhere, multidisciplinary use	Costs (PROMIS)? use once and throw away, space, technical support, need for critical mass, teaching bad habits,
High fidelity e.g., Endoscopy, urology/endovascular Ophthalmic, SimSuite	Ready to use today, configurability (easy to hard), case library, multiple instruments on the same simulator, good face validity, reasonably well validated, good assessment, reliable, multidisciplinary usage	Costs, teaching bad habits, Well reported on, well accepted by professions, summative metrics, not a full physics simulator
Human patient simulator (anesthetics)	Well reported on, widely used	Lack of standardized metrics, time-consuming to use and assess, subjective assessments which are time-consuming
Full physics virtual reality simulator VIST & ES3	Real patient data, good face validity, configurability, new procedures, new cases library, new devices, objective feedback, real-time and summative metrics	Expensive, fragile, time-consuming to produce new cases, require a lot of technical support
Real tissues Animal models, cadavers, real patients	Good to excellent face validity, devices behave the same as on real patients	Supply problems, model realism (e.g., appendix in a pig); health and safety, storage, availability just-in-time, ethical issues, performance measurement, inadvertent events (killing the animal), very expensive, specialized facilities and support (e.g., vets, animal anesthetist), hygiene/health and safety, messy

from suturing to the making and closure of incisions. These types of models are readily available in most butcher shops on the high street, are relatively inexpensive and disposable. Another advantage of this type of model is that it gives trainees appropriate exposure to what it is like to work with real tissues – including fragility and consequences of inappropriate or rough handling. Thus, for the trainee these models have good face validity and for the trainer they give a good idea of how the trainee will handle human tissue. One of the major disadvantages of working with animal tissue is that special facilities are required by health and safety (RACS 2010). Special benches and special cleaning for health, safety and hygiene

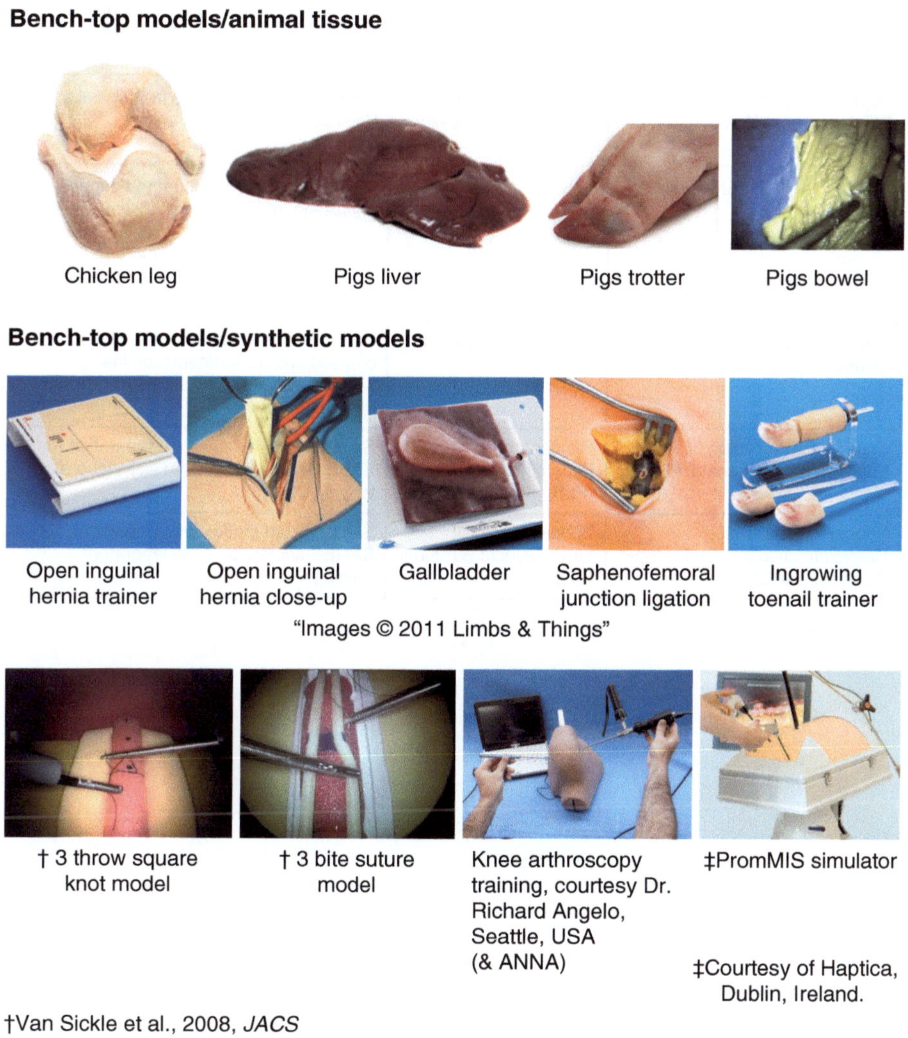

Fig. 2.1 Simulation examples

Online education/simulation models

Organization	E-learning package	Function
American College of Surgeons	ACS E-learning resource	The ACS E-learning resource provides access to webcasts, MP3 audio recordings of named lectures and panel sessions at clinical congresses
Royal Australasian College of Surgeons	Planned for	2011 – 2015 Strategic Plan: Implement e-learning strategy with Learning Management System and Knowledge Hub on web
Royal College of Physicians and Surgeons of Glasgow	NHS Scotland Knowledge Network	Fellows and members of the College have access to a wide range of e-resources through the NHS Scotland Knowledge Network
Royal College of Surgeons of Edinburgh (and University of Edinburgh)	Edinburgh Surgical Sciences Qualification (ESSQ)	Three-year M.Sc. course in Surgical Science with significant online educational resources
Royal College of Surgeons of England	School for Surgeons	In 2001 the College pioneered surgical e-learning, reconfiguring its *Surgical Training Education Programme (STEP®*, established in 1993) to incorporate an e-learning component, *e*STEP®
Royal College of Surgeons in Ireland	School for Surgeons	Virtual Grand Rounds, MRCS short courses and assignments, online discussions and debates, critical appraisal of the literature
European Association of Endoscopic Surgeons (EAES)	Fundamentals of Laparoscopic Surgeons (FLS)	Standardized modules in preparation for EAES/SAGES accredited skills laboratory training
Society of American Gastrointestinal and Endoscopic Surgeons (SAGES)	Fundamentals of Laparoscopic Surgeons (FLS)	Standardized modules in preparation for SAGES accredited skills laboratory training

Fig. 2.1 (continued)

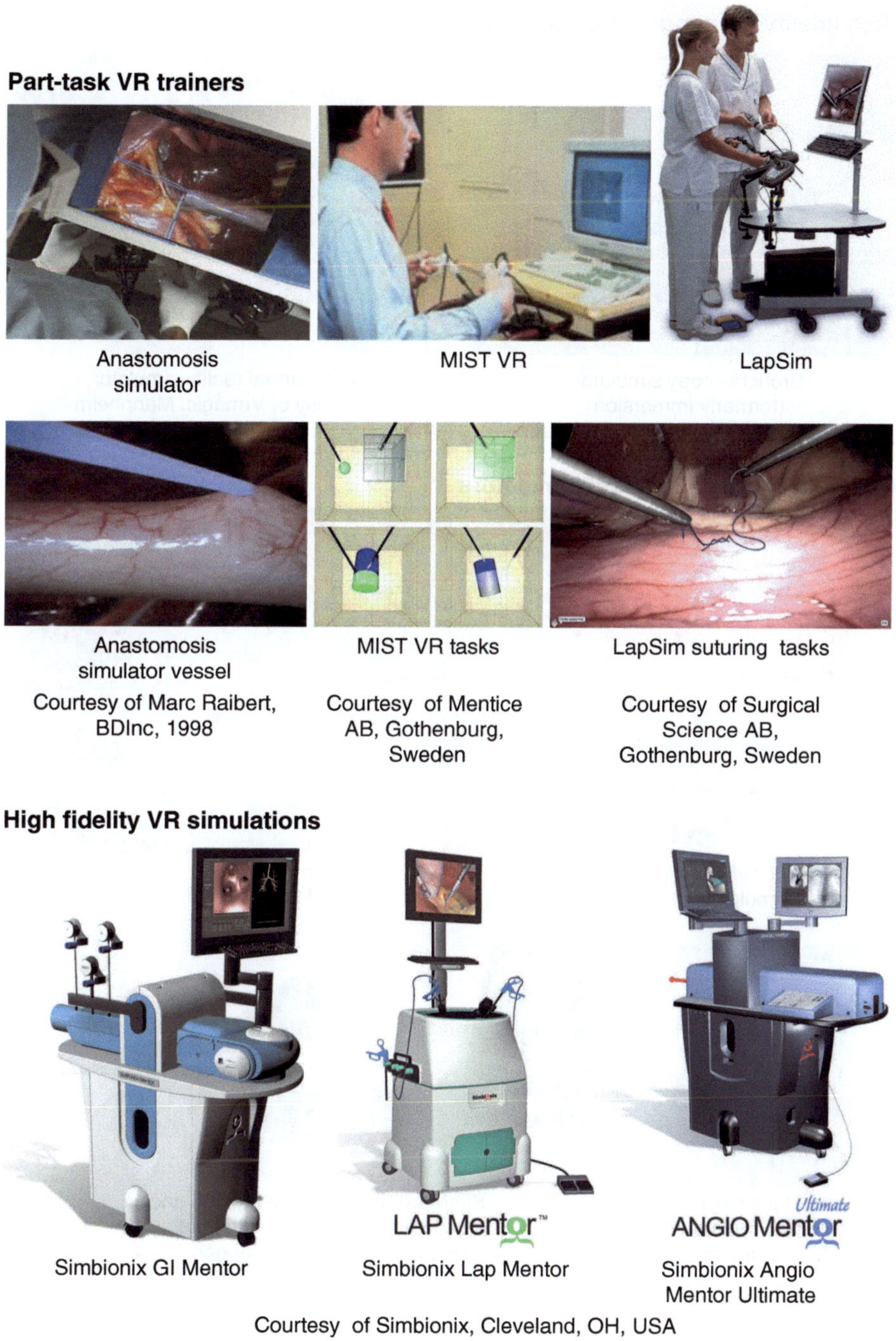

Fig. 2.1 (continued)

High fidelity VR simulations (contd.)

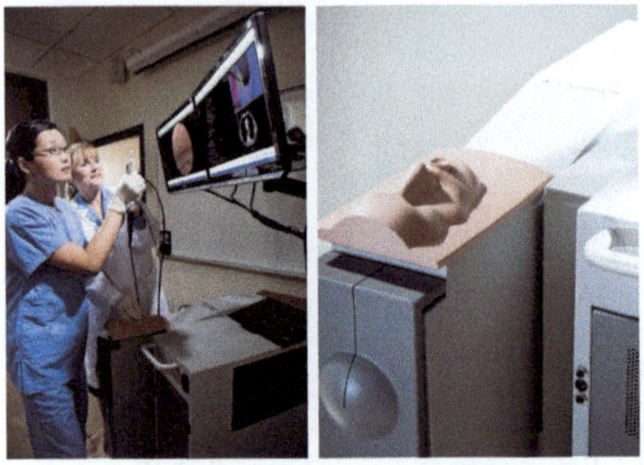

Bronchoscopy simulator
(formerly Immersion)
Courtesy of CAE, Montreal, Canada

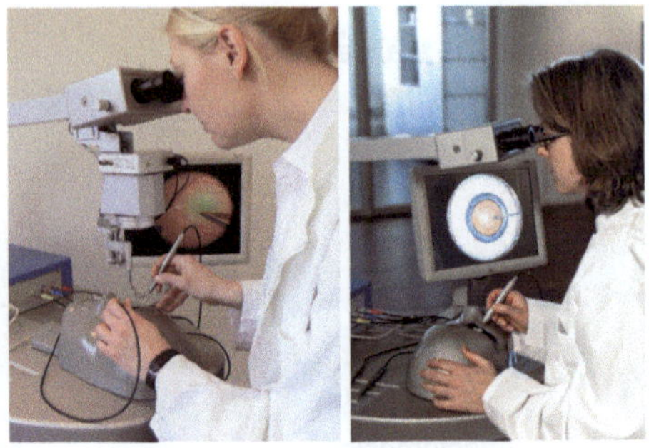

EYESI virtual reality simulator,
Courtesy of Vrmagic, Mannheim
Germany

High fidelity/human patient simulators

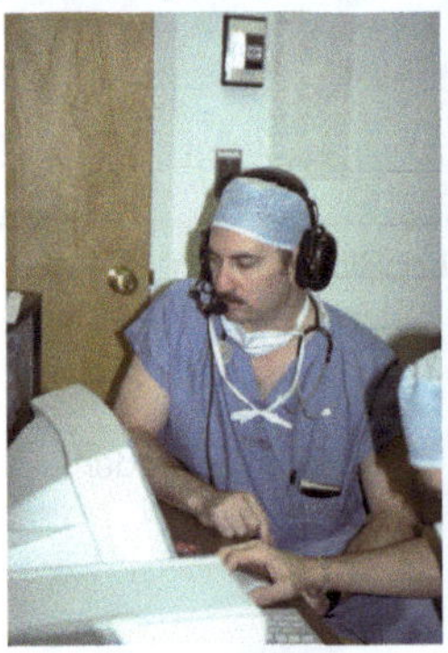

Dr. David Gaba
Pioneer of simulation in medicine

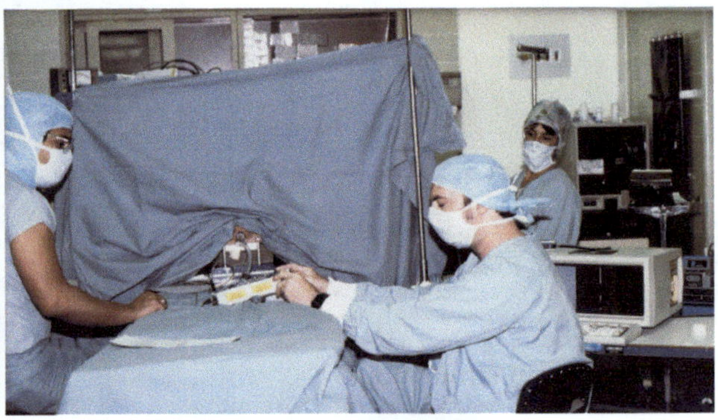

Gaba simulation
Courtesy of Dave Gaba

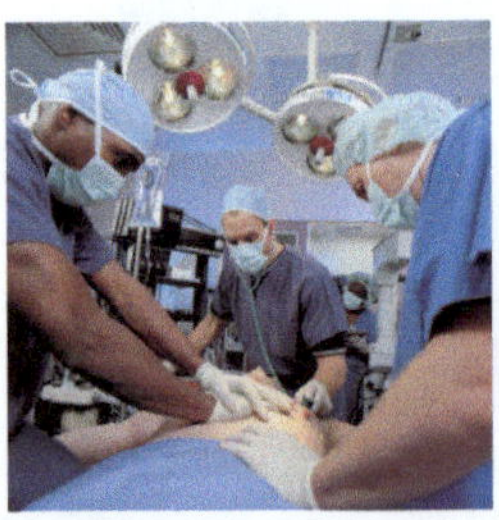

Medical Education Technologies
Inc. (METI) simulator, Courtesy
of METI, Sarasota, Fl, USA

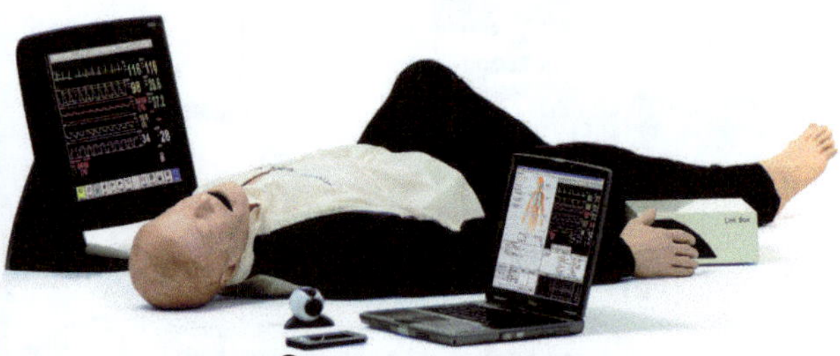

SimMan® is a portable and advanced
patient simulator for team training.
Courtesy of Laerdal, Stavanger, Norway

Fig. 2.1 (continued)

High fidelity/human patient simulators (contd.)

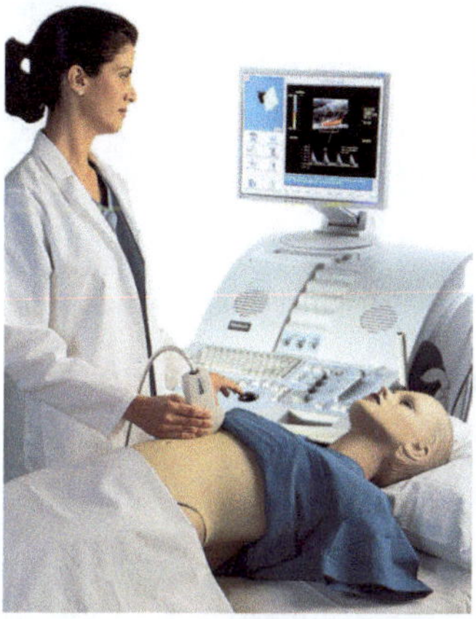

UltraSim (the first ultrasound simulator) Courtesy of MedSim; MedSim, Kfar-Sava, Israel.

SimSuite simulator

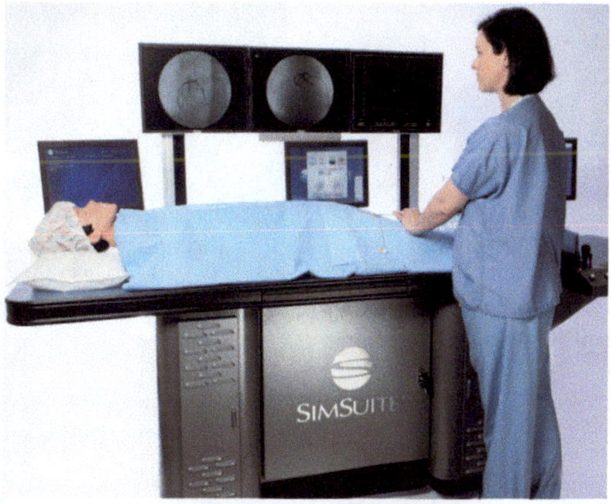

Simantha(R) Endovascular Simulator, Courtesy of Medical Simulation Corporation, Denver, Colorado

High fidelity complete operating room/cath. lab.

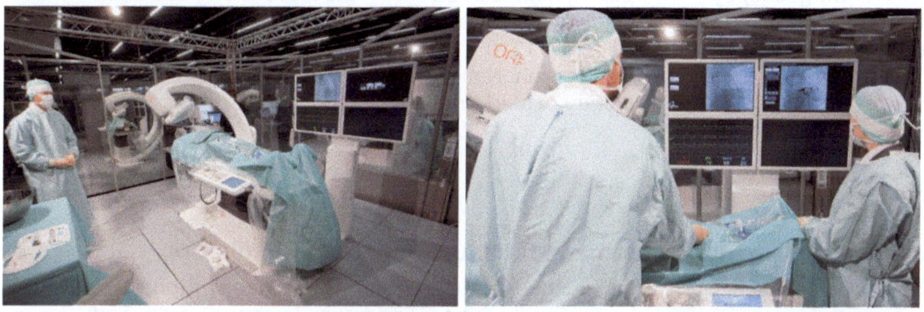

Orcamp complete operating room/cath lab. Courtesy of Orzone AB, Gothenburg, Sweden.

High fidelity/full physics virtual reality simulators

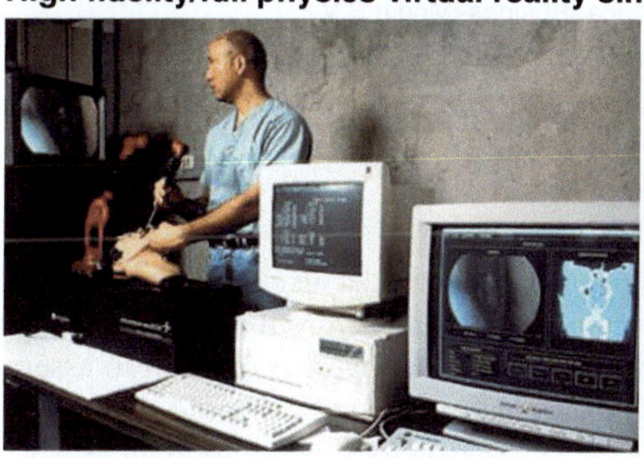

ENT Sinusoscopy Simulator (prototype) Lockheed Martin 1999

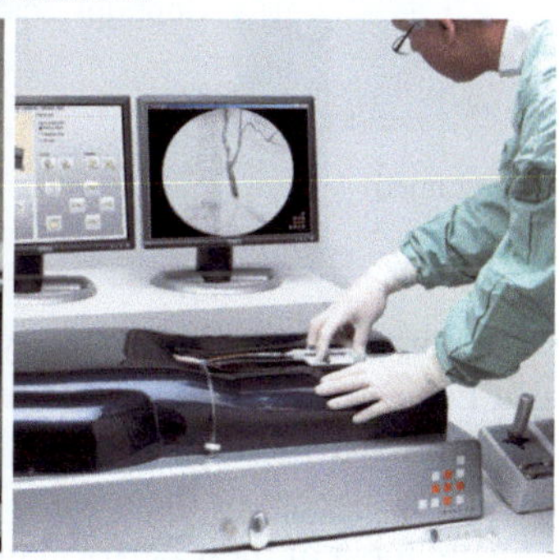

Vascular Intervention Simulation Trainer (VIST), Courtesy of Mentice AB, Gothenburg, Sweden

Fig. 2.1 (continued)

High fidelity/live tissue models as simulators

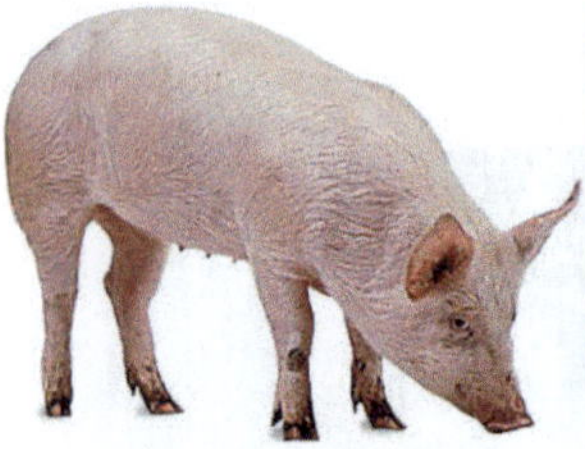

Pig model

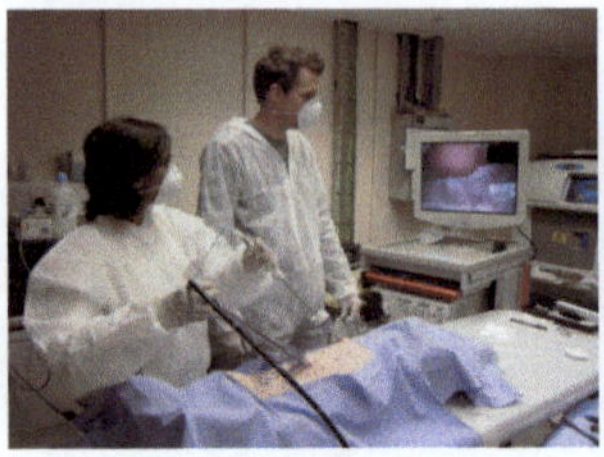

Pig operating model

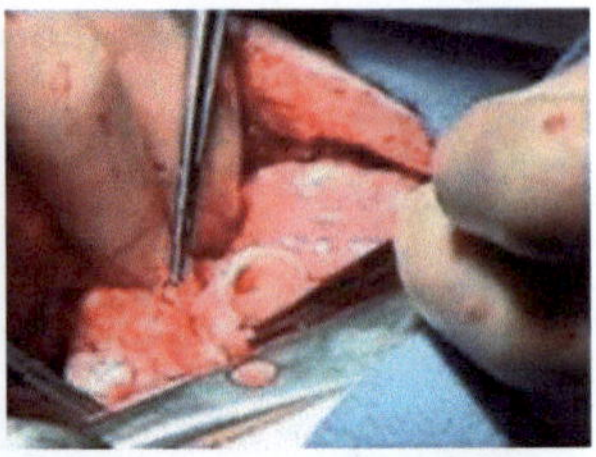

"Minor" surgery procedures

High fidelity/cadaver tissue models as simulators

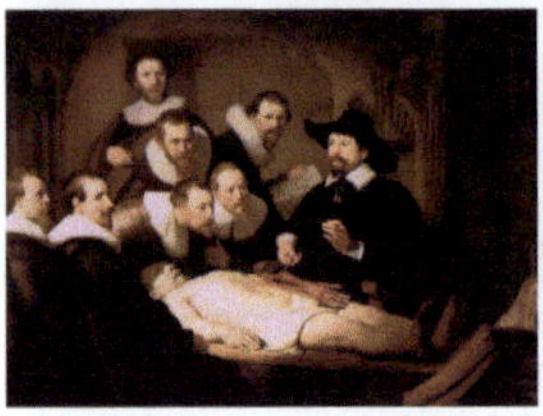

Dr. Nicholas Tulpe (City Anatomist, Amsterdam Guild of Surgeons) by *Rembrandt*, 16th January, 1632.

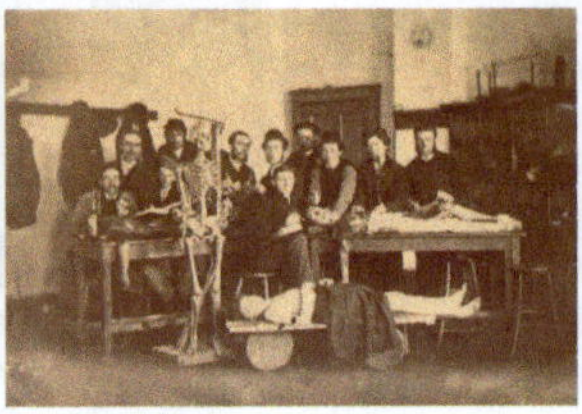

Interior of an unidentified classroom, students posing next to three cadavers and a skeleton USA, ca. 1910. Photograph. National Library of Medicine

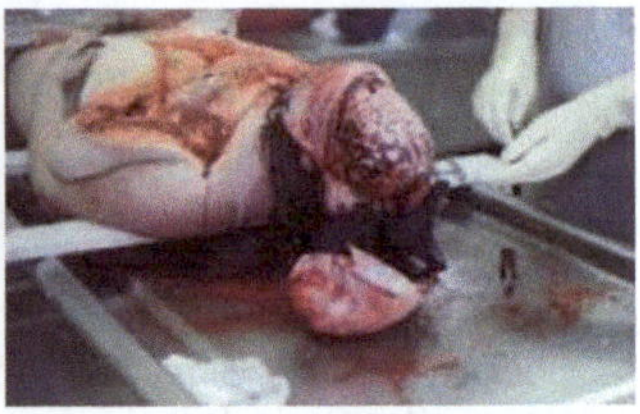

The dissection of human cadavers in medical school imparts not only the lessons of gross anatomy, but lessons on dealing with death.

Read more: Cadaver Experiences - body, life, time, human, Changes in Medical School http://www.deathreference.com/Bl-Ce/Cadaver-Experiences.html#ixzz0ZHgRgfV7

High fidelity/live human (damaged) tissue models as simulators

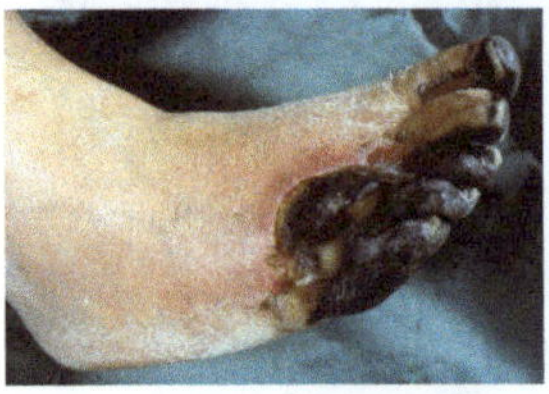

Gangrenous foot; Schneider, Rayfel; Laxer, Ronald; Ford-Jones, Elizabeth Lee; Friedman, Jeremy; Gerstle, Ted; Atlas of Pediatrics, Volume IA, Chapter 23. (2006) With Kind Permission from reproduced with permission from Springer Science+BusinessMedia B.V.

Fig. 2.1 (continued)

reasons are normally required. This type of training model also has a limited shelf life, and it can only be used a certain number of times before it becomes a health hazard. A further difficulty with this type of model is that it is difficult to assess. For optimal assessment of the trainee's performance the trainer should observe the trainee during most of their performances. The reason for this is important as when assessing the trainees performance the trainer needs to get as complete a picture as possible about their performance. In surgery it is important to assess not only the finished product of the operation, but also how it was achieved by the trainee. For example, the trainee may present a pig trotter which has a series of beautifully aligned sutures that are equally distant apart, with very neat knots and a series of suture tails that are all of the same length. However what may not be apparent is the amount of trauma caused to the tissue by the trainee inappropriately scraping and driving the needle through the tissue. While the finished product may look neat and, tidy it may hide damage to deeper level tissue. If this happened to a real patient it could lead to deep tissue infection which in surgery can have significant consequences.

How easily a training model facilitates the assessment of a trainee's performance is no small matter. Two lessons should be taken from the example cited above. The first is that the assessment of performance is very important in the training process and the second is that the look of the finished product can be deceiving. The finished model, i.e., the pig's trotter, appeared to be very well done, since the wound was closed with a series of very nice sutures. However, if only the finished product was assessed, there is no way of knowing how well or how badly the trainee performed in the process of performing the wound closure. This sort of problem does not just occur with very basic types of simulation models such as those described here but it also occurs with more advanced and very expensive simulation models. This problem will be discussed again in the context of virtual reality (VR) simulations for a carotid artery stenting.

Synthetic Models

Synthetic models for the education and training of skills in medicine have been used for some considerable period of time. However it was the introduction of minimally invasive surgery in the early 1990s that led to an increase in the demand for synthetic models for the training of laparoscopic surgical skills. One of the first companies to identify this growing market was Margot Cooper. In 1990, Mrs. Cooper established the Bristol-based company "Limbs & Things," which specialized in three-dimensional models for the minimal access surgery market. The company quickly identified a major opportunity in the development of materials, molding, and casting techniques to allow soft tissue to be simulated effectively and invested heavily in developing and refining materials for the simulation of human skin and tissue. We have used these models extensively in skills laboratories which we have worked in throughout the world. Indeed, in the National Surgical Training Centre at the Royal College of Surgeons in Ireland we used large volumes of "Limbs & Things" products for the training and assessment of surgeons in Ireland, and this has been reported on elsewhere (Gallagher et al. 2008; Kennedy et al. 2008; Carroll et al. 2009). Overall, these types of simulation products (of which Limbs & Things is just one manufacturer) are very valuable tools for any trainer to consider for the training and assessment of surgical skills. However, synthetic models are not without problems. The advantages of these products is that they are ready to use, they have good face validity in that they look like the anatomy of the surgical procedure they are supposed to simulate and there are no health and safety issues associated with their use. Consequently, they can be used in the dry skills laboratory, or in any hotel room or other place one wants to run a course. However, the tasks can be very messy. Some of the tasks illustrated in Fig. 2.1, particularly the laparoscopic cholecystectomy and the sapheno femoral junction ligation models are particularly messy as they contain fluids which leak out when the seal has been breached. Although these models could be used in a hotel room to run courses, they probably should not. Their use is more appropriate in a dedicated to dry skills laboratory. The models have other more substantive problems. For example, at the RCSI, the use of the in-growing toenail surgical model was stopped since it was believed to be anatomically incorrect. The company is receptive to feedback and will try to correct the model as soon as possible. These bench-top simulation models are quite expensive in the training situation. While the suturing pads can be used on numerous occasions, they still have a discreet "use"-life since only so many incisions can be made on a pad before it becomes unusable. Some of the surgical procedure tasks such as laparoscopic cholecystectomy or ingrowing toenail excision can only be completed once. Moreover, simple tasks such as suturing pads do not really respond the same way as human tissue or animal tissue to needle and thread dynamics and structure. For example, when teaching certain types of suturing technique such as subcuticular suturing, the synthetic tissue tends to rip which makes training this type of technique very difficult with synthetic models.

The trainer may develop their own tasks for the training of particular surgical skills. Intra-corporeal suturing is one of the most difficult advanced surgical skills that surgeons must acquire before they can perform advanced laparoscopic surgical procedures. At the Yale and Emory Universities' surgical training labs, some of the core advanced laparoscopic skills were taught to *all* trainees (Pearson et al. 2002; Van Sickle, Iii, Gallagher, et al., (2005); Van Sickle, Smith, McClusky, et al., (2005). The reasoning was that advanced intracorporeal suturing skills were the building blocks on which advanced laparoscopic surgical skills should be built. Unfortunately, there were no good simulation training models for intracorporeal suturing in existence, so the trainers developed their own. The intracorporeal suturing task was divided into two training components: the first was knot tying and the second was intracorporeal suturing by driving the needle atraumatically through the tissue. The tasks these trainers developed are illustrated in the third line of Fig. 2.1. The models developed were relatively simple and inexpensive but very effective training devices. The first model consisted of teaching trainees to tie a square knot, using both laparoscopic instruments, without dislodging the foam covered pipe from the contained sponge. This task taught the trainees two skills. The first skill was to be able to tie a square knot that did not slip inappropriately and the second was not to inflict undue trauma to the tissue. For the suturing part of the task a second simple model was devised. In this task, the trainees had to drive a needle, atraumatically, through clearly identified target areas on two plastic tubes with a middle suture which had to pass through the outer foam of the plastic tube that they used in the knot-tying task. This taught the trainees the skills of atraumatic suturing within clearly defined target areas. The assessment component for the first task was how they performed, for example, did they tie good knots which did not slip and were they able to suture on target and atraumatically. The assessment strategy for the second task was at the time a unique approach to the assessment of the task.

For the second assessment both of these tasks were placed inside a ProMIS™ hybrid, virtual reality training system also shown in Fig. 2.1 (third line). In the simulator the movement of the surgical instruments as a trainee tied the knot or performed the suture could be tracked. This provided a fairly reliable measure of how efficiently the trainee was performing the task as benchmarked against experts at intracorporeal suturing performance on the same tasks. In a validation study, the trainers were able to demonstrate that the training model worked very well in comparison to traditional intracorporeal suturing training programs (Van Sickle et al. 2008). The lessons to be learned from this account are: (1) If what you want does not exist, do not be afraid to develop a training model. (2) Do not be afraid to combine simulations as there are probably no ideal training solutions for many of the problems that exist out in the real world. The results from the study demonstrated that trainees who undertook the training program using these models performed the suturing component of a Nissen Fundoplication significantly better on real patients than those who took a traditional suture training program. The main issue when using simulation is knowing what you want to achieve and which simulation models will help you to achieve that goal. It should also be remembered that when evaluating any simulation and training product, how "pretty" it looks is only a small part of the assessment. The more important questions relating to the product assessment should be, does it train the skills it is supposed to train, what is the evidence for this and how well does it facilitate assessment of the trainee. In addition the trainer should always be mindful of the costs of achieving a training goal.

Online Education/Simulations Models

One of the most powerful education and training tools which has come into the educational and for training armamentarium of medical educationalists is the ability to deliver material via the World Wide Web (the Web). The potential of this medium for education and training is only limited by the imagination of those who are using it. There are some excellent examples of material delivered via the Web but, equally there are many disappointing examples of the way this medium has been used. Many medical education users of the Web for delivery of material seem to use it to deliver PowerPoint presentations or book chapters electronically. This is very disappointing and as stated earlier in connection with simulation; E-learning like simulation is just a very powerful tool for the efficient and effective delivery of the curriculum in medical education and training. The web should serve the same function, and indeed augment the entire training process on simulation by preparing and equipping the trainee with the knowledge and/or skills relevant to the training process.

Major surgical training organizations around the world recognize the power of the Web for training purposes. All of the Royal Colleges in the UK and Ireland, the Royal Australasian College of Surgeons, the American College of Surgeons as well as the Society of American Gastrointestinal Surgeons (SAGES) and its sister organization the European Association of Endoscopic Surgeons (EAES) have developed online training programs for surgeons in training.

The Royal College of Surgeons in Edinburgh has developed their e-learning program into a 3-year M.Sc. course in Surgical Science. SAGES and EAES are organizations which deal primarily with surgeons and physicians who practice minimally invasive procedural skills and are principally interested with the teaching and the assessment of these skills. Over about a decade they have developed a program called Fundamentals of Laparoscopic Surgery, better known as FLS (SAGES 2011). This training and education program includes two major components, one is an online e-learning component and the second is a technical skill component which can only be completed at a SAGES accredited skills laboratory. These training components are linked and the technical skills component must be completed after the online module. They have also standardized these modules for the USA. Consequently all trainees undertake the same training package, which should mean that the training program produces a fairly homogenous skills and knowledge set. Moreover, they have completely validated the technical skills training program which they are delivering. Prof. Gerry Fried (McGill University in Montréal) has completed the majority of the validation work for the technical skills component of this training package, and he has done a first class job in his psychometric and clinical validation studies of the FLS skills training package (Fried et al. 2004; Peters et al. 2004; Sroka et al. 2010). However, the problem for surgery is that laparoscopic surgical skills represent only a subcomponent of the skills a surgeon requires in his/her day-to-day professional practice.

One of the most comprehensive and elegant online education and training programs has been developed by the Royal College of Surgeons in Ireland (RCSI). Prof. Sean Tierney and Prof. Oscar Traynor developed “SCHOOL for Surgeons” (Surgical Conferencing with enHanced Opportunities for Online Learning) as part of a structured education and assessment program for trainees on the Basic Surgical Training, Irish Surgical Residency Program, and Higher Surgical Training and Programme for the Royal College of Surgeons in Ireland (Beddy et al. 2009). The program provides the trainee with regularly updated clinical material designed to promote self-directed learning; it challenges the trainees to actively seek to expand their knowledge base, and to develop analytical and clinical decision-making skills. The program is delivered using an open source virtual learning environment (Moodle), which is based on a social constructionist pedagogic model. Tierney and Traynor argue that while no program can substitute for experience at the bedside, in the clinic or in the operating theatre, SCHOOL for Surgeons can teach trainees to use a structured approach to clinical problems in order to allow them to make best use of the increasingly scarce time they spend with patients. A faculty of online tutors work with the surgical trainees during weekly program of education including, Virtual Grand Rounds, MRCS (Membergship of the Royal College of Surgeons) short courses and assignments, online discussions and debates, critical appraisal of the literature, an online journal club for discussion of important papers from major journals and training on ICT skills. This online education and training program is linked to a technical skills training program in which all of the trainees must spend a certain number of days each year in the skills laboratory. Trainees must make satisfactory progress on both units to progress in their training.

If the SAGES FLS training program could be criticized for being too specific for surgeons in general, in contrast the RCSI training program could be criticized for being too general. In personal communications with both Sean Tierney and Oscar Traynor suggestions have been made to improve this training program. The first suggestion was that the online component needs to have a more rigorous and systematic assessment process. Currently work is assessed on whether it was submitted or not, whether the answer is right or wrong or just like an essay. This seems an inefficient way to assess online performance. The second suggestion relates to linking the online education didactic component to the skills training sessions in the skills laboratory. To ensure that the skills laboratory facilities are used efficiently and effectively trainees should arrive well prepared for the skills they are about to learn. For example, if the trainees are coming to the skills laboratory to learn the skills necessary for flexible endoscopy they should know what types of conditions they would investigate using this type of technology and what types of symptoms a patient would present which would lead them to consider using this type of investigation. Prior online education and training would avoid the situation where some trainees participating in skills training have barely heard about the use of endoscopy never mind whom it should be used on and for what reasons. The majority of trainees turn up for their training at the skills laboratory well prepared. However, a small number of individuals turn up having made no preparation and tend to anchor the level of training that day to their level of "expertise." This can be very frustrating for their peers as well as the tutors who have frequently given up a day of clinical practice to pass on their expertise to the next generation of surgeons. This situation is not acceptable. The online training program should be changed so that trainees would take the module most appropriate to the next skills training session they are going to attend and they should be required to demonstrate a requisite knowledge level on the online module before being eligible to participate in the technical skills training. This may seem harsh, but training in the skills laboratory must be viewed as a high value-added component. It is certainly very expensive to organize, run, staff, and equip. As such, trainees and supervising consultants must ensure that the maximum value is elicited from the skills laboratory during training. This issue will recur in subsequent chapters when the issue of how much training constitutes enough training is discussed.

Part-Task Virtual Reality Trainers/Emulators

Col. Richard Martin Satava, first developed the idea of using virtual reality simulation to train surgeons in the late 1980s and early 1990s (Satava 1993). At that time, he was a program manager at the top-secret Defence Advanced Research Projects Agency (or DARPA, in the USA). During the 1990s, he spent millions of dollars funding research efforts into the development of virtual reality simulators for surgical tasks. Many of the simulators he funded were taken no further than prototypes or proof of concept. There were many reasons for this at the time. These included lack of enthusiasm from the medical community, absence of a viable market, and absence of low-cost high performance computing. However, the important lessons learned from these research projects were taken and applied to a wide variety of simulators that were developed around the world and subsequently taken to market. One of the most elegant surgical simulators ever built and developed during this period was the anastomosis simulator developed by BDInc., in Boston Mass. This device simulated the tissues, instruments, and images required to perform an end-to-end anastomosis. However, there were only two prototypes ever completed, and one of them currently resides in the training center of the National Capital Area Medical Simulation Centre in Washington DC. Although it looked and felt like a "real" surgical simulator little validation science was conducted on it.

In contrast, the Minimally Invasive Surgical and Trainer Virtual Reality or MIST VR (Wilson et al. 1997) looked nothing like a virtual reality surgical simulator. The first time we saw this simulator we thought it looked something like two laparoscopic surgical instruments attached to a purple motorbike engine frame. The developers of MIST VR did something rather clever when they were building this simulator. It was built in the mid-1990s, when desktop computers simply did not have the processing speed to render human tissue and surgical instrument interaction in real-time. Instead of trying to simulate the tissues in real time the MIST VR developers cleverly asked, "what skills are we trying to train and assess?" They then concentrated on developing tasks that they could present in real-time, which in turn trained and assessed the skills required to perform a laparoscopic cholecystectomy.

The first time we saw MIST VR we were pretty sure that a psychologist or a human factors person had been involved in its design and development. In contrast to MIST VR, simulators that had been developed by surgeon-engineer teams concentrated on how "pretty" the simulation looked rather than developing an effective training and assessment device. The MIST VR tasks moved in real-time, but increased in complexity as training progressed, requiring two-hand coordination of virtual tasks in three-dimensional space and on the final task required, hand-eye-foot coordination. It gives real-time feedback to the trainee on their performance as they progress through the tasks. For example if a trainee made an error on the task, the instrument they were using or the task they were working on (or both) turned red to indicate an error had been enacted. As well as real-time feedback on performance the trainees are given summative scores at the end of their training trial, both being components of an optimal training program. The tasks were also easily configurable from very easy to very difficult. These are all components of an optimal training program which has been developed with the research evidence on skills acquisition clearly informing development. Despite not really looking like a "proper" virtual reality surgical simulator MIST VR remains the best validated simulator in surgery today. Indeed, the first prospective, randomized, blinded clinical trial of virtual reality training for the operating room was completed on MIST VR. In 2001 a team of surgeons from Yale University in USA and an experimental psychologist from Ireland showed that training on MIST VR to a predetermined level of proficiency significantly outperformed a case-matched group of surgical trainees in the performance of part of a laparoscopic cholecystectomy (i.e., excision of the gallbladder from the liver bed) on real patients. The results were presented for the first time at the American Surgical Association in 2002 (Seymour et al. 2002) and was widely praised by these very senior surgeons.

This was an important milestone in the evolution and integration of simulation into surgical training as it was the first time that the clinical benefits of simulation training had been demonstrated in a robust scientific, clinical study. These results have since been replicated with other simulators (Ahlberg et al. 2007; Grantcharov et al. 2004). The Yale study is also important because it helped to define the methodology used to assess the transferability of clinical skills from the virtual training environment to the operating room (Gallagher et al. 2005). Other simulators similar in design and configuration to the MIST VR training system (currently supplied through Mentice, Gothenburg, Sweden) have since entered the market place. The LapSim™ from Surgical Science (Gothenburg, Sweden) occupies the same niche in the market as the MIST VR system. The manufacturers of the LapSim surgical training system have made special efforts to try and give their simulator more face validity than the MIST VR system. Some of the tasks bleed, almost all of the tasks look like tissue, and they move when prodded with surgical instruments. However, the issue of face validity aside, neither of these two virtual reality systems is what could be truly described as virtual reality simulators. Virtual reality emulators may provide a more accurate description of what they do.

The difference between a simulator and an emulator is that the emulator tries to imitate certain aspects of the tasks that are to be trained. In contrast, a simulator tries to represent as realistically as possible as many aspects of the simulated task as possible. In the MIST VR tasks, no attempt is made to actually simulate the tissue. The processing capacity of the computer is devoted to emulating the tasks, and the instrument–task interaction that are required to train the psychomotor hand–eye coordination required to perform a laparoscopic cholecystectomy. In contrast, the LapSim program makes some effort to make the tasks at least look tissue-like. Indeed, many surgeons have commented on the highly realistic looking LapSim tasks when compared to the MIST VR tasks. However, this "prettiness" of the tasks makes not a jot of difference to the training effectiveness of both machines. Indeed it could be argued that the MIST VR tasks are more parsimonious. The advantage about these types of "simulator" is that they are relatively inexpensive to purchase, and they include metrics on task performance built into the training modules as standard. Another advantage with these trainers is that they can be set up almost anywhere and require very little technical support. There are also no recurrent costs since the tasks are all computer-generated. However, new modules will cost extra and for the companies that manufacture these types of training devices, the hardware and to some extent the software markets must be considered as discrete.

High Fidelity Simulators

High fidelity virtual reality simulation has become more and more common with the widespread acceptance of minimally invasive surgical procedures. Two of the most successful manufacturers in this area are Simbionix (Cleveland, USA) and Immersion Medical (San Jose, USA). Simbionix is a company that originated in Israel but currently has their head office located in Cleveland in the USA. Both companies are important for different reasons. Immersion Medical is an US company which started research on the emerging medical virtual reality market, i.e., when Satava was with DARPA. The long-term impact of this has been that Immersion Medical holds the vast majority of patents relating to virtual reality simulation technology in medicine. This is particularly important in relation to the issue of haptics in virtual reality simulation. Haptics is the science and engineering that deals with the sense of touch (Monkman 1992). The emulators which were discussed in the previous paragraph have no haptic feedback. The surgical community considers this to be a particular weakness of these types of simulators and that haptic feedback is a crucial aspect of learning for the operating surgeon. Because Immersion Medical were one of the first companies to work on medical simulation they were also one of the first companies to work on haptics in simulation and to develop solutions and to patent them. In practice this means that other companies have to either find a way to give haptic feedback to the surgeon by using technology or software other than the types patented by Immersion Medical and which does not breach their patent or alternatively pay Immersion Medical a license fee for each unit sold. This issue recurs repeatedly in the medical simulation industry occasionally supported with legal representation and will almost certainly recur.

These issues aside, both companies have produced impressive high fidelity virtual reality simulators. Both companies produce, flexible endoscopy simulators, laparoscopic simulators with haptic feedback, as well as endovascular and fluoroscopically guided simulators. It is difficult to distinguish between the simulations produced by both companies since their products are very good. Although these simulators are relatively expensive, it is our opinion, they are good value for money. Most of the simulation platforms from these companies can be used to perform multiple procedures, for example, the endoscopy simulator can double as a colonoscopy simulator.

Another relatively new group of simulators are in ophthalmic surgery such as the EYESI™ (Fig. 2.1). The tasks and metrics built into this simulator are very impressive and the ophthalmic surgical community have set about the process of validating these types of simulators. What all of these simulators have in common is the ability to simulate surgical procedures that are performed within a finite volumetric space and they lend themselves to image guided intervention. However, these simulators are not without problems. Keeping them running requires some technical support and when they develop significant problems technical support from the company has to either come from Israel or the USA, which can be problematic. Another more serious problem with these simulators is the fact that they sometimes may allow technical and procedural skills which are without doubt, dangerous. For example, in some of the endoscopy simulations it is possible to push the flexible endoscope straight down through the vocal cords which in reality is never that easy on a real patient. The problem with this type of training fault is that if the trainee learns that it is this easy on the simulator there is a chance they will behave the same way toward their first patient, which could result in serious injury. This issue highlights how certain types of training on simulators could be dangerous for the patient if it goes unchecked. When supervising training on a real patient a consultant would never allow the trainee to perform in a way that exposes the patient to increased risk. However, when a trainee is training on a simulator, and at times is unsupervised, this provides opportunities for them to learn bad habits. The problem with learning bad habits is that they are very easy to acquire and they are very difficult to extinguish or unlearn. One potentially easy solution to this problem is the development of valid and reliable metrics that flag up dangerous behavior as soon as it occurs and records it for summative assessment feedback to the trainee at the end of their training session.

High Fidelity/Human Patient Simulators

It is assumed that human patient simulators are referred to as high fidelity simulations because the trainee is actually dealing with a physical mannequin that is attached to a computer. This branch of simulation, also known as full environment simulation, has been extensively developed and validated by anesthesiologists during the 1960s. Originally developed to teach airway management and resuscitative skills it was coupled with a computer to enhance the simulators capabilities and realism. One of the pioneers in this area is Prof. David Gaba an anesthetist from Stanford University, who in the late 1980s helped develop this branch of simulation into a realistic training environment with the aim of improving patient safety (Gaba and DeAnda 1988). The development of mathematical modeling programs for human physiology and drug pharmacodynamics and pharmacokinetics led to the development of mannequin and screen-based simulators. Currently the human patient simulator (HPS) based on these early models are manufactured by companies such as Medical Education Technologies Inc, also known as METI (Sarasota, USA) and Laerdal Medical AS (Stavanger, Norway). The HPS simulators can be used to stage full scale simulations whereby realistic monitoring, physiologic response to drugs, and high fidelity, pathological conditions can be encountered by trainees. This type of simulation facility affords the ability to integrate this practice into a complete curriculum, allows the trainer to alter the degree of difficulty of the simulation, and enables practice in controlled environments that can capture clinical variation that validly approximates to clinical experience. The use of the human patient simulator can add considerably to the training resources of any medical school or hospital training program. However, the mannequin is very expensive and it requires a dedicated space and technical support to ensure optimal training use.

Regular software updates are required and these are not inexpensive. It also requires a very experienced faculty of trainers to run and assess the training curriculum. This facility is probably best used as a team training environment for the emergency or the critical care scenarios. This facility might be integrated into a surgical training program and it would probably work best during medical school years, intern years, or when the trainee has acquired specific interventional procedural skills that they can implement in an operating room or emergency room environment. It would be pointless trying to teach these procedural skills during a team training exercise.

New additions to this group of simulators are continuously coming onto the market place; simulating different types of medical scenarios and clinical functionality as well as training such skills as ultrasound assessment. A relative newcomer to this group developed in the early twenty-first century is the SimSuite, supplied through Medical Simulation Corporation (Denver, USA). The manufacturers claim their simulator replicates a real-life catheterization laboratory, with a library of cases which mirror the types of cases which the interventional cardiologist would typically face in their daily practice. The manufacturer emphasizes the fact the technology replicates the real-life catheterization laboratory. It is also the case the physician can learn the appropriate devices to use for different types of cardiovascular pathology, and they may also learn how to deploy instruments such as stents. However, we are not convinced the trainee will acquire the subtle hand–eye, catheter–wire technical skills on this simulator. The reason is simple: this is not a full physics simulator, which replicates the human vascular system and catheter–wire interaction. Consequently this restricts the ability to assess trainee performance on a second-by-second business. The trainer is able to assess whether the right catheter was used, with the correct wire, with an appropriate sized balloon and stent and what percentage of the lesion was covered. However other real-time performance metrics such as advancing the catheter without wire in front of it or advancing the catheter or wire too quickly, or scraping the catheter against the vessel wall will be very difficult to assess using this simulator. Also, this is a very expensive simulator to acquire (usually leased), which requires dedicated space (permanent or temporary) and very experienced technical support to run it.

Although anesthetists and emergency room personnel are strong supporters of the mannequin type of simulation and claim to have this type of training well validated it is uncertain that this type of validation work would stand up to close scrutiny for high-stakes assessment (Bond et al. 2004). There is little doubt that training and this environment will improve team performance and enhance an understanding of how and what can go wrong in the operating room or in the emergency room situations. However, the team training environment scenario is not the optimal situation to acquire the procedural skills necessary to perform surgical procedures. While it is acceptable to indicate that someone performed well in a team, but it is quite a different matter to state that they performed well in the team, they were unable to perform the procedure well or safely. In procedural-based medicine such as surgery, interventional cardiology, and interventional radiology the unit of physician performance that is nonnegotiable is the ability of the interventionalist to perform the procedure to an adequate level, safely and in a timely fashion.

High Fidelity Full Physics Virtual Reality Simulators

These types of virtual reality simulators are probably the "holy grail" in medical simulation. They simulate in real time, the anatomy and physiology of real patients whose anatomy and pathology have been rendered from the imaged data of real patients; they simulate real interventional instruments that appear and interact with the simulated tissue almost the same as inside a real patient. The two full physics virtual simulators that we have some experience of are the ENT Sinusoscopy simulator or the ES3 system (Edmond et al. 1997) developed by Lockheed Martin and the Vascular Interventional System Training (VIST™) formerly known as the Interventional Cardiology Training System (Dawson et al. 2000). The ES3 simulator was a state-of-the-art virtual reality simulator when it was built. However, more than a decade after it was built the high-end computer platforms (two of them) that it was built on now seem antiquated. Although a very good simulator in its day it now needs to be ported down to a high-end PC computer system. The ES3 simulates the full ENT surgical procedure using the same endoscope and surgical instruments that would be used during a real procedure on a real patient. The surgical cases were developed from real patients and the instruments look, feel, and behave the same way they would inside a real patient. Unfortunately, only three prototype systems were ever built. The system that has been best funded and researched resides in the ENT department at Albert Einstein Hospital in New York. Funded by a grant from AHRQ, Prof. Marvin Fried has completed a series of validation studies that demonstrate that the ES3 is a pretty good simulation (Fried et al. 2010; Fried et al. 2007; Uribe et al. 2004). However, he continues to struggle with the antiquated computer platform that powers the ES3.

In contrast, the VIST simulator has had a much more colorful developmental history. It started out life in Dr. Steve Dawson's laboratory (CIMIT) in Harvard funded in partnership with Mitsubishi Technology. However in the late 1990s Mitsubishi withdrew their support for the project and the simulator was sold to a London-based company called Virtual Presence who in turn sold the simulator to a Swedish company called Mentice AB (Gothenburg, Sweden). One of us (AGG) purchased the first VIST system in the UK, and VIST is probably the most successful full physics simulator on the market today. It simulates a wide variety of endovascular procedures from coronary artery stenting, coronary angiography, carotid artery stenting, renal stenting, and a variety of other peripheral vascular endovascular procedures. It runs on a high-end dual processor PC system and simulates the real anatomy and pathology of a variety of patient cases, which can be completed with a range of manufacturers' devices. Because it is a full physics simulator, performance of the trainee can be assessed on a second-by-second basis and the trainee can receive intraoperative feedback on their performance as well as feedback at the end of the procedure. It has been extensively studied in the skills laboratory (Gallagher and Cates 2004a, b; Nicholson et al. 2006; Patel et al. 2006; Van Herzeele et al. 2007) with some clinical validation including a study where the data from the patient who was to be operated on was downloaded and formatted in the simulator so that the physician could rehearse performing the procedure before actually completing the procedure on the real patient, i.e., mission rehearsal (Cates et al. 2007). It is our opinion that this simulator is one of the best virtual reality simulators ever built. However, VIST is also not without its problems! The VIST requires dedicated space in a temperature controlled room, very knowledgeable technical support, and gentle handling by trainees. It is very expensive (but probably not as expensive as the SimSuite system) as are new modules. A further problem is that the system does not always run reliably. Although the system can take patient specific data, the case data must be formatted by the developers and can take up to a week before a workable model can be produced.

High Fidelity Live Tissue Models as Simulators

Surgery and interventional medical disciplines have used live animals for training for decades and this is unlikely to cease in the foreseeable future. Working on live animals under real operating room conditions, with real surgical instruments is very reassuring for surgeons. It also provides valuable information on how the instruments behave or interact with real anatomy. It is difficult to simulate inside a computer environment how a surgical instrument with an electric charge at the end of it (i.e., a cautery instrument) will behave in close proximity to moist live tissue. There are also numerous other advantages to using live animals for training purposes such as making the initial incision, operating on real beating tissue, and practicing wound closure. However, there are as many if not more disadvantages associated with training on live animals (not least of which is the ethics associated with training on live animals). There are also very significant costs associated with housing the animals, feeding them, and providing a dedicated operating room which is equipped to a similar level as a hospital operating room. Furthermore, when these animals are being operated on a vet technician, or indeed, a veterinary surgeon or an anesthetist must be present throughout the procedure. All of these aspects of animal work make training on animals, very, very expensive. Moreover, there is the whole issue of performance measurement. For example, if one is trying to train the safe and appropriate deployment of mesh for the treatment of a ventral hernia, it is very difficult to assess on an animal model how well the mesh has been placed and secured unless and until one sacrifices the animal. However, in a bench-top simulation model such as a synthetic abdomen produced by Limbs & Things, it is relatively easy to assess performance by simply removing the top of the simulator and examining how well the mesh has been stretched and tacked to the abdominal wall. Furthermore, these types of training scenarios may be run in hotel facilities and do not require dedicated operating room conditions.

Cadaver Tissue Models as Simulators

Human cadavers have always been and likely will always be an important means for discovering the intricacies of human anatomy during medical training. In 1542

Vesalius inaugurated the age of science and science-based medicine by testing published anatomical information against the facts revealed by cadaveric dissection. By placing the deceased human at the core of his investigations Vesalius had implicitly affirmed the patient centered Hippocratic cannon (Nuland 1988). Coulehan and colleagues (Coulehan et al. 1995) noted that medicine is unique in allowing the dismemberment of the whole body during professional training. In medical education the value of cadaveric dissection is still regarded as important in the education of medical students but probably not as important as it was for most of the twentieth century. Surgeons have been particularly strong advocates of cadaveric work during training. In particular, they value the development by the trainee surgeon of a touch-based topographical map of the human anatomy. Indeed touch-based learning is one of the aspects of virtual reality simulation that continues to require further development. Although the science of touch in medical simulation or "haptics" has been investigated for at least two decades considerable debate ensues as to the value of the haptics that currently exist in medical simulators. This is no small issue since the cost of adding a haptics component to a virtual reality simulation is enormous. Although the psychophysics of touch sensation has been investigated by experimental psychologists for almost two centuries (Gregory 1983) little effort was made by engineers to tap into this expertise. Instead, engineers sought the opinions of physicians who were performing the procedures, which may have been useful for qualitative insights but probably was not the optimal way to look for a solution to the problem. This issue will be dealt with in subsequent chapters when the issues of metrics identification, development, and operational definition are discussed (Chap. 5).

Surgeons have also argued that cadaveric work can also provide a good method of teaching and understanding of deep seated structures, and a framework and rational approach to understanding three-dimensional organization of anatomical structures as well as their dimensions, densities, and the strength of various tissues (Mutyala and Cahill 1996). They also point out that dissection facilitates the acquisition of manual skills which are essential to almost every branch of interventional medicine (Ellis 2001). Dissection is also a necessary exercise in the development of touch-based skills which are so important in surgery. In summary, surgeons argue that training on the human cadaver paves the way for surgeons to learn the techniques and the instrumentation of tomorrow and is key to their medical education. Of course it is not just medical students who use human cadavers for education and training purposes. Human cadavers are in much demand for postgraduate surgical training courses such as for laparoscopic colorectal procedures.

As a basic tenet of medical education we have no doubt about the value of cadaveric work for the medical student and junior doctor. Although still widely used in medical education, a review on the use of cadavers during the 1980s led to a significant reduction in instructional time. In an extensive review of the human cadaver use in medical education Aziz et al. (2002) give a number of reasons for the decrease or elimination of dissection in medical education and these are summarized in Table 2.3. Although the reasons were offered in relation to dissection and medical school education, many of these reasons are equally applicable to the training of junior and more advanced surgeons. The reasons offered by Aziz et al. include the fact that it is time consuming to prepare a cadaver for a surgical course,

Table 2.3 Reasons given for eliminating or reducing cadaver dissection in medical education

1. *Time consuming*
   Contention: dissection is overly time-consuming activity
2. *Labor intensive/shortage of anatomists*
   Contention: dissection is labor-intensive; partly due to shortage of mollified faculty
3. *Fact-filled/requires excessive rote memory*
   Contention: faculty requires students to memorize excessive often clinically irrelevant facts
4. *Cadaver unavailability*
   Contention: it is necessary to protect due to cadaver shortage
5. *Undesirable due to post-mortem changes*
   Contention: cadaveric anatomy is different from living anatomy. It misleads due to post-mortem changes
6. *Expensive*
   Contention: cadaver is costly to obtain, embalm, store, maintain, and dispose
7. *Unaesthetic*
   Contention: smells, looks ugly, repulsive, etc.
8. *Involves outdated archaic technology*
   Contention: uses "primitive" instruments; "draculasque"
9. *Potential health hazard*
   Contention: danger from the embalming fluid and infectious disease; stress provoking
   A. *Dangers of embalming fluid components* (formaldehyde, xylene)
   B. *Infectious diseases*
      (i) Transmissible spongiform encephalitis
      (ii) Human immunodeficiency virus
      (iii) Tuberculosis bacillus
      (iv) Hepatitis
   C. *Psychosocial impact* (promoting fear and anxiety)

there is a lack of appropriately trained and qualified faculty, there may be undesirable post-mortem changes in anatomy, and cadavers do in fact pose a potential health hazard. However, other factors have come to the fore more recently; these include the unavailability of cadavers for surgical training, and the expense of acquiring cadavers, both of which have not been helped by a number of very high-profile scandals involving cadavers.

Donations of human bodies for medical research have declined in recent years correlated with a marked decline in public confidence in the medical profession. With scandals such as Alder Hey and The Bristol Case (Senate of Surgery 1998) Royal Bristol Infirmary Inquiry; (Senate of Surgery 1998) people are less confident that their wishes on what will happen to their body will be carried out, so instead have not donated to medical science. Compounding this problem has been the legislation that followed the scandals, namely, The Human Tissue Act 2004 has tightened up the availability of resources to anatomy departments. The Alder Hey scandal started with the evidence from a medical witness to the Bristol Royal infirmary enquiry in 1999. Although the Bristol Royal Infirmary enquiry was investigating the deaths of children after cardiac surgery at the Royal Infirmary this witness drew attention to the large number of hearts held at the Alder Hey Children's Hospital in

Liverpool. As the details of the Alder Hay's organ retention began to come to light the public learned that the program went back decades. An investigation was opened in December 1999. However in Liverpool, it was not just Alder Hey that was affected. Walton Hospital stored the organs of 700 patients (which did not come to light until the investigation on Alder Hey was opened). This enquiry also revealed that a Dutch pathologist, Dick van Velzen systematically ordered the "unethical and illegal stripping of every organ from every child who had had a post-mortem" during his time at the hospital. To make matters worse it was revealed that this happened even to children of parents who had specifically stated that they did not want a full post-mortem on their child. When the report was published in January 2001 it revealed that over 104,000 organs, body parts, and entire bodies of fetuses and stillborn babies were stored in 210 NHS facilities. Additionally 408,600 samples of tissue taken from dead patients were also being held. To add insult to injury it also emerged that Birmingham Children's Hospital and Alder Hey Children's Hospital in Liverpool had also given the thymus glands removed from live children during heart surgery, to a pharmaceutical company for research in return for financial donations.

There is little doubt about the continued value of cadaveric dissection for the development and understanding of anatomy, of volumetric and substantial aspects of bodily structures, their dimensions, densities, and the strength of various tissues for traditional open surgery. Indeed a good case can also be made for the development of new surgical procedures by very experienced surgeons. However, the case for acquiring the skills necessary to practice minimally invasive surgery is becoming weaker as (virtual reality and bench top) simulators become more sophisticated. As we shall see in Chaps. 3 and 4 there is considerable degradation of the sensory and perceptual information that the surgeon has to use to perform minimally invasive surgical procedures on real patients (Gallagher and Smith 2003). The information they receive through surgical instruments is also degraded, as is the image that they view on the monitor. Although the image is extremely high-quality it is still a pixilated image which is orders of magnitude inferior to what the eye would perceive under natural viewing conditions. If these conditions can be realistically simulated in a virtual environment, or indeed in a bench-top simulation task, it considerably weakens the argument for training on cadavers.

High Fidelity Live (Damaged) Human Tissue Models as Simulators

When we first thought about writing this book a few years ago this category of simulation was not high on our inclusion list! In fact, we had not considered including it at all until something rather strange happened to one of us (AGG) during a lecture tour in a very highly populated far eastern country. We were running a course for very senior neurosurgeon's on carotid artery stenting using virtual reality training. We were training this procedure using a full physics, virtual reality simulator, and during these sessions we had informal discussions about the training conducted in that country. We happened to enquire how they would normally train and acquire the technical catheter-wire skills to perform such an advanced endovascular procedure. We were informed in a very matter-of-fact fashion, that they would train on patients in the hospital who were scheduled to have an ischemic limb amputated. Physicians would practice or learn their technical skills on the limb before it was amputated. We were also informed that although a full physics, virtual reality simulation was very nice to have they did not really need it. In response to this information we explained that this type of training probably would not catch on in Western medicine.

Summary

It is widely believed in medicine in general, but in interventional disciplines such as surgery in particular, that training on simulators is something new. It is not. It is also widely believed that virtual reality type simulations represent something new. They do not. Virtual reality simulation represents the most recent evolution of simulators for the acquisition of procedural skills. Medical disciplines such as surgery have had simulation type models available to them for training for centuries. These models have ranged from inanimate representations of the human body through to cadaveric dissections. However, all of them have been pioneered and developed for the purpose of improving medical knowledge and procedural skills. What has changed over the last two decades is how these training devices are construed and leveraged to deliver evidence-based training and assessment *within* a curriculum. In the coming chapters we will describe what makes for a good simulation, how to ensure that the chosen simulation is effective, efficient, and facilitates the acquisition of surgical and procedural skills. This systematic evidence-based approach to the use of simulations is new but it also builds on knowledge and research findings from the behavioral sciences that avoids reinventing the wheel. Evidence exists from prospective, randomized clinical studies that demonstrates unequivocally that simulation-based training improves operative performance. In the coming chapters we will describe and discuss how these results can be replicated in everyday surgical training environments. However, it is first necessary to understand in detail precisely what we mean when we say "training."

References

Ahlberg G, Enochsson L, Gallagher AG, et al. Proficiency-based virtual reality training significantly reduces the error rate for residents during their first 10 laparoscopic cholecystectomies. *Am J Surg*. 2007;193(6):797-804.

Aziz MA, McKenzie JC, Wilson JS, Cowie RJ, Ayeni SA, Dunn BK. The human cadaver in the age of biomedical informatics. *Anat Rec B New Anat*. 2002;269(1):20-32.

Beddy P, Ridgway PF, Beddy D, Clarke E, Traynor O, Tierney S. Defining useful surrogates for user participation in online medical learning. *Adv Health Sci Educ Theory Pract.* 2009;14(4): 567-574.

Bond WF, Deitrick LM, Arnold DC, et al. Using simulation to instruct emergency medicine residents in cognitive forcing strategies. *Acad Med.* 2004;79(5):438-446.

Carroll SM, Kennedy AM, Traynor O, Gallagher AG. Objective assessment of surgical performance and its impact on a national selection programme of candidates for higher surgical training in plastic surgery. *J Plast Reconstr Aesthet Surg.* 2009;62(12):1543-1549.

Cates CU, Patel AD, Nicholson WJ. Use of virtual reality simulation for mission rehearsal for carotid stenting. *J Am Med Assoc.* 2007;297(3):265.

Coulehan JL, Williams PC, Landis D, Naser C. The first patient: reflections and stories about the anatomy cadaver. *Teach Learn Med.* 1995;7(1):61-66.

Dawson S, Cotin S, Meglan D, Shaffer DW, Ferrell MA. Designing a computer-based simulator for interventional cardiology training. *Catheter Cardiovasc Interv.* 2000;51(4):522-527.

Edmond CV Jr, Heskamp D, Sluis D, et al. ENT endoscopic surgical training simulator. *Stud Health Technol Inform.* 1997;39:518.

Ellis H. Teaching in the dissecting room. *Clin Anat.* 2001;14(2):149-151.

Fried GM, Feldman LS, Vassiliou MC, et al. Proving the value of simulation in laparoscopic surgery. *Ann Surg.* 2004;240(3):518-525; discussion 525-518.

Fried MP, Sadoughi B, Weghorst SJ, et al. Construct validity of the endoscopic sinus surgery simulator: II. Assessment of discriminant validity and expert benchmarking. *Arch Otolaryngol Head Neck Surg.* 2007;133(4):350.

Fried M, Sadoughi B, Gibber M, et al. From virtual reality to the operating room: the endoscopic sinus surgery simulator experiment. *Otolaryngol Head Neck Surg.* 2010;142(2):202-207.

Gaba DM, DeAnda A. A comprehensive anesthesia simulation environment: re-creating the operating room for research and training. *Anesthesiology.* 1988;69(3):387-394.

Gallagher AG, Cates CU. Approval of virtual reality training for carotid stenting: what this means for procedural-based medicine. *J Am Med Assoc.* 2004a;292(24):3024-3026.

Gallagher AG, Cates CU. Virtual reality training for the operating room and cardiac catheterisation laboratory. *Lancet.* 2004b;364(9444):1538-1540.

Gallagher AG, Smith CD. From the operating room of the present to the operating room of the future. Human-factors lessons learned from the minimally invasive surgery revolution. *Semin Laparosc Surg.* 2003;10(3):127-139.

Gallagher AG, Ritter EM, Champion H, et al. Virtual reality simulation for the operating room: proficiency-based training as a paradigm shift in surgical skills training. *Ann Surg.* 2005;241(2):364-372.

Gallagher AG, Neary P, Gillen P, et al. Novel method for assessment and selection of trainees for higher surgical training in general surgery. *ANZ J Surg.* 2008;78(4):282-290.

Grantcharov TP, Kristiansen VB, Bendix J, Bardram L, Rosenberg J, Funch-Jensen P. Randomized clinical trial of virtual reality simulation for laparoscopic skills training. *Br J Surg.* 2004;91(2):146-150.

Gregory RL. Mind in science. A history of explanations in psychology and physics. *Group Anal.* 1983;16(1):88.

Haluck, R. What's Available in the Medical Simulation Field. Penn State Hershey Simulation Center , Penn State College of Medicine at the Penn State Milton S. Hershey Medical Center http://pennstatehershey.org/web/simulation/home/available. (accessed 23rd July 2011)

Kennedy AM, Carroll S, Traynor O, Gallagher AG. Assessing surgical skill using bench station models. *Plast Reconstr Surg.* 2008;121(5):1869-1870.

Lanier J, Biocca, F. An Insider's View of the Future of Virtual Reality. *Journal of Communication* 1992;42(4):150-172.

Monkman GJ. An electrorheological tactile display. *Presence: Teleoper Virtual Environ.* 1992;1(2):228.

Mutyala S, Cahill DR. Catching up. *Clin Anat.* 1996;9(1):53-56.

Nicholson WJ, Cates CU, Patel AD, et al. Face and content validation of virtual reality simulation for carotid angiography: results from the first 100 physicians attending the Emory NeuroAnatomy Carotid Training (ENACT) program. *Simul Healthc.* 2006;1(3):147-150.

Nuland SB. *Doctors; The Biography of Medicine.* New York: Vintage Books; 1988.

Patel AD, Gallagher AG, Nicholson WJ, Cates CU. Learning curves and reliability measures for virtual reality simulation in the performance assessment of carotid angiography. *J Am Coll Cardiol*. 2006;47(9):1796-1802.

Pearson AM, Gallagher AG, Rosser JC, Satava RM. Evaluation of structured and quantitative training methods for teaching intracorporeal knot tying. *Surg Endosc*. 2002;16(1):130-137.

Peters JH, Fried GM, Swanstrom LL, et al. Development and validation of a comprehensive program of education and assessment of the basic fundamentals of laparoscopic surgery. *Surgery*. 2004;135(1):21-27.

Rosen KR. The history of medical simulation. *Journal of Critical Care* 2008:23(2);157-166.

Royal Australasian College of Surgeons (RACS) Policies and Procedures; Anatomical specimens used for skills training http://www.surgeons.org/media/16948/REL_SKC_6602_P_Anatomical_Specimens_Skills_Centre_Policy.pdf. (accessed 5th July 2011).

Satava RM. Virtual reality surgical simulator. The first steps. *Surg Endosc*. 1993;7(3):203-205.

Senate of Surgery. *Response to the General Medical Council Determination on the Bristol Case: Senate Paper 5*. London: The Senate of Surgery of Great Britain and Ireland; 1998.

Seymour NE, Gallagher AG, Roman SA, et al. Virtual reality training improves operating room performance: results of a randomized, double-blinded study. *Ann Surg*. 2002;236(4):458-463; discussion 463-454.

Society of American Gastrointestinal and Endoscopic Surgeons (SAGES). Fundamentals of Laparoscopic Surgery (FLS). http://www.flsprogram.org/(accessed 5th July 2011)

Sroka G, Feldman LS, Vassiliou MC, Kaneva PA, Fayez R, Fried GM. Fundamentals of laparoscopic surgery simulator training to proficiency improves laparoscopic performance in the operating room-a randomized controlled trial. *Am J Surg*. 2010;199(1):115-120.

Uribe JI, Ralph WM Jr, Glaser AY, Fried MP. Learning curves, acquisition, and retention of skills trained with the endoscopic sinus surgery simulator. *Am J Rhinol*. 2004;18(2):87-92.

Van Herzeele I, Aggarwal R, Choong A, Brightwell R, Vermassen FE, Cheshire NJ. Virtual reality simulation objectively differentiates level of carotid stent experience in experienced interventionalists. *J Vasc Surg*. 2007;46(5):855-863.

Van Sickle K, Iii D, Gallagher AG, Smith CD. Construct validation of the ProMIS simulator using a novel laparoscopic suturing task. *Surg Endosc*. 2005a;19(9):1227-1231.

Van Sickle K, Smith B, McClusky DA 3rd, Baghai M, Smith CD, Gallagher AG. Evaluation of a tensiometer to provide objective feedback in knot-tying performance. *Am Surg*. 2005b;71(12):1018-1023.

Van Sickle K, Ritter EM, Baghai M, et al. Prospective, randomized, double-blind trial of curriculum-based training for intracorporeal suturing and knot tying. *J Am Coll Surg*. 2008;207(4): 560-568.

Wilson MS, Middlebrook A, Sutton C, Stone R, McCloy RF. MIST VR: a virtual reality trainer for laparoscopic surgery assesses performance. *Ann R Coll Surg Engl*. 1997;79(6):403-404.

Chapter 3
Human Factors in Acquiring Medical Skill; Perception and Cognition

Psychological and Human-Factor Aspects of Surgery

To a large extent, the increase in usage of laparoscopic surgery as an operative technique during the 1980s concealed many of its problems. However, had it not been for the development of laparoscopic surgery, medicine and surgery may never have taken account of 'human factors' as they relate to the practice of procedural medicine. As seen over the next two chapters, human factors are at the core of procedural medicine, particularly in relation to the problems associated with the learning and practice of modern image guided techniques. Equally, with this understanding of how human factors impinge on the practice of this type of medicine, it is a small step to consider the impact of human factors on medicine in general. Furthermore, once familiar with human factors it is relatively easy to use this knowledge to improve almost every aspect of medical education and training. Human factors analysis of laparoscopic surgery was led by three surgeons in the 1990s and early twenty-first century; Professor Sir Alfred Cuschieri from Malta but practicing surgery in Ninewells Hospital, Dundee, Scotland, Dr. Michael Patkin (FRACS) at the Royal Adelaide Hospital, Queen Elizabeth Hospital and Flinders Medical Centre, South Australia, and Professor Ramon Berguer, Dept. of Surgery, UC Davis, California, USA. Much of the work emanating from their research laboratories was instigated by the problems they saw in learning and practicing minimally invasive surgery.

The research findings in relation to laparoscopic surgery demonstrated that there were specific complications associated with the surgeon's learning curve. This resulted in a massed concerted effort from the surgical community to explain why this was and also to better understand the fundamental aspects of laparoscopy that led to this situation. It is interesting that these three individuals knew exactly where to go to look for explanations and answers, i.e., the discipline of psychology. To us it was not surprising that psychology (the scientific study of behavior and its related mental processes) and human factors had significant insights to offer into the etiology of the difficulties associated with MIS. By doing this type of analysis it is evident how the

A.G. Gallagher and G.C. O'Sullivan, *Fundamentals of Surgical Simulation*, Improving Medical Outcome - Zero Tolerance,
DOI 10.1007/978-0-85729-763-1_3, © Springer-Verlag London Limited 2012

introduction of a seemingly straight-forward technology into the operating room had enormous human-factor implications for the practitioner which in turn impacted on the care received by the patient (Gallagher and Smith 2003).

Human Factors is a discipline of study that deals with the human–machine interface in terms of the psychological, social, physical, biological, and safety characteristics of a user and of the system the user is in. It is sometimes used synonymously with ergonomics, but ergonomics is actually a subset of Human Factors. Human factors is a multidisciplinary field incorporating contributions from psychology, engineering, industrial design, statistics, operations research and anthropometry. In general, a human factor is a physical or cognitive property of an individual or social behavior which is specific to humans and influences functioning of technological systems as well as human–environment interactions. In social interactions, the use of the term human factor stresses the social properties unique to or characteristic of humans. Unfortunately, some of our colleagues have concentrated on this aspect of human factors, i.e., human interpersonal interaction in and out of the operating room as their primary focus for intervention. As we shall see this aspect of image guided surgery is probably the least worrying aspect of 'problem surgeons' and the easiest to fix. Indeed, it is likely that 'problem surgeons' attitudes have most likely developed because of some other more fundamental human factor such as skills deficit, or difficulty with managing and processing information in the operating room. It is also likely that a lack of insight and awareness of how difficult it is to operate under MIS operating conditions in comparison to open surgery conditions could have fuelled their frustration and subsequent behavior. Human factors involves the study of *all* aspects of the way humans relate to the world around them, with the aim of improving operational performance, safety, life costs and/or adoption through improvement in the experience of the end user. Put bluntly, a surgeon who has significant difficulties operating safely is unlikely to develop better technical or judgment skills on a course designed to teach better social skills in the operating room.

Human factors involves the study of factors and the development of tools that facilitate the achievement of improved operational performance. In the most general sense, the three goals of human factors i.e., (i) operational performance, (ii) safety and (iii) improvement in the experience of the end user are accomplished through several procedures in the human factors cycle, which depicts the human operator (brain and body) and the system with which he or she is interacting. First it is necessary to diagnose or identify the problems and deficiencies in the human–system interaction. After defining the problems there are five different approaches that can be used in order to implement the solution. These are:

1. *Equipment design*: changes the nature of the physical equipment with which humans work.
2. *Task design*: focuses more on changing what operators do than on changing the devices they use. This may involve assigning part or all of tasks to other workers or to automated components.
3. *Environmental design*: implements changes such as improved lighting, temperature control and reduced noise in the physical environment where the task is carried out.

4. *Training the individuals*: better preparation of the worker for the conditions that he or she will work in by teaching and practicing the necessary skills (physical, technical and interpersonal).
5. *Selection of individuals*: a technique that recognizes the individual differences across humans in every physical and mental dimension that is relevant for good system performance. Thus performance can be optimized by selecting operators who possess the best profile and characteristics for the job (Meister 1999).

To be fair, surgery and the industries that support surgery have (somewhat belatedly) made considerable efforts to investigate and develop solutions for the first four factors. However, they have been very reluctant to tackle the issue of 'selection'. We will address this issue in Chaps. 11 and 12 but it is fair to say that there are some individuals who are very bright, committed and hardworking but who simply do not seem to be able to acquire the skills to become a safe surgeon or interventionalist. We believe that for image guided interventions such as surgery these individual differences in ability to acquire the requisite skills are to do with perceptual, visual-spatial and psychomotor abilities or aptitudes which are probably acquired in the womb or shortly afterwards and therefore have profound implications for selection and who should get training. The issue of human factor aptitudes will recur in this book. Specific examples will be provided on how they impinge on normal human performance and thus on surgical performance.

Perceptual, Spatial and Psychomotor Aspects of Image Guided Surgery

Despite sensory, perceptual and cognitive processes being crucial to all medical diagnosis and decision making, they are rarely incorporated into medical education and training in sufficient detail to allow the physician enough insight into the strengths and weakness of the human being as an information processing and decision-making organism. This study of sensation in perception is one of the oldest concerns of experimental psychology. Traditionally, the term sensation refers to the basic, immediate experience that starts with physical stimulation. By perception, we generally mean, the interpreted, elaborated, organized, experience based on the raw material of sensation. Sensation and perception begin with the activity of specialized cells called receptors. In some cases, the receptors are located in complex structures called sense organs that are expressly designed to receive and respond to physical stimulation, for example, the eyes and ears for sight and sound. Receptors for other kinds of sensation are found in parts of the body that also fulfil a number of non-sensory functions, e.g., the skin and the tongue. The skin plays a key role in protecting (the body) against excessive water loss as well as insulation the body and temperature regulation. The primary function of the tongue is taste and its secondary function is speech. All receptors have a common function. They accept as their input a certain type of physical energy and produce as their output neural signals.

In other words, they transform or transduce the energy to which they are sensitive into the form of energy that is used in the nervous system, i.e. nerve impulses. Sensory systems are geared to changing rather than static to stimulation. If they are exposed to constant stimulation long enough, their sensitivity will change or adapt. Also, adaption is not a permanent phenomenon so that when stimulation changes, sensitivity changes appropriately.

Our senses are limited in their capacity to respond to stimulation. For example, light in an otherwise darkened room must reach a minimum level of intensity before we can see it. Similarly, pressure on the skin will be felt only if it is strong enough. The minimum level of physical energy required to yield a specific type of sensation is called an absolute threshold. For any type of sensation, there is no single level of stimulus intensity below which a sensation is never experienced and above which a sensation is always experienced. Instead, there will be a range of intensities that lead to a sensation some part of the time. At the bottom end of the range, there will be a level at which the subject rarely detects the stimulus and at the top, there will be a level at which the stimulus is detectable virtually all of the time. This idea of stimulus intensity is of particular importance in minimally invasive surgery when we come to discuss the issue of what the surgeon feels through their sense of touch or haptics.

From a psychological perspective many of the problems associated with MIS specifically (and image guided interventions in general) are due to the perceptual, spatial/cognitive and psychomotor difficulties encountered while learning and developing the skills necessary for laparoscopy. Many of these difficulties involve predominantly perceptual, spatial or psychomotor aspects of MIS; moreover, there is always a degree of sensory integration as an essential means of providing accurate information. A more thorough understanding of the underlying psychological problems in laparoscopic surgery may therefore provide insight into effective ways of compensating for the difficulties experienced in MIS and give clues regarding how they should be conceptualized and dealt with in other image guided intervention specialties such as fluoroscopically guided procedures. If the trainer considers the perceptual difficulties imposed on the laparoscopic surgeon as 'unfavorable' (in comparison to traditional open surgery), these difficulties are minute in comparison with the difficulties confronting fluoroscopically guided interventions. These issues will be discussed in more detail in Chaps. 11 and 12 since the consensus is that fluoroscopically guided procedures will *replace* more and more surgical procedures.

When the surgical community first started to describe the difficulties that are associated with the learning and practice of MIS, it was frequently reported that the surgeon had lost three-dimensional viewing; this description is inaccurate. A more accurate description of the considerable perceptual problems encountered in laparoscopic surgery is that the surgeon must interpret 3D information from a 2D-monitor image presented from only a single point perspective (one camera source). This is further complicated by the fact that binocular information (interpolated from the two slightly different views of the eyes) only specifies the flat 2D nature of the surgical monitor, and provides no clues to the depths of the images displayed on its picture surface (screen). In other viewing scenes (outside for instance), binocularity

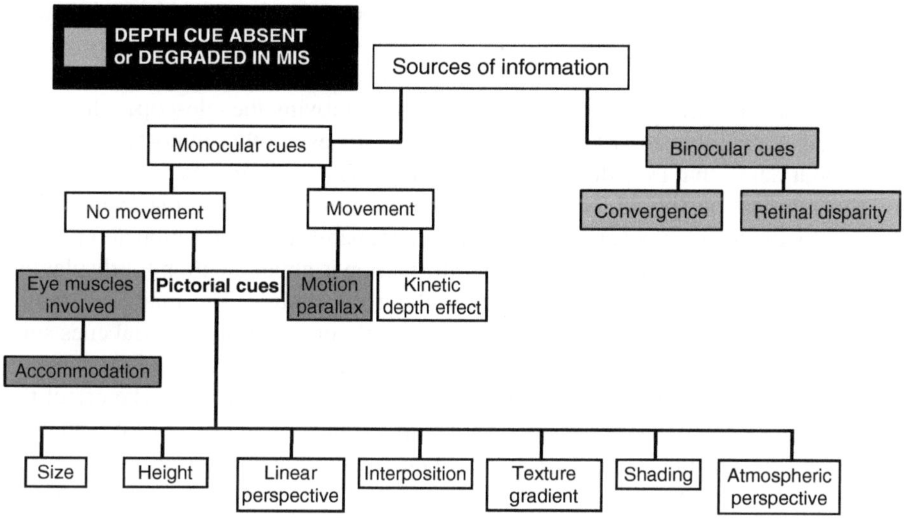

Fig. 3.1 Sources of information about an objects distance or 'depth of field'

often provides valuable information about depth. However, because of the use of only a single camera in standard laparoscopic equipment, the possible information relating to depth from stereoscopic vision (i.e. integrated information from two viewpoints) is lost in the MIS image. The result is that the MIS image can only relay monocular information to the picture surface (screen) of the monitor.

Figure 3.1 shows the range of visual cues that humans require in order to make judgments about depth in our day-to-day interactions with our environment. The human visual system and brain have evolved to optimally perceive depth under these viewing conditions. There are two primary (rich) sources of information that help the individual to judge depth of field, and these are binocular cues and monocular cues which are graphically represented in Fig. 3.1. In image guided surgery, the surgeon views tissues from the one perspective and that is the image processed by the charged coupled device which is attached to the telescope. The problem with this is that these viewing conditions deprive the brain of one of the most important sources of information on depth and that is binocular cues. The depths cues of convergence and retinal disparity provide direct information to the brain helping it to interpret the world in three dimensions. In minimally invasive surgery, this important source of information is completely lost. This means that the surgeon must rely on monocular cues for his or her information on depth of field and not even all of these cues are available to them. Because the eyes of humans and other highly evolved animals are in different positions on the head, they present different views simultaneously. This is the basis of stereopsis, the process by which the brain exploits the parallax due to the different views from the eye to gain depth perception and estimate distances to objects (Steinman et al. 2000). Motion parallax is the change of angular position of two observations of a single object relative to each other as seen by an observer, caused by the motion of the observer. Simply put, it is the apparent shift of an object against the background that is caused by a change in the observer's position. This cue to depth is also lost to the surgeon as normally in laparoscopic surgery, they have only one viewing perspective.

They can gain some information about depth by moving the telescope which will give them some monocular kinetic information. However, other important information about depth that they do have is misleading. The eye muscles and the process of accommodation (by which the eye increases optical power to maintain a clear image (focus) of an object as it draws near) are transmitting information about depth to the brain but unfortunately this depth information is about the monitor displaying the tissues rather than depth information about the tissues. The main sources of information about depth that the surgeon has to rely on are from pictorial cues such as size, relative height, linear perspective, interposition of organs and instruments and organs, lighting/shading and atmospheric or aerial perspective. The effect the atmosphere or aerial perspective has on the appearance of an object as it is viewed from a distance is that as the distance between an object and a viewer increases, the contrast between the object and its background decreases as does the contrast of any markings or details within the object.

To date, technology has been relatively unsuccessful in creating stereoscopic 3D camera systems (i.e. integrating information from two different camera sources). The results from various institutes demonstrate that current 3D cameras provide no real differences in performance in comparison to the 2D systems, and usually result in physiological discomfort and visual strain (Hanna and Cuschieri 2000; Hanna et al. 1998b). Binocular cues must therefore be only part of a vast and complex stream of information used for depth perception, and indeed different sources of information must then be more relevant when interpreting 3D information from 2D surfaces. In this way the issues involved with interpreting depth in the MIS image are more accurately encapsulated by the research associated with picture perception. Pictorial information (occlusion for instance) may provide powerful cues to the depth of the gallbladder in relation to the surrounding tissue during a laparoscopic cholecystectomy. Evidence also suggests that motion cues are likely to enhance the effectiveness of monocular information (Reinhardt-Rutland 1996). Studies that have involved driving (during which the most relevant information comes from the motion created by optic flow) indicate that permanently monocular drivers do not suffer from higher casualty rates than their binocular counterparts, and if anything appear to have superior safety records (Evans 1991; Hell 1981). It may then also be possible that trainee surgeons who interpret these other pictorial cues more efficiently will adapt faster and develop safer surgical skills. A further perceptual problem in laparoscopy arises from scaling difficulties caused by the magnification and by the severely degraded visual image of the internal anatomy, in comparison to the experience of an open operation. Despite the advances in technology the visual information displayed through monitors is still orders of magnitude inferior to the information the human visual system can directly encode from the environment. The image that the surgeon has to work with is pixilated. This can translate into difficulties for the operator that is reflected in degradation of operative performance or diagnosis. In a study assessing laparoscopic performance on a very simple bi-manual task as a function of different viewing conditions, it was found that (a) subjects who performed the task whilst looking directly at it (full binocular viewing) performed better than those subjects who performed the task under the same conditions but with one eye covered (monocular viewing), (b) who in turn performed the task better than those subjects who performed the task under full laparoscopic imaging conditions whilst looking at the monitor with both eyes (Gallagher et al. 2005b). The interesting thing about these data was not the difference in performance between binocular and monocular performance but the huge difference in performance between monocular and full laparoscopic viewing conditions. Furthermore, these results could not be explained by task complexity.

The eyes are one of the primary and richest sources of sensory information acquisition. The retina is a transparent, paper-thin layer of nerve tissue at the back of the eyeball on which the eye's lens projects an image of the world. It is connected by the optic nerve, a million-fiber cable, to regions deep in the brain. A human retina is less than a centimeter square and a half-millimeter thick. It has about 100 million neurons, of five distinct kinds. Light-sensitive cells feed wide spanning horizontal cells and narrower bipolar cells, which are interconnected by outgoing fiber bundles to form the optic nerve. Each of the million ganglion-cell axons carry signals from the amacrine cells and the ganglion cells, about a particular patch of the image, indicating light intensity differences over space or time: a million edge and motion detections. Overall, the retina can process about ten one-million-point images per second. Computer scientists have been trying to duplicate this process for some time. Their greatest success in this enterprise has not been the duplication of human vision but working out its complexity. For example, it takes robot vision programs about 100 computer instructions to derive single edge or motion detections from comparable video images. 100 million instructions are needed to do a million detections and 1,000 MIPS to repeat them ten times per second just to match the retina and this is just a recognition task (similar to our perception of stimuli).

Sensation, Perception and Memory; The Carbon-Based Information Processor (Perception)

Considerable insights into human sensory, perceptual and cognitive functioning have been gained during almost one and a half centuries of research. Helmholtz (August 31st, 1821–September 8th, 1894; Fig. 3.2) is credited as being the first in the modern era to systematically study human perception. In physiology and psychology, he is known for his mathematics of the eye, theories of vision and his ideas on the visual perception of space. Since the advent of image guided medicine, industry and academics have been trying to duplicate the human sensory system in order to facilitate surgical procedures such as image guided surgery. This goal may not be as simple to do as it sounds. Most of us take the human sensory, perceptual, cognitive and motor abilities that we have for granted; we

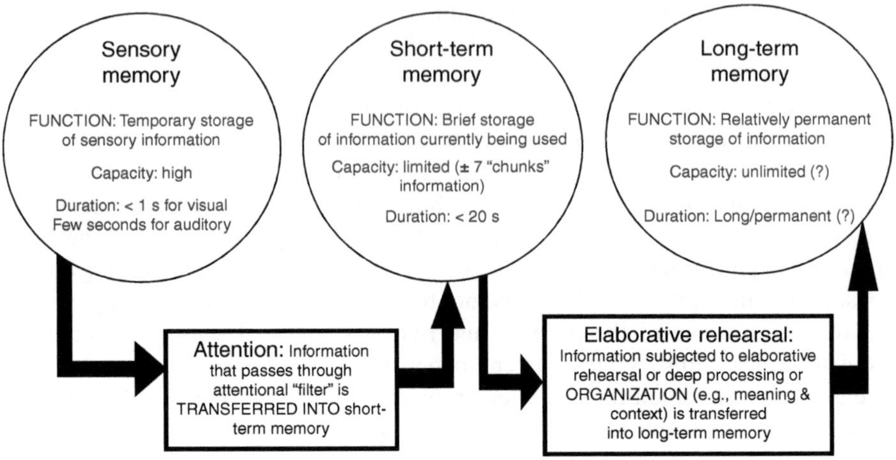

Fig. 3.2 A heuristic model of human memory processes and component functional attributes

should not. The human sensory, perceptual and cognitive information processing system is the most sophisticated multi-channel information processing system that we know. It has been speculated that modern computers demonstrate some of the processing characteristics of the human brain. However, despite current developments in computer processing and even at the developmental rate expressed by Moors law, computer processing will not catch up with human information processing capacity until the year 2030. Table 3.1 compares the functional attributes of the human brain and high-end computing. The reason industry is so interested in human visual information processing (in particular depth and pictorial cues) is that in theory it appears reasonable to speculate that the certainty of computer processing performance surpassing human information processing capacity is simply a function of engineering development and time. These developments would be extremely valuable in areas of medicine that rely heavily on human vision but are extremely prone to detection errors i.e., cytology. However, this analysis is overly simplistic and fails to take account of (1) the plasticity of the human brain and (2) the complexity of the information that the brain receives from highly evolved multi-channel sensory systems and (3) how effortlessly it deals with this information. We are not really sure how plasticity works in the human brain, but we do know that the phenomenon bestows the ability to change and to adapt very quickly in response to changes in the external environment. It seems to involve adaptations of existing brain structures rather than developing new ones, i.e., finding smarter ways of using existing neural pathways, synapses and chemical transmitters, with no apparent change in the actual anatomy of the brain. Attempts to replicate this in computers (e.g., neural networks) and camera systems have at best been disappointing. However, even with the degraded information that the laparoscopic surgeon has to work with they can by-and-large operate effectively and safely.

Table 3.1 The functional attributes of the human brain in comparison to a computer

Attribute	Carbon-based, human brain	Silicon-based, Intel Pentium 4, 1.5 GHz
Number of neurons/ transistors	20,000,000,000–50,000,000,000	4.2* 10^7
Power consumption	20–40 W	Up to 55 W
Maximum firing frequency	250–2,000 Hz	1.5 GHz
Processing of complex stimuli	0.5 s or 100–1,000 firings	If it can be do it, it takes a long time
Sleep requirement	31% of an average day	None (if not overheated)

Perhaps the fundamental difference between the computer and the brain is that computers operate by performing sequential instructions from an input program, whilst no clear analogy of this process appears in the human brain. The brain is a very efficient parallel and integrated information processing system, whereas programming for information processing in a parallel manner is extremely difficult for computer software writers. Indeed, most parallel computer systems run semi-independently, for example each system works on small separate 'chunks' of a problem. The human brain is also mediated by chemicals and analogue processes, many of which are only understood at a basic level and others of which may not yet have been discovered, so that a full description is not yet available to science. Finally, and perhaps most significantly, the human brain appears hard-wired with certain abilities, such as the ability to learn language, to interact with experience and emotions, and usually develops within a cultural context. This is different from a computer in that a computer needs software to perform many of its functions beyond its basic computational capabilities (Gray 2002; Moravec 1998).

The human brain receives information (almost effortlessly) about its environment from a variety of sources that we call senses (or sensory information). These highly efficient human functions are very sensitive. Over a century of research has suggested that sensations are innate, hardwired physiological mechanisms and perceptions which depend heavily on learning and cultural context. Furthermore, research has suggested that experience is essential for the development of some of the most elementary sensory systems (Blakemore and Mitchell 1973). Understanding sensation relies heavily on the concept of a 'threshold' which is the line between perceiving and not perceiving a 'just noticeable difference' in presenting stimuli. This is the minimum detectable difference between two stimuli. Even nineteenth century researchers realized that sensory thresholds were not an absolute fixed value. By convention a threshold has been operationally defined as the point where the subject detects the stimulus 50% of the time. This definition is necessary because of the inherent variability of the activity of the nervous system. Even when the nervous system is not being stimulated neurons continue to fire. For example, if a very weak stimulus occurs when the neurons in the visual system happen to be quiet the brain is likely to detect it. However, the stimulus is likely not to be detected if the neurons happen to be firing and so the stimulus is lost in the noise created by the firing neurons (Carlson 1994). Signal detection requires the perceiver to discriminate stimuli

Table 3.2 The acuity of each human sensory modality

Sense modality	Sensory threshold
Vision	Can see a candle flame seen at 30 miles on a dark clear night
Hearing	Can hear the tick of a watch under quiet conditions at 20 ft
Taste	Can taste one tea spoon of sugar in two gallons of water
Smell	Can smell one drop of perfume diffused into the entire volume of a 6-room apartment
Touch	Can feel the wing of a fly falling on your cheek from a distance of 1 cm

from background noise and this can be manipulated in a variety of ways from simple instructions which bias responses to sensitivity and fatigue. Table 3.2 gives some examples of the threshold sensitivity of each human sensory modality.

Touch Perception

Although we have primarily referred to visual perception and sensation here, it must also be remembered that the perceptions of touch (or as we have described in the previous chapter 'haptics') are of particular importance to the operating surgeon. Just like vision, the human perceptual system has evolved to optimally perceive haptic information directly through the skin, fingers, hand and arm and not by means of 18″ long laparoscopic instruments which pass through surgical ports in the body wall of the patient undergoing surgery. Many surgeons consider that they have lost the sense of touch when they perform laparoscopic surgery; this is an inaccurate reflection. As we shall demonstrate, our sense of touch is very sensitive and adapts to new kinds of stimulation.

Our sense of touch comes from the cutaneous sense, which gives us four basic kinds of sensation, i.e., pressure (or touch), warmth, cold and pain. Other more complex sensory experiences such as itching, wetness or tickling are based on combinations of all of these four sensations. Receptors responsible for the various skin sensations lie within the skin itself. Hairs projecting from the skin may provide an additional source of cutaneous information. For example, when a hair is moved a receptor at its base is stimulated creating a sense of touch. Receptors sensitive to different kinds of cutaneous stimulation are unevenly distributed over the body. The most pressure sensitive parts of the human body are our fingers, face and tongue. The least sensitive parts of the body are to be found on the lower extremities (Montagna 1962).

The sense of touch is important to all physicians but it is of particular importance to surgeons who use hapticaly acquired information from this sense to guide their decision-making intra-operatively. The stimulus for a touch is a mechanical force that causes displacement or deformation on the skin or hairs embedded in it. The sense of touch is subject to adaptation just as are many other kinds of sensations. Our continual and changing stimulus leads to a decrease or even complete elimination of the sensory experience of touch. If one thinks of the example of wearing a watch that one puts on for the first time, it initially feels very heavy and cold but gradually we are barely aware that we are wearing it. The skin on our fingertips are some of the most sensitive parts of the human body and of course they are of crucial importance to the operating surgeon for feeling and sensing tissues. It is understandable that surgeons are acutely aware of the loss of this information when they first operate laparoscopically. However, over time their perceptual system will adapt to the degradation of information that they receive through their fingers. This adaptation process may vary between individuals at the rate they sensitize but the vast majority of individuals will show improvement in what they can 'feel' through the laparoscopic instruments. One of the best examples of this type of sensory adaption is the ability of someone who has lost their sight learning to use their fingers to read Braille. Incredibly, it has been estimated that an experienced adult Braille reader can achieve reading rates of more than 100 words or more per minute.

Spatial Difficulties

Compounding the problem of the operating surgeon's loss of important depth cues, image and haptic degradation they also have to cope with the problem of the 'fulcrum effect' of the body wall on instrument handling. This means that when the surgeon moves the hand that is holding the surgical instrument to the right the working end of the instrument moves to the left on the monitor causing a proprioceptive-visual conflict for the brain (Gallagher et al. 1998). The issue of proprioception and its role in skills acquisition is discussed in greater detail in Chap. 4.

These spatial difficulties encountered during MIS result in cognitive mapping and hand-eye co-ordination problems. MIS presents vastly different images of anatomy due to the perspective and magnification of objects closest to the laparoscope. Sometimes this can be a positive (i.e., offering a better perspective or more light) but these may cause images that are incongruent with the surgeon's normal mental model of anatomy which was established through observations during open procedures. Spatial discrepancies are also caused by a misinterpretation of angular relationships (the azimuth angle) as the entry points of instruments do not correspond with the optical axis of the laparoscopic camera. These difficulties make the accurate planning and executing movements within the abdomen a more complex and risky endeavor (Crosthwaite et al. 1995). Another problem involving a spatial aspect of perceiving information during surgery involves camera etiquette during the laparoscopic procedure. During the laparoscopic procedure, the surgeon (usually) has no direct control over the position or orientation of the laparoscope, and instead must rely on the assistant to maintain an optimal position. Frequently unintentional camera rotation occurs which can lead to disorientation and misinterpretation of position and target organs (Gallagher et al. 2009a).

Although we move around our environment and interact with it seemingly effortlessly, there are highly complex (automated) information processing activities ongoing all of the time (even when we are asleep). The processes we have described thus far have simply concerned sensing and perceiving information in our environment. What we want to discuss now is what happens to that information once we have (or have not) it captured. During this discussion we shall also make use of the computer analogy to make comparisons with the human information processing system which has been the 'ideal' model that computer scientists have drawn inspiration from and in fact tried to simulate.

Sensation, Perception and Memory; The Carbon-Based Information Processor (Cognition)

Figures 3.2 and 3.3 show what happens to information after it is processed by the sensory and memory system. Unlike a computer, some of the information is lost before being shunted to short-term memory and conscious awareness. In Fig. 3.2 we have outlined the three widely accepted components of memory, i.e., sensory memory, short-term memory and long-term memory. Humans are not always aware of all of the information in sensory memory; however, experimentation has shown that the quantity of information that has been processed is enormous and is retrievable under certain circumstances. Information in sensory memory that has not decayed as a function of storage time or been supplanted by new incoming information and is consciously attended to is then transferred to short-term memory (STM) or working memory WM; Fig. 3.3 (Baddeley and Hitch 1974). STM and WM are very closely related but are not the same. STM is probably an atheoretical storage unit and there tends to be general agreement about its topography. WM is a newer concept, is probably an explanatory heuristic that helps to account for quite a number of memory functions (and dysfunctions). STM or WM have a much lower capacity than sensory memory and the primary function seems to be to organize and retain information that is to be transferred to long-term memory (LTM). Information that makes it through STM to long-term memory is organized further in a much more elaborated process, e.g. the 'meaning of the information'; a human face, a child's face, a 4-year-old child's face, his face looks like his mother face, the mother is my best friend. Information that enters both STM and LTM is also subject to loss as a function of interference and decay. Unlike STM the capacity of LTM is unlimited and memories are usually thought of as permanent (in theory at least, e.g., information retrieval failure occurs in Alzheimer's or brain damage and inappropriately organized information is not stored in LTM or at least cannot be located or retrieved). It is this information from LTM that is retrieved by the surgeon into STM or probably more accurately working memory at the appropriate time, place and context to apply to problem solving and then make decisions during surgery.

Figure 3.3 shows a diagrammatic representation of the components of working memory as proposed by Baddeley and Hitch (1974). Their theory proposes that two slave systems (the phonological loop and visual-spatial scratch pad) are responsible for short-term maintenance of information and the 'central executive' is responsible for the supervision of information integration and for coordinating

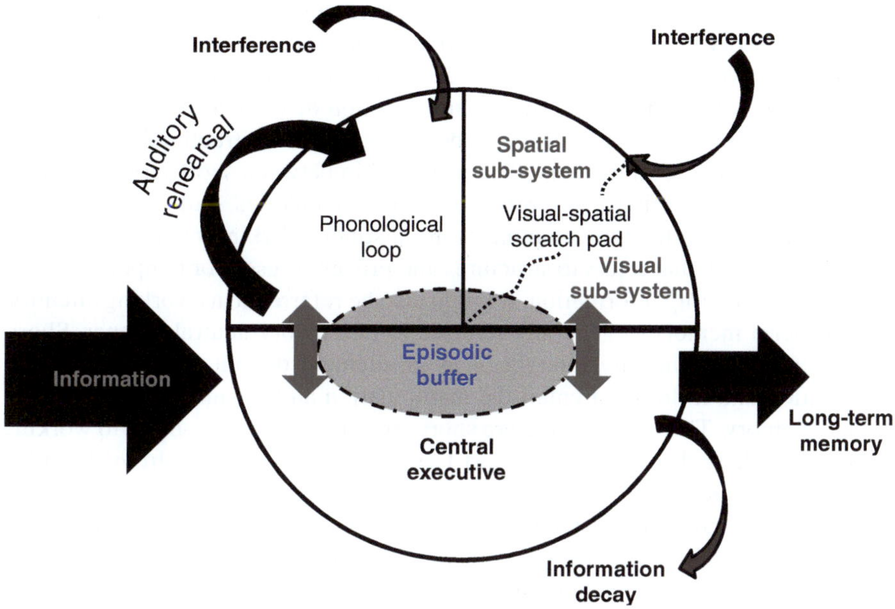

Fig. 3.3 Diagrammatic representation of working memory

the slave systems. The phonological loop stores phonological information such as the sound of language and prevents it decaying by continuously articulating its contents, thereby refreshing the information in a rehearsal loop. It can for example maintain a seven-digit telephone number for as long as one repeats the number to oneself again and again. The visuo-spatial scratchpad stores and processes visual and spatial information. It can be used, for example, for constructing and manipulating visual images and for the representation of mental maps such as that of anatomy or anatomical structures in surgery. The visuo-spatial scratchpad can be further broken down into a visual subsystem (dealing with shape, color and texture), and a spatial subsystem (dealing with location).

The central executive is one of the most interesting aspects of Baddeley's model of working memory. He ascribes 'executive' functions to it and argues that it is responsible for directing attention to relevant information, suppressing irrelevant information and inappropriate actions and for coordinating cognitive processes when more than one task must be done at the same time. Baddeley (2000) subsequently extended the model of WM by outlining a fourth component, the 'episodic buffer'. This component of working memory holds representations that integrate with phonological, visual and spatial information and possibly information not covered by the slave systems, e.g., semantic information, musical information etc. This component is episodic because it is assumed to bind information into a unitary episodic representation (or indeed a 'chunk' of information).

The models of sensory, short-term memory (or more accurately, working memory) demonstrate that information is not simply transmitted directly into a long-term memory. The models as outlined here suggest that information may reach the sensory memory, but only information that is attended to is shunted into short-term or working memory. This means that some of the information that may be perceived is lost. In the description and function of working memory outlined by Baddeley, information appears to be organized and structured before it is shunted on to long-term memory. The relationship between short-term and working memory is described differently by various theories, but it is generally acknowledged that the two components are distinct. Working memory is a theoretical framework that refers to structures and processes used for temporarily storing and manipulating information. It might also be referred to as working attention as short-term memory is generally referred to in a theory neutral manner. Short-term memory is primarily thought of as an element or unit for the storage of information and it does not entail the manipulation and organization of material held in memory. Thus, while there are short-term memory components to working memory models, the concept of short-term memory is distinct from the more hypothetical concepts proposed by Baddeley.

Short-term and working memory are generally considered to have a limited capacity. The earliest quantification of the capacity limit associated with short-term memory was the 'magical number seven' introduced by Miller (1956). He noticed that memory span of young adults was around seven elements, called chunks, regardless of whether the elements were digits, letters, words, or other units. Later research revealed that memory span depends on the category of chunks used, for example, the span is around seven for digits, around six for letters and around five for words. It is very difficult to pin down the exact capacity of short-term or working memory to a specific number of chunks because humans take advantage of prior knowledge to help organize and package new information. Chunking is the process whereby humans take advantage of prior knowledge to package information more effectively and in a way which appears to enhance storage and retrieval. For example, a sequence of digits which comprise a number of familiar dates such as 1916, 1939 and 0911 would be easier to recall than the same 12 digits in random order. Practice and frequency of use of particular information also appears to impact on our capacity to organize information and therefore our ability to store it in a retrievable form in long-term memory. Working memory also appears to be an important component in the performance of complex tasks. For example, measures of working memory capacity are strongly related to performance of other cognitive tasks such as reading comprehension, problem-solving (Conway et al. 2005), and also with any measures of IQ (Engle et al. 1999).

Others have argued that the capacity of working memory is better characterized as the ability to mentally form relations between elements, or to grasp relations in given information. Engle et al. (1999) have argued that working memory capacity reflects the efficiency of executive functions, most notably the ability to maintain a few task-relevant representations in spite of distracting irrelevant information. The results from task performance seem to reflect individual differences in ability to focus and then maintain attention, particularly when other events are serving to capture attention. Research also suggests that there is a close link between the working memory capacity of a person and their ability to control information from the environment that they can selectively enhance or ignore (Fukuda and Vogel 2009). Such attention allows for the person to shift *their* focus in regard to their goals in relation to information and spatial locations or objects they are interested in rather than attending to information that might otherwise capture their attention due to sensory saliency. Baddeley (2000) has elaborated on the central executive. He describes it as a mechanism that consists of four components: the capacity (i) to focus attention, (ii) to divide attention, (iii) to switch attention and (iv) to provide a link between working memory and long-term memory. According to this view, the central executive represents a capacity limited provider of attention that coordinates the two capacity limited subsystems (i.e., phonological loop and visual-spatial scratch pad). Furthermore, it appears that the ability to override sensory capture of attention differs greatly between individuals and this difference closely links to their working memory capacity. The greater a person's working memory capacity, the greater their ability to resist sensory capture. The limited ability to override attentional capture is likely to result in the unnecessary storage of information in working memory. This suggests that having a poor working memory not only affects attention, but also that it can limit the capacity of working memory even further (Fukuda and Vogel 2009).

The kind of behavior that results from this functional aspect of working memory (attention capture/ignore) can be seen regularly in the operating room, mostly in junior surgeons in training but also in more senior colleagues (where it is a matter of some concern to observe it at all). The situations that seem to trigger these types of responses in surgeons usually occur when things start to go wrong in the operating room. Frequently, what will happen is that a minor event will occur, e.g., a small (or maybe not so small) hemorrhage, that the surgeon should really ignore and prioritize to continue operating. However, the operating surgeon has difficulty ignoring the minor hemorrhage and this seems to affect his/her performance on the task in hand. So much so, that as the minor hemorrhage becomes more serious and needs to be dealt with, the surgeon appears unable to deal with either. What can be observed in these situations is a disintegration of the surgeon's performance when what is required is a systematic and level-headed approach to dealing with both problems. Here we have a very clear example of how a simple human factor such as being able to attend to or ignore information directly impacts on operating performance and thus on patient safety.

The Brain

Although the human brain represents only 2% of the body weight, it receives 15% of the cardiac output, 20% of total body oxygen consumption, and 25% of total body glucose utilization (Siegel et al. 1999). The brain mostly utilizes glucose for energy and hypoglycemia can result in loss of consciousness. The energy consumption of the brain does not vary greatly over time, but active regions of the cortex consume somewhat more energy than inactive regions: this observation forms the basis for the functional brain imaging methods PET and fMRI (Gusnard and Raichle 2001). These are nuclear medicine imaging techniques which produce a three-dimensional image of metabolic activity. Psychologists have been investigating brain function for centuries and these techniques have allowed neuroscientists to confirm or refute the hypotheses they have had relating to brain function. Historically, particular brain functions such as sensation, perception and cognition could only be inferred from quantitative experimental manipulations or from brain injured patients. Although this approach has proved particularly fruitful (and accurate) and has thrown considerable light on brain mechanisms, the functions of these latter activities and their anatomical origins always had to be inferred. However, with the advent and now widespread availability of PET and fMRI, correlations can now be observed between these activities and cerebral blood flow and/or tissue oxygen metabolism. These observations enable more robust speculation about anatomical locus and topography of brain function.

Biological Basis of Memory

Much is known about the biological and anatomical basis of memory mostly from neuropsychological studies of normal subjects but also from brain injured patients and from animal studies. In contrast, anatomical insights into working memory are of much more recent vintage. Early work on the anatomical basis of working memory usually involved animal studies. Fuster (1973) recorded the electrical activity of neurons in the pre-frontal cortex of monkeys while they were doing a delayed matching task. In this study, monkeys observed an experimenter place food under one of two identical looking cups. A screen/shutter was then lowered for a variable delay period screening off the view of the cups from the monkey. After a delay the shutter opens and the monkey is allowed to retrieve the food from under the cup. Successful retrieval (after training) on the first attempt required holding the location of the food in memory over a period of delay. Fuster found neurons in the prefrontal cortex that fired mostly during the delay period. This suggested that these neurons were involved in representing the food location while it was hidden from them during the delay period.

More insights into memory or cognitive function have been developed in the latter part of the twentieth century particularly with new brain imaging techniques (e.g., PET and fMRI). Localization of brain function in humans has become much easier with the advent of these imaging methods. Research has confirmed that areas of the prefrontal cortex are involved in working memory functions. However, brain imaging studies have revealed that working memory functions are not just limited to the prefrontal cortex (E. E. Smith and Jonides 1999). A number of studies reviewed by Smith and Jonides (1999) show that the areas of activation during working memory tasks are scattered over a large part of the cortex. The results of these studies also showed that there is a tendency for spatial tasks to recruit more right hemispheric areas, and for both verbal and object working memory to recruit more left hemisphere areas. Furthermore, there is an emerging consensus that most working memory tasks recruit and network prefrontal cortex and parietal areas (Honey et al. 2002).

Much has been learned over the last two decades about where in the brain working memory functions are carried out, but much less is known about how the brain accomplishes short-term maintenance and goal directed manipulation of information. The persistent firing of certain neurons in the delay period of working memory tasks shows that the brain has a mechanism for keeping representations active without external input. One proposal is that short-term memory involves the firing of neurons which depletes the Readily Releasable Pool (RRP) of the neurotransmitter vesicles at presynaptic terminals (Tarnow 2009). The pattern of the depleted presynaptic terminals represents the long-term memory trace and the depletion itself is the short-term memory. After the firing has slowed down, endocytosis causes short-term memory to decay. Endocytosis is the process by which cells absorb molecules (such as proteins) from outside the cell by engulfing it with their cell membrane. It is used by all cells of the body because most substances important to them are large polar molecules that cannot pass through the hydrophobic plasma membrane or cell membrane. Endocytosis is required for a vast number of functions that are essential for the well-being of cells including regulation of nutrient uptake, cell adhesion and migration, receptor signaling neurotransmission and receptor down-regulation (Miaczynska et al. 2004) and so is a realistic candidate for involvement in memory processes.

Brain Capacity and Workload for Performing Surgery

Human beings (whether they are qualified surgeons or not) are highly complex and sensitive information gathering and processing organisms. Some ideas about how complex they are can be gleaned from computer scientists' efforts to duplicate human performance. For example, in contrast to the human perceptual and cognitive system, current computers are only able to solve formalized problems due to their more limited pattern recognition capability. Furthermore, a human, as well as processing incoming information from different sensory modalities, can utilize another level of cognition to help understand context such as in arbitrary text, something even the most powerful and best software is not able to discern. If it is not clear by now how complex and sophisticated the human being is as an information processing system, perhaps the following example may help to elucidate this complexity. Developments in computer vision reveal that one million instructions per second (MIPS) can extract simple features from real-time imagery, e.g., tracking a white line or a white spot on a speckled background; 10 MIPS can follow complex grey-scale patches; 100 MIPS can follow moderately unpredictable features like roads; 1,000 MIPS will be adequate for coarse-grained three-dimensional spatial awareness (illustrated by several mid-resolution stereoscopic vision programs) and 10,000 MIPS can find three-dimensional objects in clutter which has been shown for high-resolution stereo-vision demonstrations (which can accomplish the task while an hour or so at 10 MIPS). However, this is at the very edge of computer capability which is some way off simple human capabilities. Furthermore, we perform these simple tasks many thousands of times daily (usually without conscious awareness) as we navigate our way through the world that we live in. These are precisely the same skills and abilities that a surgeon uses to perform image guided surgery.

The human information processing system (from sensing to perceiving and then 'thinking') is the most ecologically functional system for dealing with tasks that we encounter in the environment that we live in. We experience the world through our senses and our knowledge stems from our experience and subsequent learning and meaning applied to sensations (experienced). Our attempts to approximate these functions using computers have taught us two things (1) how far off we are at replicating the functional ability of the human brain and sensory system and (2) how complex, sophisticated and elegant the human system is.

Brain Workload and Performance

Not surprisingly the seeming effortlessness of human sensing, perceiving, remembering and thinking do not occur without a cost. The human brain is a vitally important component of a fully functioning interconnected ecological system. As we have indicated earlier, the brain for its size appears to utilize a disproportionate amount of glucose and oxygen. This observation has led neuroscientists to speculate that there should be robust correlations between problem-solving and cortical metabolism. What neuroscientists had been hoping to find was that problem-solving workload could be located to discrete parts of the brain. In contrast, what they have found is that task performance rather than being correlated with their specific brain region is scattered across brain regions and hemispheres (Parks et al. 1988). Similar findings of regionally diffuse metabolism correlated with performance have also been reported Boivin et al. (1992). Another consistent finding that has emerged from these studies looking at the correlation between metabolic rates and task performance is an inverse relationship between metabolic rates and performance. What these results seem to indicate is that individuals who are better at the tasks seem to have lower rates of brain metabolism. For example, Boivin et al. (1992) found that individuals who scored low on verbal fluency scores were negatively correlated with brain metabolism. Similarly, Charlot et al. (1992) reported that participants with low mental imagery ability tended to show an overall elevation of cortical activity (as measured by blood flow) during imagery tasks, whereas participants with good imagery ability tended to show regional activity decreases. On preliminary analysis, these findings may seem counterintuitive, because glucose utilization reflects task engagement and on the basis of this logic, one would expect participants who are more engaged to perform better on the task. However, another interpretation of these results is that individuals who were not very talented at these tasks had to work harder to perform them.

Whichever of these two explanations turns out to be correct is somewhat immaterial for surgery as both have profound implications even as they stand. The surgeon who has to operate using minimally invasive technology has to work with considerably degraded sensory and perceptual information in comparison to the surgeon who operates with the traditional open technique. What this means is that the brain must work harder to make sense of the information that the surgeon is sensing and processing in order to allow them to perform the surgery, safely and efficiently. In turn this means that the brain will have a higher oxygen and glucose metabolic rate than during the performance of the same surgical procedure performed by the open technique. It could also account for the consistent reports by many laparoscopic surgeons about their considerable levels of fatigue after operating for a day minimally invasively in comparison to doing the same procedures in the traditional open way. These reports are probably indicative of the considerably increased workload of the brain during the performance of MIS procedures. Furthermore, if brain metabolic rates are inversely correlated to, ability to perform the task, proficiency, talent (or aptitude) this compounds the problem even further for some surgeons. It means that a brain of a less well trained or talented surgeon, which is already being required to work very hard to perform a procedure minimally invasively, will have to compensate even further to perform at an equivalent level to a better trained or more talented colleague. To be frank, we are not sure that this is a realistic possibility or if anything strengthens the case even further for selection of aspiring surgeons, based partly on aptitude. Although these questions have not been asked in relation to surgical performance, they have been asked in experimental studies and so can provide some indication of what we might expect to find.

One neuroimaging study of individual differences showed that the match between an individual's cognitive abilities and the resources necessary to perform a task are important for neural efficiency considerations. Using a sentence-picture verification paradigm, Reichle and colleagues manipulated the use of either verbal or visual strategies in individuals with varying verbal and visual-spatial skill (Reichle et al. 2000). They found that participants with higher verbal abilities, as measured by reading span, had lower activation volumes in typical language regions (e.g., Broca's area) when engaging in verbal strategies. Similarly, individuals with higher visual-spatial skills, as measured by mental rotation ability, had lower activation volumes in typical visual association regions (e.g., parietal cortex) when engaging in spatial strategies. Thus, individuals with greater ability in a certain domain showed more efficient neural processing in the cortical regions that supported that domain, when using a strategy that evoked that specific type of processing. This means that requiring surgeons to perform complex spatial tasks with degraded sensory information such as in MIS means that the surgeons we choose should be 'naturally' good at spatial tasks to begin with. If they are not, they will have limited extra spatial capacity/ability to draw on when the surgical tasking they are performing becomes more difficult.

Summary

The human body is a highly efficient device for the capture of information from our environment through highly developed sensory systems that modern computer systems have only started to approximate but not yet match. Much of this information is degraded when the surgeons operates minimally invasively, particularly information about depth of field and the quality of input perceived through the eyes and hands. The degraded information that is captured and shunted from sensory memory into short-term memory is then subjected to loss by processes of decay and interference from new information or previously stored information. Information that does survive is organized and then stored in long-term memory. The organizational process appears to be a primary function of the working memory central executive and in particular the episodic buffer. The working memory central executive also appears to function as what most of us call attention. It seems to fulfil a supervisory and organizational role in determining what new information we attend to, integrating new information with prior knowledge retrieved from long-term memory and prioritizing how we select and act on this information. Working memory appears to draw on resources from a large part of the cortex but with a tendency for spatial tasks to make demands on the right hemisphere and verbal tasks to recruit more left hemisphere areas. All of these working memory activities are associated with increased brain oxygen and glucose metabolism. However, there appears to be an inverse relationship between brain metabolism and performance when ability or aptitude are controlled i.e., those who are better at a task (because of training, ability, or talent) have a lower brain metabolic rate than those who experience more difficulties with the tasks. The implications of these findings for training and selection cannot be ignored by surgery.

References

Baddeley A. The episodic buffer: A new component of working memory? *Trends Cogn Sci.* 2000;4(11):417-423.

Baddeley AD, Hitch G. Working memory. In: Bower GH, ed. *The Psychology of Learning and Motivation*, vol. 8. New York: Academic Press; 1974:47-90.

Blakemore C, Mitchell DE. Environmental modification of the visual cortex and the neural basis of learning and memory. *Nature*. 1973. doi:10.1038/241467a0. 467–468.

Boivin MJ, Giordani B, Berent S, et al. Verbal fluency and positron emission tomographic mapping of regional cerebral glucose metabolism. *Cortex*. 1992;28(2):231-239.

Carlson NR. *Physiology of Behavior*. Needham Heights: Allyn and Bacon; 1994.

Charlot V, Tzourio N, Zilbovicius M, Mazoyer B, Denis M. Different mental imagery abilities result in different regional cerebral blood flow activation patterns during cognitive tasks. *Neuropsychologia*. 1992;30(6):565-569.

Conway ARA, Kane MJ, Bunting MF, Hambrick D, Wilhelm O, Engle RW. Working memory span tasks: a methodological review and user's guide. *Psychon Bull Rev*. 2005;12(5):769.

Crosthwaite G, Chung T, Dunkley P, Shimi S, Cuschieri A. Comparison of direct vision and electronic two- and three-dimensional display systems on surgical task efficiency in endoscopic surgery. *British Journal of Surgery*, 1995:82(6);849-851.

Cuschieri A. Whither minimal access surgery: tribulations and expectations. *Am J Surg*. 1995;169(1):9-19.

Engle RW, Kane MJ, Tuholski SW. Individual differences in working memory capacity and what they tell us about controlled attention, general fluid intelligence, and functions of the prefrontal cortex. In: Miyake A, Shah P, eds. *Models of Working Memory: Mechanisms of Active Maintenance and Executive Control*. Cambridge: Cambridge University Press; 1999:102-134.

Evans L. *Traffic Safety and the Driver*. New York: Van Nostrand Reinhold Company; 1991.
Fukuda K, Vogel EK. Human variation in overriding attentional capture. *J Neurosci*. 2009;29(27):8726.
Fuster JM. Unit activity in prefrontal cortex during delayed-response performance: neuronal correlates of transient memory. *J Neurophysiol*. 1973;36(1):61-78.
Gallagher AG, Smith CD. From the operating room of the present to the operating room of the future. Human-factors lessons learned from the minimally invasive surgery revolution. *Semin Laparosc Surg*. 2003;10(3):127-139.
Gallagher AG, McClure N, McGuigan J, Ritchie K, Sheehy NP. An ergonomic analysis of the fulcrum effect in the acquisition of endoscopic skills. *Endoscopy*. 1998;30(7):617-620.
Gallagher AG, Ritter EM, Lederman AB, McClusky DA 3rd, Smith CD. Video-assisted surgery represents more than a loss of three-dimensional vision. *Am J Surg*. 2005b;189(1):76-80.
Gallagher AG, Al-Akash M, Seymour NE, Satava RM. An ergonomic analysis of the effects of camera rotation on laparoscopic performance. *Surg Endosc*. 2009a;23(12):2684-2691.
Gray P. *Psychology*. 4th ed. New York: Worth Publishers; 2002.
Gusnard DA, Raichle ME. Searching for a baseline: functional imaging and the resting human brain. *Nat Rev Neurosci*. 2001;2(10):685-694.
Hanna GB, Cuschieri A. Influence of two-dimensional and three-dimensional imaging on endoscopic bowel suturing. *World J Surg*. 2000;24(4):444-449.
Hanna GB, Shimi SM, Cuschieri A. Randomised study of influence of two-dimensional versus three-dimensional imaging on performance of laparoscopic cholecystectomy. *Lancet*. 1998b;351(9098):248-251.
Hell W. Research on monocular depth perception between 1884 and 1914: Influence of the German Unfallversicherungsgesetz and of the jurisdiction of the Reichsversicherungsamt. *Perception*. 1981;10(6):683-694.
Honey G, Fu C, Kim J, et al. Effects of verbal working memory load on corticocortical connectivity modeled by path analysis of functional magnetic resonance imaging data. *Neuroimage*. 2002;17(2):573-582.
Meister D. *The History of Human Factors and Ergonomics*. Mahwah: Lawrence Erlbaum Associates; 1999.
Miaczynska M, Pelkmans L, Zerial M. Not just a sink: endosomes in control of signal transduction. *Curr Opin Cell Biol*. 2004;16(4):400-406.
Miller GA. The magical number seven, plus or minus two: some limits on our capacity for processing information. *Psychol Rev*. 1956;63(2):81-97.
Montagna W. *The Structure and Function of Skin*. New York: Academic Press; 1962.
Moravec H. When will computer hardware match the human brain. *J Evol Technol*. 1998;1(1).
Parks RW, Loewenstein DA, Dodrill KL, et al. Cerebral metabolic effects of a verbal fluency test: a PET scan study. *J Clin Exp Neuropsychol*. 1988;10(5):565-575.
Reichle ED, Carpenter PA, Just MA. The neural bases of strategy and skill in sentence-picture verification* 1. *Cogn Psychol*. 2000;40(4):261-295.
Reinhardt-Rutland AH. Remote operation: a selective review of research into visual depth perception. *J Gen Psychol*. 1996;123(3):237-248.
Siegel G, Agranoff B, Albers R, Fisher S, Uhler M, eds. *Basic Neurochemistry: Molecular, Cellular and Medical Aspects*. Philadelphia: Lippincott; 1999.
Smith EE, Jonides J. Storage and executive processes in the frontal lobes. *Science*. 1999;283(5408):1657.
Steinman SB, Steinman BA, Garzia RP. *Foundations of Binocular Vision: A Clinical Perspective*. New York: McGraw-Hill Medical; 2000.
Tarnow E. Short term memory may be the depletion of the readily releasable pool of presynaptic neurotransmitter vesicles of a metastable long term memory trace pattern. *Cogn Neurodyn*. 2009;3(3):263-269.

Chapter 4
Human Factors in Acquiring Medical Skills; Learning and Skill Acquisition in Surgery

Mouret first performed laparoscopic cholecystectomy in the late 1980s. Previously, laparoscopic techniques were part of gynecological practice and it was not until the development of a video computer chip allowed the magnification and projection of images on to television screens that laparoscopic surgery became integrated into general surgery (Johnson et al. 1992). The main difference between laparoscopic and traditional open surgery is that there is no need for a single large incision; instead a number of small stab incisions are made in the patient's abdomen through which surgical instruments are passed via trocars. The surgeon views the operative site by means of a monitor image obtained by a CCD miniature camera attached to a laparoscope. Since its introduction into general surgery it has developed rapidly in both application and complexity and the laparoscopic cholecystectomy has now replaced the open cholecystectomy as the procedure of choice for the removal of the gall bladder (Centres 1991).

However, as we have seen in Chaps. 1 and 3, the widespread introduction of laparoscopic or minimally invasive surgery (MIS) in the 1980s had a number of unforeseen consequences. Introduced on a wave of enthusiasm surgical procedures such as laparoscopic removal of the gallbladder (laparoscopic cholecystectomy or LC) became the treatment of choice almost overnight. This was understandable given the benefits MIS conferred on both patients and hospitals. For the patient it meant that they were in and out of hospital quickly after having major surgery performed, e.g., LC in one or two days rather than more than a week. They also had reduced pain and scarring and returned to work more quickly (Peters, Ellison, Innes et al., 1991). The advantages for the hospitals were better bed occupancy rates. However, MIS imposed considerable difficulties on the surgeon. For example, the tissue being worked on could no longer be seen directly. Instead, the surgeon viewed the image captured by a single or triple chip charged coupled device camera on a monitor. Although the image was of extremely high quality, it was orders of magnitude poorer than would be viewed by the eye under natural viewing conditions (Reinhardt-Rutland 1996). There was also considerable decrement in depth cues.

As we have discussed in Chap. 3, laparoscopic surgeons need to form visual impressions of a 3-D structure – consisting of organs and instruments – from a

A.G. Gallagher and G.C. O'Sullivan, *Fundamentals of Surgical Simulation*, Improving Medical Outcome - Zero Tolerance,
DOI 10.1007/978-0-85729-763-1_4, © Springer-Verlag London Limited 2012

2-dimensional television monitor. While this is often described as loss of binocularity, it is simpler and more accurate to call it loss of pictorial perception. So-called primary cues – binocular disparity and convergence, accommodation, and motion parallax – are present in abundance. The difficulty is that they (and other cues related to lighting and texture) yield a conclusion that is inimical to surgery: they specify that the structures in view form a single surface, virtually flat and usually vertical. A surgeon has to set aside that conclusion in order to register the information carried by subtler 'pictorial' cues; and to reconstruct the structure that they specify despite the incompleteness of the information provided by these cues. Individuals differ in this ability and such differences could clearly contribute to performance variability for pictorially guided laparoscopy. Most reports on the difficulties experienced by surgeons indicate the loss of tactile feedback because they must perform surgery with 18-inch long surgical instruments. As we have discussed in Chap. 3, this conclusion is inaccurate. Tactile feedback is still present but it is considerably degraded. Other difficulties include unintentional camera rotation by the camera holder and having to learn how to use an angled laparoscope, e.g., 30° or 70° (Gallagher et al. 2009). These difficulties can be corrected by increased care and attention and by proceeding with caution. In addition, one of the most important difficulties that the laparoscopic surgeon has to overcome is the 'fulcrum effect' of the body wall on instrument handling. When the surgeon moves his or her hand to the right, the working end of the instrument moves to the left inside the patient and on the monitor resulting in fundamental visual-proprioceptive conflict. This cannot be overcome with increased care and attention due to the attentional demands of surgery (Gallagher et al. 1998) but only with extended practice. All of these difficulties mean that the minimally invasive surgeons must operate at the very edge of their perceptual, cognitive and psychomotor faculties (Reinhardt-Rutland and Gallagher 1995). As MIS became more commonly practiced for procedures such as LC, it became clear very quickly that the laparoscopic approach was associated with a significantly higher complication rate (Peters et al. 1991), particularly during the early part of the surgeon's career. The Southern Surgeons Club (Moore and Bennett 1995) found that the probability of a bile duct injury was a function of the laparoscopic surgeons experience (Fig. 4.1). Risk was greatest during the first 10 cases that the trainee performed (approximately 2 in 50) and dropped off dramatically as the surgeon become more experienced at performing the procedure. Indeed, the probability of a bile duct injury had reduced from 1.7% during the first ten cases performed to 0.17%.

A number of reports that have shown that training junior surgeons during operating time adds considerably to the length and therefore to the cost of the procedure (Bockler et al. 1999). In the US it has been conservatively estimated that each operating room (OR) costs $30 per minute to run (excluding staff salaries). In an already hard-pressed health sector hospital, chief executives are finding the extra expense of surgical training increasingly unacceptable. Consequently, there is considerable pressure on surgeons to conduct as little training as possible during OR time. Most complications during MIS occur early in the surgeon's career, i.e., first 50–100 laparoscopic procedures (Gigot et al. 1997; Moore and Bennett 1995). It has also

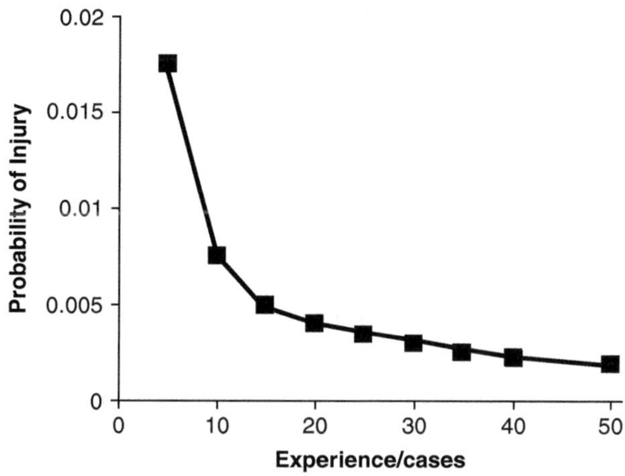

Fig. 4.1 This graph shows the probability of a bile duct injury as a function of surgeon experience/cases of laparoscopic cholecystectomy performed by them

been demonstrated that complications are also significantly more likely to occur if the surgeon performs a given procedure infrequently or if that procedure is performed infrequently in a hospital (Lerut 2000). The implications of these findings could have dramatic consequences for surgeons. Possible consequences of these types of data could include withdrawal of operating privileges for some hospitals and surgeons who perform too few of that type of procedure per year. This would mean that expertise would come to be concentrated in a smaller number of centers of excellence, which in turn would have implications for training junior surgeons and re-accrediting senior surgeons.

This evidence would seem to indicate that certain surgeons have difficulty acquiring and practicing the 'new' skills required for minimally invasive surgery. Furthermore, the surgical community seems to infer that the problem is simply a matter of acquiring the appropriate skill set. However, a small number of surgeons who were aware of the literature on human factors have realized that the answer probably is not that simple. Here we have two different approaches to solving the problem of higher complication rates associated with laparoscopic surgery. The traditional surgical approach was to recommend more, better or more specialized training. Indeed, this is what happened during the late 1990s and early part of the twenty-first century. Specialist units were set up to train the skills required for minimally invasive surgery. Trainers in these units developed different types of training tasks that encouraged the trainees to interact with and to learn the technology associated with the practice of minimally invasive surgery. Around the world these units became very well-known for their types of training, training tasks and new minimally invasive approaches to traditional open surgical procedures. For example, one of the surgical tasks that was commonly used in many of these surgical training units was intracorporeal suturing. We have discussed one example of a systematic training programme for the acquisition of these skills in detail in Chap. 2. While these tasks and training programs appeared to have achieved their goal, this was more by accident than design. In essence, this approach was too crude and gave very little insight into the underlying human factor reasons for the difficulty in acquiring the skills for minimally invasive surgery. Analysis of the underlying human factors is essential if tasks and training methods are to be developed which educate and assess these skills within an efficient and effective programme.

It is interesting to look at the efforts of Prof Sir Alfred Cuschieri and his team in Dundee. At the outset they seemed to grasp that a deeper level of analysis and understanding of the difficulties associated with the acquisition of minimally invasive surgical skills was required for the development of a long-term solution to the problem. One of the objectives of this book is to increase the fundamental understanding of the human factors involved in learning and practice of minimally invasive procedural medicine such as surgery. If the problem is understood in a holistic sense, efficient and effective solutions can be built taking this understanding into account. One of the concerns that we have with virtual reality simulation for training surgical skills is that the simulators are really no better than the novel laparoscopic surgical training tasks that were developed for training minimally invasive surgical skills. Moreover, we believe that virtual reality or simulation per se holds far greater potential than is currently being harnessed. Although we have applied our analysis to the skills required for the learning and practice of minimally invasive surgery, this analysis can be applied to any set of clinical skills in procedural medicine.

Psychomotor Skill

One of the ideas that we have tried to communicate in Chap. 3 is that important units of behavior such as sensing, perceiving and thinking do not occur in isolation. The human being (whether they are qualified in medicine or not), whilst going about their everyday life, is a unitary, integrated, highly complex biological system. The same is true for the practice of skilled performance such as in surgery. The accurate integration of spatial, perceptual, and psychomotor information is of fundamental importance in nearly every aspect of everyday life (such as running for a bus, catching a ball, reaching for an object across a table, threading a needle or indeed performing surgery). For instance, computation of direction and distance has to be made before reaching to the vicinity of a target object; not only in terms of global assessment before acting, but also by prospective evaluation of what is going to happen next and throughout the period in which the action takes place. Such anticipation relies on an implicit hypothesis about the stability of both the spatial position of the target object and the spatial position of the agent (Brooks et al. 1995). Thus both perception and action take place within a spatial framework (probably integrated in working memory).

Most of us are aware that we are constantly receiving information about objects and events in our external (and internal) environment. Yet few of us give more than a moment's thought to the information we continually receive about the position and movement of our own bodies. Proprioception is the general term used for the sensory system that provides such information. Unlike the six exteroceptive senses (sight, taste, smell, touch, hearing and balance) by which we perceive the outside world, and interoceptive senses by which we perceive pain and movement of internal organs, proprioception is the third distinct sensory modality that provides feedback solely on the status of the body internally. Proprioception is actually made up of two subsystems, i.e., the kinesthetic and vestibular systems. Although these two systems are anatomically distinct, they are closely coordinated in their operation, probably in a cognitive manner.

Kinesthetics

Psychomotor skill refers to the ability to accurately perform, learn or adapt to situations requiring fine and complex sequences of motor activity (Adams 1990). The process is dependent on the body's sensory information regarding the position and movement of its limbs. Fine motor skills are the coordination of small muscle movements which occur, e.g., in the fingers, usually in coordination with the eyes. In relation to the motor skills of hands (and fingers), the term (surgical) dexterity is commonly used and is widely accepted as an important attribute of the aspiring or practicing surgeon. Fine motor skills are those that involve a refined use of the small muscles controlling the hand, fingers, and thumb. As with many things, we tend to take for granted many human functional attributes until we try and replicate them. This is also true of the human hand. Figure 4.2 shows one of the best efforts to duplicate the functionality of the human fingers, thumb and hand. The 'Shadow Dexterous Hand' has been designed to have a range of movement equivalent to that of a typical human being. The four fingers of the hand contain two one-axis joints connecting the distal phalanx, middle phalanx and proximal phalanx and one universal joint connecting the finger to the metacarpal. The little finger has an extra one-axis joint on the metacarpal to provide the hand with a palm curl movement. The thumb contains one one-axis joint connecting the distal phalanx to the proximal phalanx, one universal joint connecting the thumb to the metacarpal and one one-axis joint on the bottom of the metacarpal to provide a palm curl movement. The wrist contains two joints, providing flex/extend and adduct/abduct. To mimic the hand, the Shadow Dexterous hand has 24 joints altogether, with 20 degrees of freedom. However, even with this degree of sophisticated engineering, its functionality comes nowhere close to the range and sensory sensitivity of the original model, i.e., the human hand.

Kinesthesia (or movement sensitivity) refers to the specialized sensor groups that provide information about the angles of the joints, the length of muscles, the degree of muscle tension, and the rates at which all these values change. Kinesthetic information is thus primarily gained from body movements whether self-generated or externally imposed (Clark and Horch 1986). Kinesthesis contributes to such basic abilities as walking, reaching and grasping. It is also critical for such highly skilled

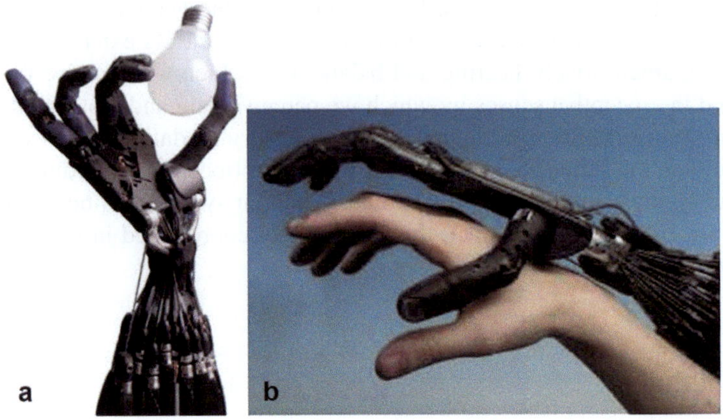

Fig. 4.2 The Shadow Dexterous Hand (http://www.shadowrobot.com/hand/) has been designed to have a range of movement (approaching) equivalence to that of a typical human being (27 DOF) with 20 degrees of freedom

activities as playing a musical instrument, signing your name or anything that requires precise control over the position and movement of body parts. The receptors for kinesthesis are located in the muscles and tendons and in the linings of the joints. These receptors respond to mechanical force, such as that exerted by the pull of a tendon, stretch of the muscle or the bending of a joint.

Vestibular System

The vestibular system refers to the overall position and motion of the body in space. In particular, it focuses on the orientation and movement of the head relative to gravity. Vestibular information can indicate such things as whether we are standing upright and whether we are falling to the left or to the right. It therefore plays an important part in maintaining balance and a number of other reflexive actions. One of the most important reflexes which is triggered by vestibular sensation is compensatory eye movements. An example of this compensatory action takes place every time we walk. When walking, as well as forward propulsion we shift from one foot to the other and our head bobs about so that we maintain a clear and focused view of our environment. It is our vestibular system that 'smoothes' out the images that we encounter. It does this by registering the direction and extent of head movements, and then uses this information to make automatic corrective eye movements in the direction opposite to the head movements. The result is a stabilization of the visual world. The two chains of anatomical structures that underlie the vestibular sense are the vestibular sacs which tell us about the orientation of the head when it is at rest and the semicircular canals which provide information about the rotation of the head. These structures are located in the innermost cavity of the ear although they are unrelated to hearing. Like other sensory systems, the vestibular system is especially attuned to changes in stimulation, e.g., for speeding up or slowing down rather than constant motion. For example, we are only aware of a lift leaving one floor and arriving at another, and in an aircraft we are only aware of takeoffs and landings and not the great speeds maintained during the flight travel (Carlson 1994).

Hand–eye coordination such as those required in surgery (whether open or minimally invasively) is the coordinated control of eye movement with hand movement, and the processing of visual input to guide reaching and grasping along with the use of proprioception of the hands to guide the eyes. It is a way of performing everyday tasks and in its absence most people would be unable to carry out even the simplest of actions such as picking up a book from a table or playing a video game. Studies have shown that when eyes and hands are used for search exercises, the eyes generally direct the movement of the hands to targets (Liesker et al. 2009). Furthermore, the eyes provide the initial information of the object, including its size, shape, and possibly grasping sites which are used to determine the force needed to be exerted by the fingertips for engaging in a given task. For shorter tasks, the eyes often shift on to another task in order to provide additional input for planning further movements. However, for more precise movements or longer duration movements, continued visual input is used to adjust for errors and to create more presision. For sequential tasks, it has been observed that eye gaze movements occur during important kinematic events like changing the direction of a movement, or when passing perceived landmarks. This is related to the task search oriented nature of the eyes and their relation to movement planning of the hands, and the errors between motor signal output and consequences perceived by the eyes and other senses which can be used for corrective movements. Furthermore, the eyes have been shown to have a tendency to 'refixate' upon a target in order to refresh the memory of its shape, or to update for changes in its shape or geometry. In tasks that require a high degree of accuracy it has been shown that when acting upon greater amounts of visual stimuli, the time it takes to plan and execute movements increases linearly as per Fitts's law (Lazzari et al. 2009). This law proposes a model of human movement for human–computer interaction and ergonomics which predicts that the time required to rapidly move to a target area is a function of the distance to and the size of the target. Fitts's law is used to model the act of pointing, either by physically touching an object with a hand or finger, or, virtually, by pointing to an object on a computer display using a pointing device. Fitts's law is an unusually successful and well-studied performance model and experiments that reproduce Fitts's results and/or that demonstrate the applicability of it in different situations are not difficult to perform. The data measured in such experiments invariably fit a straight line with a correlation coefficient of approximately 0.95 or higher which indicates that the model or 'law' is very good at accounting for the data.

Psychomotor Performance and Minimally Invasive Surgery

The vast majority of the motor difficulties in MIS are a result of the unique nature of the laparoscopic intervention and instrumentation. Several studies have demonstrated the effects of viewing monocular images (such as those on the surgical monitor display) on the performance of visually guided kinematic skills including moving, reaching and grasping. For example, Servos (2000) found that prior to the onset of movements, individuals greatly underestimated the distance and size of objects whilst under monocular viewing. Research by Haffenden and Goodale (2000)) have further indicated that under monocular viewing conditions, the relationship between individuals' estimation of the reach and grip necessary to obtain an object, and the objects size and distance specified by pictorial cues, required a period of learning and adaptation before an effective association could be formed. Thus, as a result of the MIS intervention, the interpretation of the monocular display (as on the surgical monitor) is likely to initially create psychomotor difficulties due to the distorted effects of depth and distance on subsequent movements. Marotta and Goodale (1998) illustrated that increased attention to evaluation in the field could be used as an effective cue to an object's distance and size, indicated by more accurate limb trajectories and grip estimation.

However, one of the greatest obstacles to the development of MIS skill is caused by the Fulcrum effect (Gallagher et al. 1998), which creates substantial difficulties in psychomotor coordination that result in a perceived inversion of movements. The Fulcrum effect (Gallagher et al. 1998) is directly caused by the unarticulated MIS instrumentation being limited to a fixed axis of movement through the wall of the body. The result is a first-order paradoxical movement (Patkin and Isabel 1993), similar to those experienced when operating a lever (such as the rudder of a boat or reversing a trailer). Consequentially, when the surgeon moves his/her hand to the right, the working end of the instrument within the body cavity moves to the left (and vice versa). This natural fulcrum affects both the horizontal and vertical movements displayed on the monitor. Thus as with perception, motor adaptation requires readjustments that seem to involve a period of learning. von Holst (Von Holst and Mittelstaedt 1950) stated that a fundamental aspect of motor adaptation involved establishing stable relationships' between the self-initiated movements of the body and the resulting changes in the patterns of information encoded by the sense organs, i.e., in surgical terms what they see or feel (and occasionally smell). The term reafference was used to refer to the feedback stimulation that resulted from self-produced movements, whilst the sensory information observed from changes in the external world was termed exafference. Effective perceptual-motor activity was then dependent on the individual's ability to distinguish between exafferent and reafferent stimulation. Von Holst (Von Holst and Mittelstaedt 1950) believed that the process of differentiation was mediated by efferent impulses (signals that initiated the movements) which in turn left behind an image or representation (the efferent copy) of the signal to be stored for comparison. According to von Holst, every movement by the body produces an efferent copy for comparison with the reafferent signal, thus enabling the individual to distinguish it from a change in the environment (exafferent information). Jeannerod (1999) also stated that movement and action were highly effective ways of differentiating the self from others.

Traditionally the assessment of visuomotor adaptation has involved creating a conflict between the actual visual scene, and the information experienced through the individual's visual reafferences. Motor and visual-motor studies generally require that a subject makes one or more movements of the hand and/or arm from a specific starting position to a target. Direction, amplitude and accuracy constraints are placed upon the movement by varying the target's location and size. Dependent variables include aiming error, reaction time and movement time (Fitts and Peterson 1964; Keele 1968; Wallace et al. 1978). A number of experimenters have used variations of visuomotor discordance to investigate the problems of adaptation. Harris (1963) showed the deterioration in performance of a drawing task when inverted by a mirror. However, Smith (1970) demonstrated that humans could adapt to writing in a mirrored reflection. The negative effects of inversion on the proprioceptive system during a simple movement task have also been documented by Mather and Lackner (1980).

Of course, in laparoscopic surgery, the visual discordance created by the fulcrum effect is the *normal* viewing condition, and it should really have come as no surprise to the surgical community that it would cause significant difficulties in developing the skills necessary for the practice of MIS. Gallagher et al. (1998) quantitatively demonstrated the detrimental impact of the 'fulcrum effect' on the performance of novice subjects during a simulated laparoscopic cutting task. The two studies showed that for laparoscopic novices the normal laparoscopic condition resulted in a significantly degraded technical performance. The influence of the fulcrum effect as an obstacle to motor adjustment in MIS was further demonstrated by the statistically significant improvement in novice performances, when the image on the monitor was inverted around the Y-axis (resulting in a left-right movement by the hand being displayed as such on the screen). Research by Held and colleagues have demonstrated the necessity for active movements in the process of motor adaptation (Held and Gottlieb 1958; Held and Rekosh 1963). The experiments involved measuring the adaptation of self-produced activity in comparison to passive movements whilst under conditions of displaced visual viewing. The results indicated that only the self-movement group had adapted, as illustrated by a compensating shift in the accuracy task as a result of the visual displacement. Thus, even though all the participants received the same visual input concerning hand movement, the passive condition alone was insufficient to produce adaptation due to the lack of connection between the sensory output and visual input (i.e., no formation of an efferent copy). Held and Rekosh (1963) concluded that the process of adaptation was dependent on individuals adjusting their judgments of spatial relationships according to the modified reafferent information. These findings therefore demonstrate the necessity for active psychomotor practice in order to effectively adapt to the discordance difficulties imposed by MIS. The research indicates that whilst adaptation is possible (Crothers et al. 1999) it requires a prolonged period of learning, practice, and attention (Gallagher et al. 1998). Furthermore, if adaptation was simply just 'more practice' the tasks developed by laparoscopic surgical training units around the world would have been sufficient to solve the problem. However, they were not. These training units simply produced trainees who on graduation had considerable variability in skill levels including some who were no more skilled than when they entered the training program.

Theories of Psychomotor Learning

Newell (1991) has proposed that a behavior could be identified as skilled or a skill when it was

1. Directed toward the attainment of an identifiable goal;
2. Organized so that the goal was reliably achieved with economy of time and effort; and
3. Acquired through training and practice.

Research on motor skills has primarily focused on the hand as the effector system for manipulative skills (such as the instrumentation in MIS), and the trunk and limbs as the principle effectors of whole body skills (Adams 1987). Another important effector includes the ocular-motor (eye-movements) system, which is involved in spatially orientated behavior, specifically tracking and localization (Courjon et al. 1981). These varied effector systems have different physical properties that must be taken into consideration in any theoretical analysis of control mechanisms (Annett 1969). The skeletal effectors are essentially lever systems in which the angle at the joint is controlled by balanced groups of muscles, the agonists and the antagonists. The eye, in contrast, has low inertia that enables it to make fast saccades to pre-selected locations, an essential requirement for spatially directed behavior (Newell 1991).

The combination of the properties of object (size, distance, structure etc), the type of movement required, and the effector systems involved are all important in determining the kind of control that is needed for the task (Lee et al. 1995). Generally motor skills are dependent on two kinds of control laws, characterized as feedforward and feedback information. In a feedforward system, output (i.e., muscular activity) is controlled by a program or set of stored instructions that are initiated by a starting signal in much the same way as a home computer runs through a series of actions when a particular program is set up and initiated. In a feedback system, a target value for one or more variables is set (the set point) and the output is controlled by a signal proportional to the difference between the currently sensed value and the set point. Fitts (Fitts and Peterson 1964) used simple positioning tasks (placing a peg in a hole) to illustrate how the two types of control can operate in one movement; an initial pre-programmed ballistic or "open loop" phase, followed by a controlled or closed loop second phase of sensory adjustment. The pre-programmed phase represents typical feedforward control in which a pattern of motor impulses may be computed on demand or may be drawn from a memory bank (Annett 1969). The initial entry and movement of the laparoscopic instruments toward the target area of the operation is an example of a feedforward controlled movement in MIS; whilst the slower and continually adjusted movements to accurately obtain the target (e.g., tissue on needle for suturing) represent actions under the control of feedback information. A skill such as performing a laparoscopic procedure must therefore (by its very definition) be specifically learned and invariably taught. However, the process of skill acquisition is not simply a matter of continual practice. For example, early studies from trainee Morse telephonists showed that the number of signals correctly transcribed per minute rose steadily over the first three to four months of practice remained roughly constant (at a plateau) for the next two months, and then began to rise again (Annett 1996). The later acceleration in learning was accompanied by a change in technique (i.e., receiving and writing down whole words rather than transcribing each individual letter).

It is therefore recognized that practice results in both quantitative and qualitative changes in performance (Chaiken et al. 2000). Indeed, this plasticity of skilled behavior created many problems for the early theories of performance and resulted in the abandonment of the linear information-processing models of the 1950s. The fundamental concept of a capacity-limited processing channel that accounted for choice reaction time data (Hick 1952) and the trade-off between speed and accuracy in rapid movement tasks (Fitts and Peterson 1964) collapsed when it was demonstrated that extended practice changed the relationship between stimulus information and performance (Annett 1969). Given the quantitative changes that occur with practice, several researchers have attempted to define the process in more complex mathematical terms. Fitts (Fitts and Peterson 1964) indicated that for simple repetitive skills, the logarithm of time for each repetition was a linear function of the logarithm of the number of practice trials. Thus a log-log linear law of learning could be formed, and its apparent simplicity suggested that there might be a single underlying learning process. Newell and Rosenbloom (1981) maintained that a power function provides a better fit to skill acquisition data. The power law of practice was based on results from both motor and mental skills, and proposed that the central principle component of learning involved "chunking" the information. Information was said to be chunked when it was dealt with as a single unit.

However, Annett (1996) indicated that the log-log linear law was most probably not representative of a single slow acting process, but rather a population of ways of learning that are successively drawn upon until exhausted. Thus, in the early stages, relatively rapid progress can be made by imitating the method of a skilled model or taking advice of a trainer, whereas much later in practice, when major sources of improvement have been exhausted, repetition may refine perceptual and temporal judgments or facilitate the connections between task elements. These studies and theories suggest that the development of MIS skill is likely to come from a relatively short initial period of rapid improvement, followed by a much longer period of sensory refinement and adjustment which seems to fit well with the data shown in Fig. 4.1. Adams (1971) closed loop theory of motor learning represents one of the most influential and holistic approaches to the process of skill adaptation. The model was based on the premise that the combination of sensory feedback and knowledge of results (KR) were used as a means of correcting motor errors. The theory poses that a motor trace (a record of the individual's movement) for the required action response is stored and compared to a perceptual trace (a record of sensory feedback). He suggests that sensory feedback is a function of error and is used to adjust movements until the desired goal is achieved. Repeating the movement brings the anticipatory arousal of the perceptual trace to which the ongoing motor feedback is

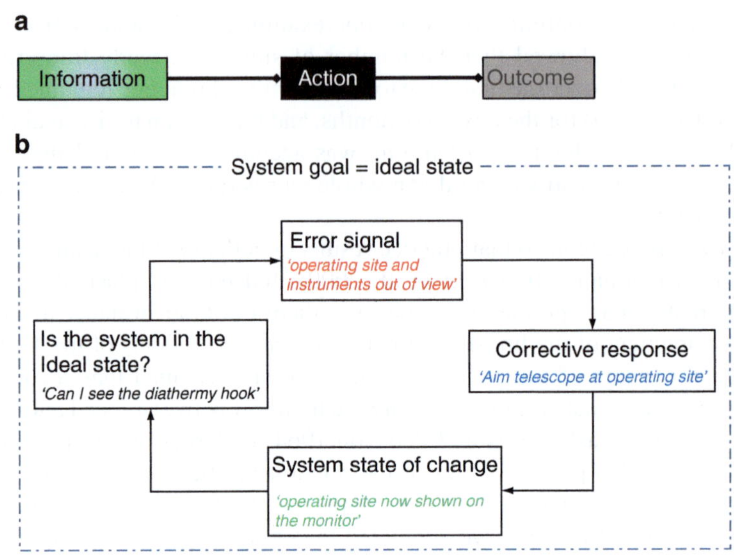

Fig. 4.3 **(a)** Operation of a simple open-loop control system, **(b)** Operation of a simple closed-loop control system for the simple skill of holding the camera and the laparoscope during an MIS procedure

continually reconciled. A positive relationship is formed when the perceptual trace confirms the implicated goal of the movement sequence. Practice strengthens the perceptual trace such that the sensory consequences of the motor outputs are anticipated. Frequently one will observe a very experienced (and usually talented) laparoscopic surgeon insert both of his operating instruments and 'check' that tissues and organs are located in depth of field at the distances and locations he remembers. It also accounts for why the same surgeon progresses cautiously around the triangle of Calot during a laparoscopic cholecystectomy, i.e., anatomy included the cystic duct, the common hepatic duct, and the cystic artery which can be easily damaged during the surgical procedure. This anatomy can present unusual configurations. Injury to the bile duct can lead to bile leak and liver damage and cause a painful and potentially dangerous infection requiring corrective surgery.

Systems, in general, may be characterized as Open Feedback or Closed Feedback and we have given examples in Fig. 4.3a, b. Open systems have outputs which are conditioned by information inputs but the outputs or outcomes themselves have no influence on the inputs. It is possible to think of an open feedback system in terms of the simple schematic shown in Fig. 4.3a. An open loop control system is not aware of its own performance, so that past action does not have any influence on future behavior, nor does it monitor and respond to current performance. All in all it is a very passive system.

By contrast, most processes have a structure in which the actions or behavior are shaped and influenced by past and current performance, which feeds back into system behavior to bring about some adjustment and change. The human body contains a number of excellent examples, one of which is the temperature regulation system. The body is designed to operate at 36.4°C, so that if exercise is taken which raises body temperature then perspiration occurs, leading to the appearance of moisture on the skin's surface which evaporates, thereby cooling the body. Conversely, if the body temperature falls below 36.4°C, muscle activity is in the form of shivering which causes the body's temperature to rise. This process, known as homeostasis, is fundamental to the control of the body and many other biological systems. The feedback in the system operates to make use of the current value of some quantity to influence the behavior of the system as a whole. We can represent the feedback in this system as a Closed Loop control system and we have given a schematic example in Fig. 4.3b.

The goal of the control system is to attain and maintain the 'ideal state'. The example provided in Fig. 4.3b is of a trainee surgeon or a senior medical student holding and navigating the laparoscope for the operating surgeon. The 'ideal state' is for the operating surgeon to clearly see the tissues and structures being operated on with an electrocautery instrument. The operating surgeon 'instructs' (error signal) the trainee that they cannot see the operating site nor the working end of the instruments. The trainee's response is to correct the aim of the telescope so that it is pointing at the operating site (corrective response). This means that the operating surgeon can now clearly visualize the operating site and the working end of the surgical instruments. Thus the trainee will maintain this view until required to change it by new information. All real-life systems exhibit some or all of the characteristics of this feedback process, where information continually arrives and is acted upon to produce an effect which shapes and influences the activity or inactivity to maintain an ideal state. All feedback within systems may be classified into one of two forms: positive (or reinforcing) feedback and negative (balancing) feedback. The feedback either acts to increase the probability that the exhibited behavior will continue to move the system in the same direction as the initial impetus, or else the feedback operates to decrease the probability that the exhibited behavior will continue, thus countering the initial impetus for change in the direction.

The closed loop theory of motor learning has been used to explain the processes involved in learning, developing, and maintaining laparoscopic ability through experience and practice based on the empirical findings of Crothers et al. (1999). The analysis of the results in terms of Adams' theory explained why surgeons perform significantly better than the novice under normal MIS conditions. The surgeons had already adapted to the contradiction between the perceptual trace (sensory feedback) and the motor trace caused by the fulcrum effect, and had thus stored the correct motor output necessary to perform the procedure. In contrast, the novice group was just starting the process of adaptation by correcting for the error between output and feedback. The theory further accounted for why the inversion of the monitor image around the y-axis had such a detrimental effect on surgeons' performance. The surgeons, through substantial experience and practice (>50 MIS operations), had become automated in their movement patterns. Automation occurs when the motor output can be pre-selected based on its expected sensory outcome. The perceptual traces as a result of significant experience eventually become so strong that the task can be performed without the need for feedback (previous conscious movements have become automatic). Inverting the image resulted in a disruption of the surgeons' automated processing and caused paradoxical feedback to their learned patterns. The inverted condition means that the surgeons must concentrate on adapting their motor outputs to be counter-intuitive to their adapted patterns and so compensate for the fulcrum effect. The fast rate of learning found for the group illustrated that the surgeons already knew how to perform the procedure, but needed to adapt their movement patterns once more. The process of motor learning also explained why the *Y*-axis inverted condition caused a significant improvement in novice performance, inverting the MIS image compensated for the perceptual and cognitive problems posed by the 'fulcrum effect'. Thus, the novice group was presented with a more 'natural' representation of their actual movements, as conflicting feedback between the perceptual and motor traces had been eliminated (i.e., moving the instrument right resulted in the monitor image of the working end moving to the right).

Schmidt (1975) extended Adam's closed loop theory to account for a more generalized (one-to-many) memory construct through the concept of the "schema". Schmidt's theory suggested that the choice of motor outputs was related to their expected sensory consequences obtained from previous response specifications, sensory consequences, and outcomes; that is, whether or not the sensory consequences would signal a desired state of affairs. The various sources of information are then consolidated into a 'recognizable schema' or 'chunk' that encodes the relationships between sensory consequences and outcomes, and a recall schema that relates outcomes to response specifications. Horak (1992) used a simulated neural network to represent Schmidt's recall schema in the learning of a uni-dimensional ballistic skill (such as throwing an object at a target under varying distances). The results demonstrated that the network learned to match its variable force output to the different inputs representing the variations of target distances, by changing the weights of interconnections between its elements (analogous to individual neurons) according to performance outcomes. In a sense, the network discovers the rule relating perceived target distance to appropriate force output in much the same way as suggested by Annett's (1969) account of the role of knowledge of results in learning.

The significance of the models of Adams (1971) and Schmidt (1975) of motor learning and adaptation is that they offered theoretical frameworks which were testable and refutable, which is the starting point for science. Another strength was that they demonstrated that the development of a skill did not simply rely on habit (continual repetition), but involved a substantial cognitive component (such as the evaluation of differences between the motor and perceptual traces and formation of schemas). Indeed, the role of cognition in the development of skill had received modest attention compared to the study of sensory information for most of the twentieth century. The theories, however, implicated the necessity of cognitive processing to encode, compare, evaluate and adjust movements within a developing framework of performance. As a result the 1980s saw a surge in empirical studies investigating the role of cognition in psychomotor learning and indicated several cognitive concepts that are likely to help explain the development of MIS skill.

Although closed loop models of learning seem to provide a reasonably good account of skill acquisition and to facilitate the duplication of similar processes by computer scientists, on closer scrutiny they are overly simplistic. One of the problems of closed loop theory of learning is that it ultimately reduces skilled performance to a response chain in theory. By this we mean that each movement or component of a movement is assumed to be triggered by perceived error feedback. Yet many movement sequences can be performed effectively when feedback is removed. Complex movements can often be performed effectively (or at least significantly reduced) without proprioceptive or other forms of feedback. For example, during intracorporeal suturing performed robotically by the surgeon they have *no* tactile or haptic feedback and yet most surgeons can learn to suture safely with this device. Even under laparoscopic conditions this is a difficult task but robotically the surgeon has to ensure that they do not break the needle or thread or damage the tissue they are suturing. Another difficulty with the closed loop theory is that it predicts incorrectly that the more knowledge of results a learner receives the more effectively they will perform. However, in a study by Winstein and Schmidt (1989), they observed results that contradict this prediction. In this study, two groups of subjects were trained to reproduce target movements with their arm. One group of subjects had knowledge of results on 100% of the training trials and the other group of subjects was given knowledge of their results on 50% of their training trials. During training the performance levels of both groups did not differ and neither was there a difference between the groups in an immediate retention trial in which knowledge of results was withheld from both groups. However, in delayed retention tests given a day later, the group that was given knowledge of results on only 50% of the training trials performed best.

Another problem with the closed loop theory of learning is that it is possible for humans to accurately perform novel movements that they have never performed before. For example, it is possible for someone who has only ever played soccer to start playing rugby and play well, despite the fact that they have never played the game before and it has entirely different rules and shape of ball. Closed loop theory cannot explain the accurate performance of the novel movements required to play rugby in the absence of prior sensory feedback. An integral part of closed loop theory learning is the formation of a perceptual trace for learned movements. The difficulty with this hypothesis is that it would be impossible to conceptualize of a separate perceptual trace and memory store of every movement ever performed.

Before the birth of the proceduralization concept, theories of motor learning have been influenced by the open-loop versus closed loop system distinction (Adams 1971; Schmidt 1975). The original formulation of the closed-loop view on motor performance and learning build on the momentum of internal feedback from executed movements, which allow for error detection and adjustment of actions through the process of contrasting perceptual traces against memory representations (Adams 1971). Motor learning was accordingly seen as dependent on repetition, accuracy, refinement and synchronization of a series of called-up movement units (i.e., open-loop structures) that are regulated by closed-loop structures.

In response to this view, a different open-loop perspective emerged, namely the one of motor programs (Schmidt 1975). The learning of motor skills was thereby seen in terms of the build-up, modification, and strengthening of schematic relations among movement parameters and outcomes. This learning results in the construction of "generalized motor programs" (i.e., a sequence or class of automated actions) that are triggered by associative stimuli, habit strengths and re-enforcers, and can be executed without delay (Anderson et al. 1996; Schmidt 1975; Winstein and Schmidt 1989). The advantage of Schmidt's theory was that he proposed that motor programs do not contain the specifics of movements, but instead contain a generalized rule for a specific class of movements. He predicted that when learning a new motor program, the individual learns a generalized set of rules that can be applied to a variety of contexts. Schmidt proposed that, after an individual makes a movement, four things are available for storage in short-term memory: (a) the initial movement conditions, such as position of the body and the weight of the object manipulated; (b) the parameters used in the generalized model program; (c) the outcome of the movement in terms of knowledge of results; and (d) sensory consequences of the movements, i.e., how it felt, looked and sounded. This information is stored in short-term memory only long enough to be abstracted into two schemas: (1) the recall schema (motor) and (2) the recognition schema (sensory).

The *recall* schema is used to select a specific response. Each time a person makes a movement with a particular goal in mind, they use a particular movement parameter such as movement force and they then receive input about the movement accuracy. After making repeated movements using different parameters causing different outcomes in the nervous system, these experiences create a relationship between the size of the parameter and the movement outcome. Each new movement added contributes to the internal system to refine the rules associated with that action class. After each movement, sources of information are not retained in the recall schema but only the rule that was created from them. The recognition schema is used to evaluate the response. The sensory consequences and outcomes of previous similar movements are coupled with the current initial conditions to create a representation of the expected sensory consequences. This is then compared to the sensory information from the ongoing movement in order to evaluate the efficiency of the response and performance modified on the basis of this feedback.

Observational Learning

In medicine, an important part of a surgeon's training is observing experienced surgeons performing operative procedures. Whilst previous studies have demonstrated the importance of action in motor adaptation, there is also good evidence to suggest that simply observing activities improves the formation of skill. Ferrari (1996) suggested that observational learning involved two complementary types of observation: the observation of the process, which allows one to imitate and to understand a modeled demonstration; and self-observation, which allows one to deliberately regulate one's own motor learning and performance. The deliberate self-regulation of action, in turn, assures a more efficient and effective learning of the skilled behavior. Some other major influences on observational learning include the properties of the model (e.g., level of skill, social status etc.); the nature of the task (e.g., its familiarity, salience, complexity, functional value etc.); and observer determinants. These include self-regulation of learning, self-efficacy beliefs, comprehension of the demonstration and feedback, all of which have been found to improve skill acquisition and performance (Druckman and Bjork 1992).

Bandura's (1982) theory of observational learning essentially states that individuals acquire new motor skills by attending to salient aspects of the modeled performance and by coding the received information into cognitive representations that can later be recalled. These representations allow the learner to produce novel motor performance through observation by using these representations as an internal standard against which to monitor the correctness of their produced movements. Research by Jeannerod (1999) has demonstrated support for Bandura's theory by illustrating similarities in cortical stimulation between individuals performing a motor task and those observing the activity. These findings support the efficacy of laparoscopic trainees observing operations as a means of accurately shaping and representing MIS skill. These results also highlight the importance of observing effective and reliable performance of the task to avoid developing inappropriate representations of the model. However, in procedural medicine this can sometimes be problematic as some very senior physicians may have acquired their seniority and rank on the basis of good, management ability, science (papers and grant income) and patient care but are not quite as technically proficient. Unfortunately some of this influential group are blissfully unaware of this fact and indeed some are firmly of the belief that they are technically highly skilled. Whilst this may not be a problem for their consultant peers who recognize the quality of technical skills for what they are, it most certainly can be a problem for more junior colleagues who equate seniority and career success with technical proficiency. A young colleague informed us one day of his experience learning how to perform laparoscopic cholecystectomy with a fairly senior academic surgeon. It was not until this colleague moved to his next rotation that he discovered it was not part of the 'normal' surgical procedure to puncture the gallbladder.

How do we recognize technical skill? As in other domains, experts in motor skill achieve a higher quality of performance by achieving more efficient movements with less wasted motion or power (Cheng 1985) and by appreciating ever more specialized prototypic situations or conditions to which specialized actions are attended (Anderson 1982; Ericsson and Kintsch 1995). However, experts do not excel when they cannot use their superior knowledge of the activity (i.e., when the elements of a situation or task are not arranged in a meaningful pattern). Norman et al. (1989) examined the diagnostic skill in dermatology at five levels of expertise. As expertise increased, correct diagnosis was associated with shorter response times while errors were associated with longer response time (suggesting greater deliberation for erroneous responses). Atypical slides continued to account for a constant proportion of error at all levels of expertise, suggesting that experts do not use more elaborate classification rules. These findings are comparable to the reported results of Crothers et al. (1999) illustrating the considerable degradation in performance of *y*-axis image inversion on the performance of experienced laparoscopic surgeons (due to the disruption of their 'fulcrum effect' automation).

While experts may not be proportionally more likely to recognize marginal cases, they have more knowledge with which to judge possible alternatives. However, if experts proceed habitually, they may fall victim to what Langer and Piper (1987) termed premature categorization. Premature categorization was found to occur when experts did not actively use contextual cues to help interpret novel instances or similarities but rather relied on prototypical instances with which they are familiar (Gick and Holyoak 1987).

Acquiring Technical Skills: Efficient Learning and Performance Strategies

Phases of Learning Skill

Motor learning involves the acquisition of a sequence of highly coordinated responses that are systematically related to one another and each response or component response is intricately related in a chain-like manner. Sensory motor learning involves the sensory systems such as seeing and hearing both in directing the motor pattern on and in providing feedback including knowledge of results. Motor learning, in contrast to other areas of learning such as conditioning and rote memorization, appears to be an ongoing process of refinement and improvement.

There are at least two ways to conceptualize the stages in motor learning. The first involves tasks or situations that consist of a series of levels. Consider the skill of typing. The first stage in acquiring this skill requires learning finger control and location of the keys. During this stage, the learner shows rapid improvement in terms of both speed and accuracy although the novice typist may feel that their initial progress seems slow. The next stage of their learning involves moving from letter to word habits and from word to phrase habits. During each stage, initial improvement in performance tends to be followed by a plateau showing little improvement until the learner moves to the next higher stage. What appears to be going on here is the cognitive consolidation of skill acquisition and neuropsychological evidence of this process has now started to emerge from imaging studies (Dudai 2004).

Another way to represent the stages of motor learning was provided by Fitts and Posner (1967). They focused on the stages that the individual passes through in the process of skill acquisition. They identified three clear stages.

Cognitive: In the first stage the learner needs to know what the elements of the task are in terms of expected performance. During this stage of learning, the novice draws upon reasoning abilities and past experiences which appear to relate to the performance of the task. This information (and 'rules') will be modified as they gain experience with the task.

Associative: The associated stage commences as other prior cognitive activities begin to drop out. Major errors are greatly reduced during this stage and the learner refines responses. In the initial cognitive stage, the learner places great emphasis on what responses are required and in what order. The learner tends to concentrate on how best to coordinate and to integrate those respondents and identify which ones are redundant or inefficient.

Autonomous: The third stage of motor learning refers to extremely advanced levels of performance. At this stage errors have been greatly reduced and the learner seems to perform the task automatically, i.e., their skills have become automated. It is at this stage that less attention is required to perform the task and so these attentional resources can be devoted to the performance of other activities at the same time. Once a skill has become automated, we can say that it has become programmed. The learner has established a sequence of highly coordinated movements that are integrated in time and are characterized by a rhythmic structure of their own. These highly integrated motor programs are acquired during advanced stages of motor learning and are very robust against interference from other tasks and also from extinction. Examples of the former come from evidence of highly skilled individuals being able to perform apparently incompatible tasks at the same time, e.g., a professional typist can work effectively and efficiently whilst reciting nursery rhymes from memory. Another example is the ability to ride a bicycle on holidays despite not having practiced or used the skills for many years. It is as though the basic elements of the skills have become so highly integrated that they were retained as an intact unitary skill.

The process of skill automation is a particularly important one for minimally invasive or endovascular surgeons. As described in Chap. 3, these types of interventions make unique and challenging demands on the surgeon which is especially true when they are operating on a patient. One particular aspect of cognition that has received minimal consideration in the surgical literature is 'attention' but it is of paramount importance to the surgeon while learning a new task or set of skills. In our review of working memory in Chap. 3, we have touched on this subject. Attention usually refers to the ability to concentrate mental powers upon an object such as careful observing or listening, or the ability to concentrate mentally. It has been known for at least half a century that human beings have a limited attentional capacity (Broadbent 1958). This means that we can only attend to a finite amount of information or stimuli at any given time. Figure 4.4 shows a diagrammatic representation of attentional resources used by a master surgeon, a junior surgeon and a novice surgeon for different aspects of operative performance. All three surgeons must allocate some of their attentional resources (consciously or unconsciously) to psychomotor performance and judgments about depth and spatial relationships. They must also attend to the patients vital signs on instrument read-outs. However, the distribution of this resource allocation differs depending on the experience of the surgeon. When a novice is acquiring a new skill such as those required for laparoscopic surgery, he/she must use more of these attentional resources to consciously

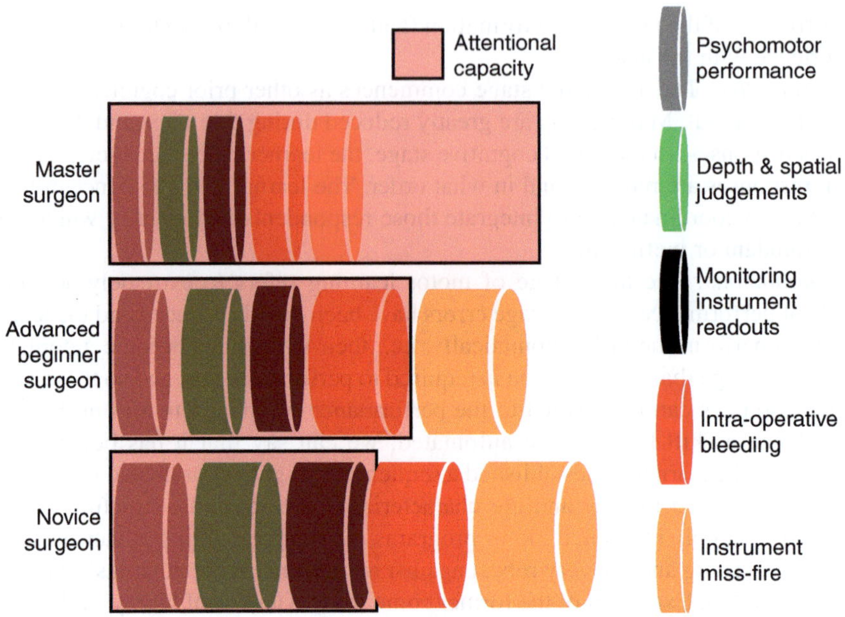

Fig. 4.4 Hypothetical model of attentional resource allocation of three surgeons with different levels of experience and skill during a laparoscopic surgical procedure

monitor what their hands are doing and where in space they are doing it while trying to remember the details of the surgical task they are performing and the order these tasks are to be performed. Consequently, if they are learning these skills whilst performing surgery on a patient, much of their attentional resources (which are limited) are already used up. When an intra-operative event such as bleeding occurs, they may not have the attentional resources available to even notice the event. The more experienced junior surgeon would notice due to the fact that some of their skills have automated and require less conscious attention. However, if a second intra-operative event occurs, they could quickly exceed their available attentional resources whereas the master surgeon simply attends to and deals with these events.

It has been quantitatively demonstrated that this is one of the fundamental problems posed by the fulcrum effect on instrument handling in the acquisition of laparoscopic skills (Gallagher et al. 1998) and that this situation improves with training, practice and experience (Crothers et al. 1999). This happens because basic skills such as simple hand–eye coordination that are being learned will eventually 'automate' as these skills can be practiced proficiently with minimal attentional demands. These attentional resources are thus free to attend to other aspects of the task such as surgery, while the rest of the team are doing and mentally rehearsing how the surgery will proceed. This automation process is represented in Fig. 4.5. There are two collateral pressures impinging on the reduction of attentional resources. The first is the skill level of the surgeon, the second is the experience they have gained. Experience or the learning curve of the surgeon is what most surgical

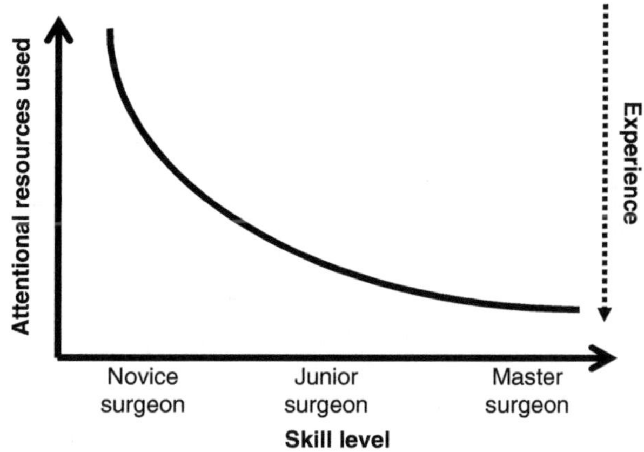

Fig. 4.5 Hypothetical model of attentional resources used as a function of task demands, attained skill level and operative experience

disciplines have concentrated on. However, the surgeon's learning curve will interact with their innate ability. The more innate visio-spatial, perceptual and psychomotor ability the learner has, the faster they will acquire the surgical skills thus automating faster and requiring fewer attentional resources to monitor basic aspects of the task they are performing, e.g. surgery, Figure 4.5 should be familiar to most surgeons as it appears to resemble the 'learning curve' associated with skill acquisition shown in Fig. 4.1. This is because the learning curve has been used as a proxy indicator for skill level and thus attentional automation are almost always linked to operative experience. However, as many surgeon educators are all too aware, the number of procedures performed by a learner is at best a crude predictor of actual operative performance. A better predictor is objective technical skills performance. The goal of any surgical training program should be to help the junior surgeon automate these basic psychomotor skills before they operate on a patient. This is one of the major advantages of simulation; it allows the trainee to automate in a risk-free environment and the trainer to monitor the automation process. Establishing when automation has been achieved will be dealt with later in Chap. 8.

Observational Learning

Perhaps the very fact that observational learning is so obvious helps explain why it was a relatively neglected area of research by psychologists until the late part of the twentieth century. Observational learning is the tendency of humans and many animals to learn by imitation. One explanation for the widespread importance of observational learning is its efficacy which means that learners can frequently avoid the tedious trial and error procedures that are characteristic of instrumental conditioning. Another advantage is that they will also know whether the efforts of the actor have been successful or not. Factors which appear to influence the effectiveness of observational learning are, for example, the status of the model (i.e., a consultant,

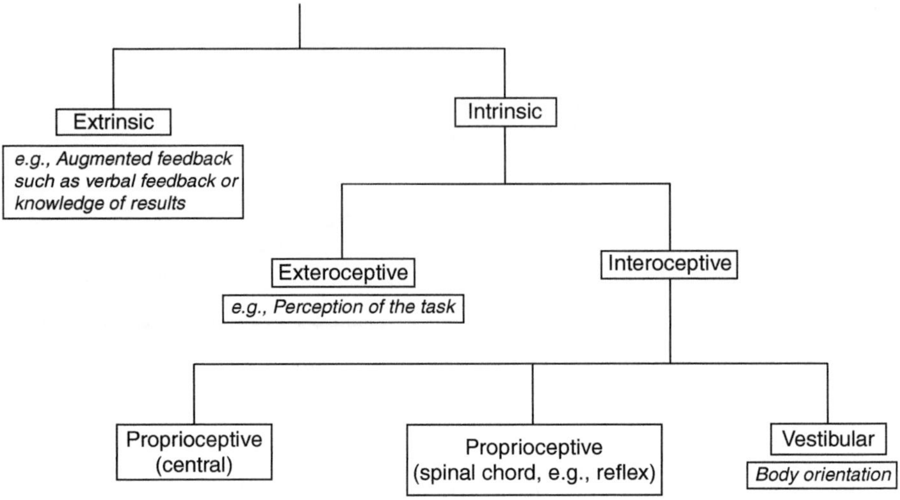

Fig. 4.6 Different types of feedback that may be used for regulation of performance

modeling the skills to be learned will be more effective than those of a peer) and levels of reinforcement. This means that the trainee is more likely to repeat performance characteristics that have a successful outcome or which have been rewarded. We will return to the issue of observational learning in Chap. 9 when we discuss the issue of didactic education and training and Chaps. 10 and 11 when we discuss how better use could be made of online learning.

Feedback: Knowledge of Results

For the operating surgeon proximal feedback on their performance is crucial. Figure 4.6 shows the different types and sources of feedback the surgeon can access to regulate and modify their performance. Extrinsic feedback from their environment is available from a wide variety of sources such as their trainer, knowledge of their results etc. Feedback can also come from a number of intrinsic sources such as perception of the task (visual, tactile, haptic, auditory and olfactory). It can also come from interoceptive information sources which provide information on the movement of internal organs and whether the body is moving with the correct effort. Proprioceptive information also comes from the final chords (reflects) type actions. Lastly, the surgeon can access information from the vestibular system which provides information on body orientation and location in space. One of the most valuable and efficient sources of feedback information is from the visual system. This is not really a problem in open surgery, but for any type of image guided surgery it becomes an issue if the surgeon cannot see images in real time. In image guided interventional medicine such as MIS, visualization in real-time is of crucial importance. Visualization of a dynamic process milliseconds after it's occurrence requires rapid information processing. Traditionally our reference point for real-time imaging has come from the film and TV industry. Image presentation is measured in Frame rates at which an imaging device produces unique consecutive images called frames. The term applies equally to computer graphics, video cameras, film cameras, and motion capture systems. Frame rate is most often expressed in frames per second (FPS) and in progressive scan monitors as hertz (Hz). In the United Kingdom, the TV and film industry generally uses 25 FPS and in the USA 30 FPS and these are regarded as real time. The reason real-time imaging is considered crucial by surgeons who operate with image guidance is that they need feedback on the impact of the working end of the instrument on tissues while they are operating. If they do not receive this information in real time and are operating close to vital structures such as an artery, they could inadvertently cause very serious and even life-threatening injuries. It is this speed of image processing that has delayed the expansion of tele-robotic surgery over great distances especially in deep space travel.

Real-time rendering is one of the interactive areas of computer graphics. It means creating synthetic images fast enough on the computer so that the viewer can interact with a virtual environment and is vital for high-fidelity virtual reality simulation. The most common place to find real-time rendering is in animated movies or video games. The rate at which images are displayed is also measured in frames per second (fps) or Hertz (Hz). In this instance, the frame rate is the measurement of how quickly an imaging device produces unique consecutive images. If an application is displaying 15 fps, it is considered real time.

Feedback: Metrics (Augmented Knowledge of Results)

Metrics are a standard set of measurements by which a plan, process or product can be assessed and that quantify these elements of performance. In terms of training in surgery, metrics are best considered as an extrinsic augmented form of feedback, which gives detailed information on knowledge of results. As indicated above, this type of information helps to optimize the learning experience and allows the trainee to acquire the desired skills in a more efficient manner. We shall discuss this very important issue of metrics in some depth in Chap. 5, but it is fair to say that valid and reliable metrics which are easily accessible should be an integral part of any good simulation that purports to train medical skills. The formulation of metrics requires breaking down a task into its essential components (task deconstruction) and then tightly defining what differentiates optimal from suboptimal performance. Unfortunately this aspect of simulation has been given all too little attention by the simulation industry. Drawing on the example from the MIS community almost all of the VR simulators use time as a metric. Unfortunately time analyzed as an independent variable is at best crude and at worst a dangerous metric. For example, in the laparoscopic environment being able to tie an intracorporeal knot quickly gives no indication of the quality of the knot. A poorly tied knot can obviously lead to a multitude of complications. There are only a few reports in the literature that use objective end product analysis (Hanna et al. 1997) due to the difficulty in acquiring this type of information. For example, Fried and Satava have reported the metrics for the entire endoscopic sinus surgery procedure in Otolaryngology Clinics of North America (Satava and Fried 2002). There is no magic solution to the issue of metrics and it is almost certain that good metrics will have to be procedure specific. For example, time may not be the most crucial metric for MIS simulations (within reason), but for fluoroscopically guided procedures in interventional radiology or cardiology, time and resultant radiation exposure are very critical. Whatever the metrics or procedures used, a finding that appears with regularity is that performance variability and errors appear to be key indicators of skill level, i.e., senior or experienced operators perform well, consistently and make few errors (Gallagher and Satava 2002; Van Sickle et al. 2005). The most valuable metrics that a simulation can provide are on errors. The whole point of training is to improve performance, make performance consistent and reduce errors. One of the major values of simulators is that they allow the trainee to make mistakes in a consequence-free environment, before they ever perform that procedure on a patient. The errors that each simulator identifies and provides remediation for will certainly be procedure specific, and the absence of error metrics should cause trainers to question the value of the simulator as a training device. Well-defined errors in simulation allow trainees to experience the operating environment and include risks such as bleeding without jeopardizing a patient. Thus trainees can learn what they have done wrong, and NOT to make the same mistakes *in vivo* when operating on patients in the future. Learning is optimized when feedback is proximate to when the error is committed. If simulators are to be used for high stakes assessment such as credentialing or certification, then the metrics for that simulator must be shown to meet the same psychometric standards of validation as any other psychometric test. This is a matter of some gravity because metric-based assessment of physician performance could make the difference between an individual progressing to the next stage of their career (or not) and whether an experienced physician can continue to practice. We address the issue of metric validation in some detail in Chap. 7 and come to some rather stark conclusions about respected validation evidence.

Training Schedule

There is no research available which outlines the schedule of initial training required to attain stable performance in the operating room. Extensive research has been conducted to determine the effects of practice schedules on the acquisition of simple motor skills (Catania 1984). Among the possible variables affecting the acquisition of motor skills none has been more extensively studied than the practice regime.

Distribution of practice refers to the spacing of practice sessions either in one long session (massed practice) or multiple, short practice sessions (interval practice). Metalis (1985) investigated the effects of massed versus interval practice on the acquisition of video-game-playing skill. Both the massed and interval practice groups showed marked improvement, however, the interval practice group consistently showed more improvement. Studies conducted in the 1940s and 1950s attempted to address the effects of massed as compared to interval practice. The majority of these studies showed that interval practice was more beneficial than massed practice and this is what Gallagher et al. (2005) counseled in their review of skill acquisition factors in surgery. Moulton et al. (2006) assessed the validity of this advice and confirmed its accuracy. At present, new MIS skills are taught in massed sessions often lasting one or two days. The surgeons are often considered trained in this new technology after such a short course and the issues of competence and supervision of the newly trained surgeons are relegated to the individual hospital. Why is interval practice a more effective training schedule than massed practice? A likely explanation is that the skills being learned have more time to be cognitively consolidated between practices. Consolidation is the process that is assumed to take place after acquisition of a new behavior. The process assumes long-term neurophysiological changes that allow for the relatively permanent retention of learned behavior. Scientific evidence for this process is now starting to emerge (Louie and Wilson 2001).

Random vs Blocked Training

In the massed versus distributed learning example we have discussed above, the same amount of training was given but the period of time in which it was given was varied. Another variant on training schedule is whether different tasks should be learned individually, practiced in blocks, or whether the tasks are practiced in a random order. It might be assumed that it would be easier to learn each task in a blocked design. However, this is not the case. Although performance is better during the acquisition phase with the blocked design training conditions, when tested on the transfer task, performance is actually better in randomly ordered conditions. In a study by Jordan and colleagues (2000), they investigated four different types of training programmes intended to help laparoscopic surgeons automate to the 'fulcrum effect'. All subjects received 10 two-minute training trials under one of four practice conditions. Three other groups had blocked training trials which were: (1) full binocular viewing conditions; (2) *Y*-axis inverted viewing conditions; and (3) normal laparoscopic viewing conditions. The fourth group received the same amount of training as the other three groups but the image and a practice on was randomly alternated between *Y*-axis inverted viewing conditions and normal laparoscopic viewing conditions for the ten training trials. All of the subjects were required to complete the exact same task that they had trained on but under normal laparoscopic viewing conditions. In this test, the group who trained under the randomly alternating imaging conditions outperformed the other three groups, i.e., they made significantly more correct responses and significantly fewer objectively assessed errors.

This type of training programme, although highly effective, may not suit all learners or tasks to be learned. Randomly alternating practice appears to be most effective when used with skills that require different patterns of coordination, and thus different underlying model programs (Hall and Magill 1995). In addition, characteristics of the individual such as the level of experience may also influence the effectiveness of random practice. For example, Goode and Magill (1986) found that random practice may be inappropriate until learners understand the dynamics of the task being learned.

Task Configuration and Training Strategies

When someone is learning a new set of skills such as hand–eye coordination of laparoscopic instruments, some thought should be given as to the type and difficulty of the tasks that trainees should practice first. Skill acquisition should be as free from frustration as possible. When attempting to acquire difficult skills, if the trainee experiences a high failure to success ratio they are unlikely to persist with training. We continually see this when we are trying to train residents to suture and knot-tie intracorporeally. Training tasks should start simple and gradually progress in difficulty. This is known in the behavioral science literature as '*shaping*'. This term simply means that successive approximations of the desired response pattern are reinforced until the desired response occurs. What is accepted as 'consistently' must be explicitly defined for the specific task. (This issue will be revisited when we discuss performance criterion levels.) To be fair, many of the simulators that currently exist for training laparoscopic skills do indeed use shaping as their core training methodology. Tasks are configurable from easy, medium and difficult settings and tasks can be ordered so that they become progressively more difficult. However, it is not clear whether the software engineers were aware that this was what they were doing when they wrote the software. Also, this is only one training strategy that could be used.

Another training strategy is '*fading*' and is used by a number of simulators such as the GI Mentor II (Simbionix, Cleveland, USA) and Endoscopic Sinus Simulator (ES3, Lockheed Martin). This strategy involves giving trainees major clues and guides at the start of training. Indeed, trainees might even begin with abstract tasks that elicit the same psychomotor performance as would be required to perform the task in vivo. As tasks become gradually more difficult, the amount of clues and guides are gradually faded out until the trainee is required to perform the task without support. For example, the ES3 simulator on the easy level requires the trainee to navigate an instrument through a series of hoops, the path of which mirrors the nasal cavity. The abstract task teaches the trainee the optimal path without having to worry about anatomical structure. The intermediate level requires the trainee to perform the same task; however, on this setting, the hoops are overlaid on simulated nasal cavity tissue and anatomical landmarks. The third and more difficult level gives no aid. This aid has in effect been faded out.

A very effective training strategy, i.e., '*backward chaining*' (Catania 1984) does not appear to have been used by any of the simulation companies. While shaping starts at the very beginning or basic steps of a skill or psychomotor task and gradually increases the complexity of the task requirement, backward chaining starts at the opposite end of the task, i.e. the complete task minus one step. This training strategy was developed for tasks that are particularly difficult and frustrating to learn. A good example of a task that would fit this category is intra-corporeal suturing and knot-tying and the procedure is broken down into discrete psychomotor performance units (task deconstruction).

A number of researchers have done this for their teaching curriculum but then proceeded to require trainees to perform the complete task (Rosser et al. 1998). The problem with this approach is that the trainee has a high failure to success ratio resulting in frustration, which in turn usually means that they give up trying to learn suturing. Backward chaining specifically programs a high success to failure ratio thus reducing or eliminating learner frustration. Using the example of tying a laparoscopic sliding square knot, tasks would be set up so that the trainee does the last step first, i.e., tying the final square knot. Trainees would continue to do this until they could do it proficiently every time. The next training task would involve trainees cinching or sliding the knot down into place and then squaring it off. Both steps would continue to be practiced until they are being performed consistently. The next training task would involve the square knot to a slip knot and then the two previous steps. This process would continue all the way back to the first step, i.e., the formation of 'C' loop and the wrap and so on. The benefits of this approach to training is that only one new step is being added with each backward step or 'chain' and that the forward chained behaviors have already been mastered, ensuring a high level of task success and a low level of frustration. In the box-trainer environment, this approach would have been very time consuming with the trainer having to prepare the backward chained task configuration; in addition, the task is difficult to assess. These difficulties disappear in virtual space. Furthermore, at least three VR companies currently have suturing tasks that could be configured this way (Mentice AB, Sweden, SimSurgery AS, Norway, Surgical Science AB, Sweden).

Simulation Fidelity

In the fields of modeling and simulation, fidelity refers to the degree to which a model or simulation reproduces the state and behavior of a real world object, feature or condition. Fidelity is therefore a measure of the realism of a model or simulation. While one of the advantages of training on a high-fidelity, full procedural simulator may be additional knowledge accrual, this should not be interpreted as a mandate that all types of computer-based simulation must be high-fidelity. In reality, there are many other means of conveying this knowledge-based information that will be equally or more effective with considerably less cost. The main function of a simulator is in fact for technical skills training, and knowledge should be acquired prior to training on the simulator. As simulator fidelity increases so does the price with some current high-fidelity devices costing between $100,000 to over $1 million.

Thus end users of surgical simulation must assess how much fidelity is required to achieve the greatest return on investment. The data from the MIST VR clinical trials clearly demonstrate that a low-fidelity simulator can consistently improve intra-operative performance. However, this does not mean that simulation fidelity is unimportant. Consider, a straight-forward laparoscopic cholecystectomy performed by a surgical resident under the direct guidance of an attending/consultant surgeon in the operating room. This is not a particularly high-risk situation and the probability of a life-threatening or life-altering complication is very low (Derossis et al. 1999). Conversely, an endovascular surgeon performing a carotid angioplasty and stenting procedure carries more risk. Results from the only multi-specialty prospective randomized trial on this procedure performed by experienced physicians showed that the risk of stroke or death at 30 days was as high as 4.6% (Yadav et al. 2004). In a high-risk procedure such as carotid artery angioplasty and stenting, the fidelity of the simulator should be maximized in attempts to replicate the exact procedure as closely as possible, to take every procedural step possible to minimize patient risk.

Another important point to make about fidelity of a simulator is that fidelity goes beyond computer graphics and presentation. Unfortunately many surgeons are over-awed by, and place too much emphasis on, the pure graphics aspect of the simulator. In a high-fidelity simulation, the tissue and instruments should behave as closely as possible to how they do in a patient. The instruments must not behave as if there is a predefined path for them and tissue behavior should also be as realistic as possible. A high-fidelity simulator must allow the trainee to err and learn from these mistakes and their performance must be meaningfully quantified, with well thought out metrics that distinguish between those who are good at the procedure and those who are not. If surgeons ignore or fail to appreciate this issue, we risk spending large amounts of resources for simulators which will not meet our needs.

Transfer of Training and Skills Generalization

Although these two learning phenomena are related and both refer to the process of skill acquisition, they are fundamentally different. *Skills generalization* refers to the training situation where the trainee learns fundamental skills that are crucial to completion of the actual operative task or procedure. *Skills transfer* refers to a training modality that directly emulates the task to be performed in vivo or in the testing condition. A practical example of the difference between skills generalization and transfer can be taken from the game of golf. Every golf pro will have beginning golfers practice swinging without even holding a club. This would be skills generalization. The swing is crucial to executing any golf shot, but swinging without a club does not directly relate to a shot. An example of skills transfer would be a golfer repeatedly hitting a sand wedge out of the right side trap near the 18 green. If during the next round the golfer finds himself in that trap, the practiced skills will directly transfer to his current situation. In the world of simulation, a good example of skills generalization is the MIST VR laparoscopic surgical training system.

This system teaches basic psychomotor skills fundamental to performing a safe laparoscopic cholecystectomy (LC) as well as many skills required in advanced laparoscopic procedures. The VR tasks do not resemble the operative field, but it has been clearly demonstrated that subjects who trained on the MIST VR performed a two-handed LC faster with fewer intra-operative errors (Seymour et al. 2002). It has also been demonstrated that these skills improve laparoscopic intra-corporeal suturing (Pearson et al. 2002). These are two good examples of skills generalization, which represents a very powerful, but misunderstood learning and training methodology. Simulators which rely on skills transfer might include mannequin type simulators such as TraumaMan™, (Simulab Corp, Seattle, USA), high-end VR simulators such as both the Lap Mentor and GI Mentor II (Simbionix, Cleveland, USA), the VIST (Mentice AB, Gothenburg, Sweden), and the ES3 (Lockheed Martin, Bethesda, MD). The simulated procedures look and feel similar to the actual procedures and will train skills that will directly transfer to the performed procedures.

A common mistake made by many trainers is that only simulators that provide a high-fidelity experience improve performance. This is inaccurate as is clearly demonstrated by the Yale VR to OR study mentioned above which used a skills generalization-based VR trainer. The question that should be asked is 'does the simulator train the appropriate skill to perform the procedure? It should also be noted that as fidelity increases, so does price. One of the most sophisticated VR simulators in the world is the VIST system (Mentice AB, Gothenburg, Sweden) which simulates in real time a full physics model of the vascular system (with fluid dynamics). However, it costs $300,000 per unit. Not all training programs can afford this level of simulation. Trainers must look beyond face validity of simulators and ask more important questions such as 'does it work? (i.e., train the appropriate skills), how well does it work? and how good is the evidence? This may involve trainers developing realistic expectations of what simulators should look like, which in turn will involve a genuine understanding of what simulations should be capable of achieving in a training program.

Whole vs Part Training

Simulation has been available in some form in medicine for at least four decades. Anesthetists were one of the early groups in medicine to recognize the advantages of this training methodology. They also have been very strong supporters of the group training for the whole procedure. In contrast, laparoscopic surgeons have attempted to use part task emulators and virtual reality simulators. The difference in approach between these two groups of physicians to solving the problem of training may have more to do with the resources available to them than what they would have preferred. Anesthetists pioneered the use of full body mannequins (or high-fidelity simulation) while laparoscopic surgeons required simulations of instrument tissue interactions in real time. This latter type of simulation required huge computer processing capacity, which until relatively recently was very expensive (even if it was available in the 1990s). In the second decade of the twenty-first century, this is less of an issue and we have seen some surgical simulations move to a full procedure, e.g., laparoscopic cholecystectomy, produced by Simbionix. However, the issue of whole versus part training is not simply a matter of the types of simulations that are available, but more to do with training effectiveness and efficiency. We shall discuss this matter in more detail in Chaps. 8 and 10.

At this point, it is fair to say that research has shown that whole-task training is the preferred method if the task is simple and can be reasonably approximated by the simulation. However, if the task is dangerous or highly complex and can be easily divided into subtasks, part-task training is the better choice. Context-dependent methods are favored over context-independent methods for recall and recognition. If the acquired knowledge and skills must be selectively applied in a variety of situations, context independent presentation methods are recommended.

Summary

Skill acquisition for the practice of MIS has been an issue for trainee surgeons which has been repeatedly found to be associated with increased complication rates during the learning phase. A considerable volume of well-founded scientific knowledge currently exists about the anatomy and neuropsychology of skill acquisition structures and processes which academic surgery has yet to fully embrace. This knowledge should help drive the design and implementation of efficient and effective training programs. It should also inform the design of simulations that support and help to deliver skills training as part of the curriculum. One of the most important parts of that curriculum (no matter how or on what type of simulation platform it is delivered on) is feedback. This is a crucial aspect of an objective, effective and efficient learning process. It occurs as a natural consequence of our interaction with our environment. Unfortunately, we may miss the feedback or the delay between performance and feedback may be so large that the contiguous relationship that did in fact exist is lost, as is the opportunity for learning. Simulation affords the opportunity to the surgical trainer and trainee to augment feedback on performance and ensure that it is delivered to the trainee in a timely, salient and effective manner during training. This feedback is called metrics which we will deal with in detail in Chap. 5.

References

Adams JA. A closed-loop theory of motor learning. *J Mot Behav*. 1971;3(2):111-149.

Adams JA. Historical review and appraisal of research on the learning, retention, and transfer of human motor skills. *Psychol Bull*. 1987;101(1):41-74.

Adams JA. The changing face of motor learning. *Hum Mov Sci*. 1990;9(3-5):209-220.

Anderson JR. Acquisition of cognitive skill. *Psychol Rev*. 1982;89(4):369-406.

Anderson JR, Reder LM, Simon HA. Situated learning and education. *Educ Res*. 1996;25(4):5.

Annett J. *Feedback and Human Behaviour*. Baltimore: Penguin Books; 1969.

Annett J. On knowing how to do things: a theory of motor imagery. *Cogn Brain Res*. 1996;3(2):65-69.

Bandura A. Self-efficacy mechanism in human agency. *Am Psychol*. 1982;37(2):122-147.

Bockler D, Geoghegan J, Klein M, Weisharpmann Q, Turan M, Meyer L. Implications of laparoscopic cholecystectomy for surgical residency training. *JSLC*. 1999;3(1):19-22.

Broadbent DE. *Perception and Communication*. New York: Pergamon Press; 1958.

Brooks V, Hilperath F, Brooks M, Ross HG, Freund HJ. Learning "what" and "how" in a human motor task. *Learn Mem*. 1995;2(5):225.

Carlson NR. *Physiology of Behavior*. Needham Heights: Allyn and Bacon; 1994.

Catania A. *Learning*. Englewood Cliffs: Prentice-Hall; 1984.

Centres R. Cholecystectomy practice transformed. *Lancet*. 1991;338(8770):789-790.

Chaiken SR, Kyllonen PC, Tirre WC. Organization and components of psychomotor ability* 1. *Cogn Psychol*. 2000;40(3):198-226.

Cheng PW. Restructuring versus automaticity: alternative accounts of skill acquisition. *Psychol Rev*. 1985;92(3):414-423.

Clark FJ, Horch KW. Kinesthesia. In: Boff K, Kaufman L, Thomas J, eds. *Handbook of Perception and Human Performance*. 1st ed. New York: John Wiley; 1986.

Courjon JH, Jeannerod M, Prablanc C. An attempt at correlating visuomotor-induced tilt aftereffect and ocular cyclotorsion. *Perception*. 1981;10(5):519-524.

Crothers IR, Gallagher AG, McClure N, James DT, McGuigan J. Experienced laparoscopic surgeons are automated to the "fulcrum effect": an ergonomic demonstration. *Endoscopy*. 1999;31(5):365-369.

Derossis AM, Antoniuk M, Fried GM. Evaluation of laparoscopic skills: a 2-year follow-up during residency training. *Can J Surg*. 1999;42(4):293.

Druckman D, Bjork RA. *In the Mind's Eye: Enhancing Human Performance*. Washington: National Academies Press; 1992.

Dudai Y. The neurobiology of consolidations, or, how stable is the engram? *Annu Rev Psychol*. 2004;55:51-86.

Ericsson KA, Kintsch W. Long-term working memory. *Psychol Rev*. 1995;102(2):211-244.

Ferrari M. Observing the observer: self-regulation in the observational learning of motor skills* 1. *Dev Rev*. 1996;16(2):203-240.

Fitts PM, Peterson JR. Information capacity of discrete motor responses. *J Exp Psychol*. 1964;67(2):103-112.

Fitts PM, Posner M. *Human Performance*. Belmont: Brooks/Cole Publishing Co; 1967.

Gallagher AG, Satava RM. Virtual reality as a metric for the assessment of laparoscopic psychomotor skills. Learning curves and reliability measures. *Surg Endosc*. 2002;16(12):1746-1752.

Gallagher AG, McClure N, McGuigan J, Ritchie K, Sheehy NP. An ergonomic analysis of the fulcrum effect in the acquisition of endoscopic skills. *Endoscopy*. 1998;30(7):617-620.

Gallagher AG, Ritter EM, Champion H, et al. Virtual reality simulation for the operating room: proficiency-based training as a paradigm shift in surgical skills training. *Ann Surg*. 2005;241(2):364-372.

Gallagher AG, Al-Akash M, Seymour NE, Satava RM. An ergonomic analysis of the effects of camera rotation on laparoscopic performance. *Surg Endosc*. 2009;23(12):2684-2691.

Gick ML, Holyoak KJ. The cognitive basis of knowledge transfer. In: Cormier SM, Hagman JD, eds. *Transfer of Learning: Contemporary Research and Applications*. San Diego: Academic Press; 1987:9-46.

Gigot JF, Etienne J, Aerts R, et al. The dramatic reality of biliary tract injury during laparoscopic cholecystectomy. *Surg Endosc*. 1997;11(12):1171-1178.

Goode S, Magill RA. Contextual interference effects in learning three badminton serves. *Res Q Exerc Sport*. 1986;57(4):308-314.

Haffenden AM, Goodale MA. Independent effects of pictorial displays on perception and action. *Vision Res*. 2000;40(10-12):1597-1607.

Hall KG, Magill RA. Variability of practice and contextual interference in motor skill learning. *J Mot Behav*. 1995;27(4):299-309.

Hanna GB, Frank TG, Cuschieri A. Objective assessment of endoscopic knot quality*. *Am J Surg*. 1997;174(4):410-413.

Harris CS. Adaptation to displaced vision: visual, motor, or proprioceptive change? *Science*. 1963;140(3568):812.

Held R, Gottlieb N. Technique for studying adaptation to disarranged hand-eye coordination. *Percept Mot Skills*. 1958;8:83-86.

Held R, Rekosh J. Motor-sensory feedback and the geometry of visual space. *Science*. 1963;141: 722-723.

Hick WE. On the rate of gain of information. *Q J Exp Psychol*. 1952;4(1):11-26.

Horak M. The utility of connectionism for motor learning: A reinterpretation of contextual interference in movement schemes. *J Mot Behav*. 1992;24:58-66.

Jeannerod M. To act or not to act: perspectives on the representation of actions. *Q J Exp Psychol A*. 1999;52(1):1-29.

Johnson C, Jago R, Frost R. Laparoscopic cholecystectomy. In: Johnson C, Taylor I, eds. *Recent Advances in Surgery*. London: Churchill Livingstone; 1992.

Jordan JA, Gallagher AG, McGuigan J, McClure N. Randomly alternating image presentation during laparoscopic training leads to faster automation to the "fulcrum effect". *Endoscopy*. 2000;32(4):317-321.

Keele SW. Movement control in skilled motor performance. *Psychol Bull*. 1968;70(6):387-403.

Langer EJ, Piper AI. The prevention of mindlessness. *J Pers Soc Psychol*. 1987;53(2): 280-287.

Lazzari S, Mottet D, Vercher JL. Eye-hand coordination in rhythmical pointing. *J Mot Behav*. 2009;41(4):294-304.

Lee TD, Swinnen SP, Verschueren S. Relative phase alterations during bimanual skill acquisition. *J Mot Behav*. 1995;27(3):263-274.

Lerut T. The surgeon as a prognostic factor. *Ann Surg*. 2000;232(6):729.

Liesker H, Brenner E, Smeets JBJ. Combining eye and hand in search is suboptimal. *Exp Brain Res*. 2009;197(4):395-401.

Louie K, Wilson MA. Temporally structured replay of awake hippocampal ensemble activity during rapid eye movement sleep. *Neuron*. 2001;29(1):145-156.

Marotta JJ, Goodale MA. The role of learned pictorial cues in the programming and control of grasping. *Exp Brain Res*. 1998;121(4):465-470.

Mather JA, Lackner JR. Adaptation to visual displacement with active and passive limb movements: effect of movement frequency and predictability of movement. *Q J Exp Psychol*. 1980;32(2):317-323.

Metalis SA. Effects of massed versus distributed practice on acquisition of video game skill. *Percept Mot Skills*. 1985;61(2):457-458.

Moore MJ, Bennett CL. The learning curve for laparoscopic cholecystectomy. The southern surgeons club. *Am J Surg*. 1995;170(1):55.

Moulton CAE, Dubrowski A, MacRae H, Graham B, Grober E, Reznick R. Teaching surgical skills: what kind of practice makes perfect?: A randomized, controlled trial. *Ann Surg*. 2006;244(3):400.

Newell KM. Motor skill acquisition. *Annu Rev Psychol*. 1991;42(1):213-237.

Newell A, Rosenbloom PS. Mechanisms of skill acquisition and the law of practice. In: Anderson JR, ed. *Cognitive Skills and Their Acquisition*. Hillsdale: Lawrence Erlbaum Associates; 1981:1-55.

Norman GR, Rosenthal D, Brooks LR, Allen SW, Muzzin LJ. The development of expertise in dermatology. *Arch Dermatol*. 1989;125(8):1063.

Patkin M, Isabel L. *Ergonomics and Laparoscopic General Surgery. Laparoscopic Abdominal Surgery*. New York: McGraw-Hill; 1993.

Pearson AM, Gallagher AG, Rosser JC, Satava RM. Evaluation of structured and quantitative training methods for teaching intracorporeal knot tying. *Surg Endosc.* 2002;16(1):130-137.

Reinhardt-Rutland AH. Remote operation: a selective review of research into visual depth perception. *J Gen Psychol.* 1996;123(3):237-248.

Reinhardt-Rutland AH, Gallagher AG. Visual depth perception in minimally invasive surgery. In: Robertson SA, ed. *Contemporary Ergonomics.* London: Taylor and Francis; 1995:531-536.

Rosser JC Jr, Rosser LE, Savalgi RS. Objective evaluation of a laparoscopic surgical skill program for residents and senior surgeons. *Arch Surg.* 1998;133(6):657.

Satava RM, Fried MP. A methodology for objective assessment of errors: an example using an endoscopic sinus surgery simulator. *Otolaryngol Clin North Am.* 2002;35(6).

Schmidt RA. A schema theory of discrete motor skill learning. *Psychol Rev.* 1975;82(4):225-260.

Servos P. Distance estimation in the visual and visuomotor systems. *Exp Brain Res.* 2000;130(1): 35-47.

Seymour NE, Gallagher AG, Roman SA, et al. Virtual reality training improves operating room performance: results of a randomized, double-blinded study. *Ann Surg.* 2002;236(4):458-463; discussion 463-454.

Smith WM. Visually-guided behaviour and behaviourally-guided vision. *Ergonomics.* 1970;13(1):119-127.

Van Sickle K, Iii D, Gallagher AG, Smith CD. Construct validation of the ProMIS simulator using a novel laparoscopic suturing task. *Surg Endosc.* 2005;19(9):1227-1231.

Von Holst E, Mittelstaedt H. The reafference principle. Interaction between the central nervous system and the periphery. In: *Selected Papers of E. von Holst: The Behavioral Physiology of Animals and Man*, vol. 1. London: Methuen; 1950:39-73.

Wallace SA, Newell KM, Wade MG. Decision and response times as a function of movement difficulty in preschool children. *Child Dev.* 1978;49(2):509-512.

Winstein CJ, Schmidt RA. Sensorimotor feedback. In: Holding D, ed. *Human Skills.* 2nd ed. Chichester: John Wiley & Sons; 1989:17-47.

Yadav JS, Wholey MH, Kuntz RE, et al. Protected carotid-artery stenting versus endarterectomy in high-risk patients. *N Engl J Med.* 2004;351(15):1493.

Chapter 5
Metrics for the Measurement of Skill

Objective Assessment in Surgery

The 'Bristol Case' (Senate of Surgery 1998) and the "To Err is Human" (Kohn et al. 2000) report have revealed a major deficiency in the area of surgical education, training, and assessment. Analysis revealed that there is no uniform or consistent training in surgical skills, either at a local or national level. Surgical training continues in the traditional mentoring method, where students are exposed to patient care with the guidance of an experienced surgeon teacher. The experience is unstructured, being dictated by the random admission of patients rather than a consistent exposure to all the fundamental surgical problems. Likewise, there is no objective method to assess surgical technical competence. Although many factors influence surgical outcome, the skill of a surgeon in the operating theatre is very important. Darzi et al. (1999) reiterate the contention of Spencer that a skillfully performed operation is 75% decision-making and 25% dexterity (Spencer 1978). They do however concede that in some surgical specialties such as minimally invasive surgery dexterity becomes more important. We believe that this is an over simplification of the role of technical skill in operative performance and it is very difficult to achieve an overall performance ratio that can be attributed to cognitive or decision-making aspects of performance and technical performance. We believe that it does not make sense to try and separate these aspects of performance since they are inextricably linked and interwoven. For example, a surgeon may see a patient and ask the appropriate questions during a consultation, request the appropriate laboratory investigations and then formulate the correct diagnosis and decide to perform the correct intervention. However, this effort will have largely been in vain, if they are unable to perform the appropriate surgical procedure in a timely, efficient and safe manner. It could be argued that the most important part of this exercise was the work-up of the patient, making the correct diagnosis and then deciding on the appropriate intervention. It is entirely possible that the same surgeon could refer this patient on to a colleague to perform the surgical procedure. However, if this happened on a frequent enough basis for surgical procedures that were relatively

A.G. Gallagher and G.C. O'Sullivan, *Fundamentals of Surgical Simulation*, Improving Medical Outcome - Zero Tolerance,
DOI 10.1007/978-0-85729-763-1_5,

straightforward, one would have to question whether the individual making the referral was still a practising surgeon. Alternatively, simply asking someone with excellent surgical technical skills to perform the procedure is also not a realistic option. Even the most gifted technician must have the surgical wisdom on an ongoing basis to perform even the most straightforward surgical procedure. In the straightforward surgical procedure, this wisdom is rarely called upon. However, the potential for something to go wrong during an operative procedure is ever present. The wisdom and the skill that an operating surgeon has acquired during training and mentorship are not necessarily essential during every moment of every surgical procedure they perform. However, on the infrequent occasions that they are required both are essential.

It is not clear why surgeons have emphasized the importance of cognition (e.g. knowledge and decision making) in the practice of surgery over technical skills as common sense would seem to suggest that the technical performance of the surgeon would be crucial to the outcome for the patient. Indeed, it has been our experience that most of our surgical colleagues are dismissive of the role of technical skills in bad outcomes. However, at odds with this is the emergence of evidence linking technical skills to injury. In one study by Regenbogen et al. (2007), they investigated the pattern of technical errors among 444 randomly sampled malpractice claims that had been settled. The reason that they chose malpractice claims that have been settled was because there was a clear outcome and decision as to where the blame or fault lay. In the 444 malpractice claims they found that 258 injuries were due to error; 52% of these involved technical errors and 65% were linked to manual errors by the surgeon. In defence of these findings, most of our surgical colleagues would argue that these errors were probably associated with junior surgeons or occurred during a complex surgical procedure. What Regenbogen and colleagues did in fact find was that most of the technical errors occurred during routine operations that were being performed by experienced surgeons. We are not surprised by this finding. In a study conducted at the American College of Surgeons annual congress in 2002 (Gallagher et al. 2003), 210 very experienced laparoscopic surgeons had their laparoscopic surgical skills assessed. They completed the exact same task twice on a virtual reality simulator, and twice in a box trainer. The task was relatively simple as the goal of this study was to assess the strength of the relationship between the performance of the task in the real world and performance of the same task in virtual environment. The surprising finding from the study was that 15 of these very experienced surgeons could complete no part of the tasks. It was also found that of those surgeons who were able to complete the tasks 10% of them were performing significantly worse than colleagues, and some of them scored more than 20 standard deviations from the mean. The suspicion of the researchers at the time of this study was that there might have been a fault with the tasks that were chosen, how they were presented or indeed it might have been the fault of the simulator. However, with the passage of time and considerably more experience in the objective assessment of technical skills in surgery and other disciplines in medicine, these explanations now seem less attractive. The inevitable conclusion from this type of study is that some of the surgeons assessed in 2002 may not have been technically very skilled. The problem for surgery is that until relatively recently they have had formal assessment of surgical knowledge but there has been no requirement for the assessment of technical operative skill.

Early Metrics in Surgery

Robert Liston (1794–1847) who was appointed to the Chair in Surgery (UCL) in 1835 was as famous for his compassion as a healer as he was for his skill as a surgeon (Fig. 5.1). He was an abrupt, abrasive man but was charitable to the poor and tender to the sick that he cared for. He cared for patients who many of his surgical colleagues at the Edinburgh Royal Infirmary had previously dismissed as incurable. This did not make him popular with his colleagues and he eventually left Edinburgh for London. During the nineteenth century, prior to the introduction of anesthesia, the speed of surgery was directly correlated with the success of the operation. A shorter operating time meant less pain and less opportunity for the patient to bleed to death. Liston, who was famous for his operating speed (without anesthesia), completed the first surgical procedure in the UK carried out under Ether anesthesia. He

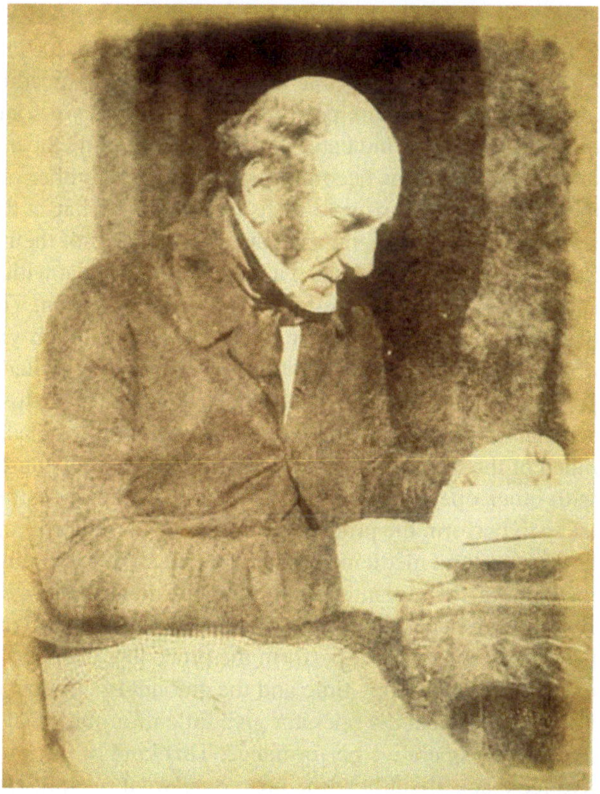

Fig. 5.1 Robert Liston (1794–1847) who was appointed to the Chair in Surgery, University College London (UCL) in 1835

amputated the leg of Frederick Churchill in about 28 s which was considerably faster than his normal 150 s. (Presumably the increase in speed was due to the decrease in the patient flailing around during the operation). As we can see from this example, even in the nineteenth century, measurements such as time were used as a metric for the assessment of the skill of the surgeon. A metric is a means of deriving a *quantitative measurement* (preferably interval or ratio scale) or *approximation* for otherwise *qualitative phenomena* such as skill (Reber and Reber 1985).

The Illusion of Metrics

Medicine in the twenty-first century is still struggling with the same issue, i.e., how to assess skill. Unlike the nineteenth century, operating time in the twenty-first century has become at best a very crude metric for skill as it gives no indication of the quality of performance. Indeed, this was also true in Liston's time, but apparently conveniently ignored. For example, in another one of Liston's most famous cases, it is always reported that he amputated the leg of the patient in about 2 1/2 min. What is less frequently reported is that the patient subsequently died from gangrene; Liston accidentally amputated the fingers of his operating assistant who also subsequently died of gangrene and he sliced through the coat of an observer who, although not injured, collapsed and died of fright (Gordon 2001).

Simply reporting the time taken to perform a procedure gives no indication of the quality of the procedure performance. However, we continue to use time to perform the procedure as an indicator of the skill level of the operator. We also use the amount of time someone has been in training and the number of times they have completed the procedure as surrogate measures of skill. That is the equivalent of a surgeon's skills in Liston's era being evaluated on the basis of their blood stiffened Frock coats: Surgeons at that time equated a blood stiffened coat with a busy and hence successful surgical practice and by inference, a skilled surgeon. The problem with these types of information is that they are incomplete and only provide crude surrogate information on the skill of the operator. For example, a skilled and efficient operator may perform a procedure quickly but so also might an unsophisticated operator. Anesthesia, a better understanding of hemostasis and fluid replacement, may have mitigated much of the temporal urgency during surgical procedures but this has been replaced with other operating factors which still impose constraints on the amount of time taken to perform the procedure, i.e., the use of fluoroscopy. Compounding this problem, procedural medicine has become much more sophisticated and complex involving the surgical implantation of fragile medical devices, e.g., pacemaker implantation. A good understanding of the skill of the operator is still required to determine whether the operator is ready to perform the procedure unsupervised. Metrics such as procedure time, fluoroscopy time and the amount of contrast used whilst conveying some information about the operator give little information of value that is reliably predictive of their operative performance. This kind of information provides only summative feedback about how the procedure went overall. However, for optimal learning and practice the operator needs feedback that is proximate to their performance (Catania 1984). For example, an operator would be unwise to advance a catheter into the ostium of a vessel with as little as a 0.5 s delay in visual feedback or to make an incision with a similar delay.

The Evolution of Metric-Based Assessment in Surgery

Objective Structured Assessment of Technical Skill (OSATS)

During the last decade of the twentieth century, considerable effort was made on the objective assessment of surgical skills. For example, Reznick and colleagues (Martin et al. 1997) have developed and reported validation studies on Objective Structured Assessment of Technical Skill (OSATS) to objectively assess the technical capabilities of Surgical Residents. OSATS was one of the first widely accepted approaches. It was developed along the same lines as the Objective Structured Clinical Examination (or OSCE). OSATS was originally developed for a bench station test and consists of a task specific checklist (CL) and global rating scale (GRS). The GRS has seven items, each evaluated on a global five-point Likert-scale where the lowest, middle and highest scorers are defined by explicit descriptions of performances. It has been widely reported that these GRSs are reliable, have a high inter-rater reliability and have demonstrated construct validity. Since first reported OSATS has been modified and tested in many different surgical areas such as open surgery, cardiac surgery (Hance et al. 2005) and gynecology (Larsen et al. 2006). Although widely accepted by the surgical community, OSATS has a number of methodological problems which are discussed in some detail in Chap. 7. Users of OSATS have consistently used a correlation coefficient or an alpha coefficient as measures of inter-rater reliability (IRR). We explain in some detail in Chap. 7 that methodologically this is unacceptable practice as a correlation coefficient is a measure of association not a measure of agreement. Therefore, citing a correlation coefficient as a quantitative measure of agreement is at best misleading and at worst inaccurate. There are a number of reasons for this. The first is that a correlation will be higher if there is a substantial range or spread in the scores of the group on which it is based than it does if the members of the group score closer together. Thus when interpreting reliability of a test or device one should ensure that the two groups of scores have about the same amount of variability. Furthermore, when users do report measures of agreement these are calculated for the entire group, and not for the individuals being assessed (Larsen et al. 2006). This is also methodologically inappropriate. The IRR is probably best construed as a measure of objectivity, transparency and a fairness check for *individuals* being assessed and thus is a quality assurance indicator. Although it is important that the overall IRR threshold is >0.8, it is even more important that this applies at the level of the individual assessment because if all individual assessments reach >0.8 IRR this guarantees the group result will have reached at least this level, but not vice versa.

One of the greatest problems in the objective assessment of surgical performance is asking experienced surgeons to score performance that has not been clearly operationally defined, or where there is ambiguity in the response scale that is being used. Because of potential ambiguity in responding, the Likert-type scale may introduce too much unexplained variation, both random and systematic. For example, in one of the original OSATS scales which was designed to assess confidence of movements and instrument handling, point 3 on the scale is described as "competent use of instruments, although occasionally appeared stiff or awkward". In another example where authors are assessing respect for tissue, they describe point 1 on the scale as "frequently used unnecessary force on tissue or risk of damage by inappropriate use of instruments or instruments out of sight". The problem with these descriptions is that there is no uniform and global understanding and implicit definition between surgeons of what 'competent use of instruments' or 'inappropriate use of instruments' means. Most surgeons probably have a fair idea what these concepts mean but for reliable assessments these potential subpopulation sources of variation should be minimized. Performance to be assessed should, where possible, be unambiguously defined so as to make it easy for the assessor to decide whether or not the performance was adequate. In doing this it is arguably better to simplify the response scale while, with appropriately worded statements, ensuring a common understanding of the event. Despite this, the users of OSATS have consistently reported superior results with the GRS rather than the checklist. This seems counterintuitive to our own experience because of the difficulties in trying to train consultant assessors to score performance with >0.8 IRR using a Likert scale. In the method described in this chapter, we advocate the use of clearly defined measures of performance that are scored as having occurred or not. Using this method, it is much easier to establish an IRR ≥0.8 with a minimum of training for the assessors.

In the quest for assessment strategies of surgical performance, it is important that individuals who observe performance agree on the occurrence/non-occurrence of key behaviors. This is essential to ensure that evaluation of the desired behaviors remains consistent and is not subject to the development of a single observer's bias. The main reasons for this are (1) assessment will only be useful if it can be achieved with some consistency, (2) if a single observer is recording performance his/her data may simply reflect a change in that observer's definition over time, i.e., she/he may become biased or less stringent over time. In order to evaluate reliability, one needs either (a) at least two observers or (b) observations on repeated occasions; (3) agreement between observers because it tells us something about how we have defined the behavior of interest.

Imperial College Surgical Assessment Device (ICSAD)

Other investigators have attempted to develop mechanical or computerized techniques to measure surgical skill more objectively than OSATS, such as motion analysis of surgical tools during surgery using electromagnetic tracking (Smith et al. 2002).

There is no magic solution to the issue of metrics and it is almost certain that good metrics will have to be procedure specific. For example, time may not be the most crucial metric for minimally invasive surgery (within reason), but for radiographically guided procedures in interventional radiology or cardiology time and resultant radiation exposure are very critical. The Imperial College surgery group led by Professor Lord Ara Darzi has been researching economy of hand movement for a number of years with an electromagnetic tracking system they have developed, the Imperial College Surgical Assessment Device (ICSAD) (Smith et al. 2002). They found that senior or very experienced surgeons have a smoother instrument path trajectory in comparison to less experienced surgeons. The elegance of this approach is that the system could be used to assess open as well as MIS skills.

The ICSAD device is based on a design that was originally used for tracking laparoscopic instruments in virtual reality simulators. It uses orthogonal electromagnetic fields to sense 3D position and orientation (Ghazisaedy et al. 1995; Meyer et al. 1992; Nixon et al. 1998; Raab et al. 1979). The electromagnetic transmitter contains three orthogonal coils that are pulsed in a sequence; the receiver also has three orthogonal coils that measure the electromagnetic field produced by the transmitter. The strength of the received signals is compared to the strength of the sent pulses to determine the position and compared to each other to determine the orientation. The measurements produced by this setup are rather noisy; therefore an additional filtering is required. Working range of both systems is claimed to be up to 10 ft from the transmitter, but the accuracy of the systems decrease as the distance between the transmitter and the receiver increases. Also, due to the dependence of the measurements on the local electromagnetic field, the tracking systems are sensitive to the ambient electromagnetic environment. If there is either a metal or other conductive material or equipment that produces an electromagnetic field near the tracker's transmitter or receiver, the transmitter signals are distorted and the resulting measurements contain both static and dynamic error. The manufacturers of the tracking systems suggest that there should be no metal components near the transmitter and receiver, which is often not possible to achieve particularly when measuring surgical skills. The operating room is crammed with high-quality steel, other metals and materials that could conduct an electromagnetic signal. Given these limitations it is probable that assessment tools such as ICSAD may only be of use in the skills laboratory as it may be difficult to capture a reliable signal in the operating room. Another problem with ICSAD is that it only provides (noisy) measurements of hand movements but provides no contextual information. Without contextual information the data generated by ICSAD could be from a surgeon performing a laparoscopic cholecystectomy or an automobile mechanic working on a carburettor. This means that measurement conducted with ICSAD requires two levels of measurement, the first being the tracking of hand movements and the second the scoring (or recording at least) of surgical performance. Both of these measurements would require some sort of assessment of what the surgeon actually does, e.g., clipping the cystic artery. This information would also have to be supplemented with information on whether the clips were applied correctly or whether they damaged other anatomical structures in the process (i.e., perforate the gallbladder).

Awareness of these shortcomings may help to explain why the group at Imperial College London uses OSATS so frequently in their studies. But, as we have briefly indicated here and go into greater detail in Chap. 7, OSATS has a number of methodological shortcomings which significantly undermine its utility. Although a useful assessment tool, ICSAD has not been widely used outside the Imperial College London surgical skills research laboratory.

Advanced Dundee Endoscopic Psychomotor Tester (ADEPT)

Performance on an Advanced (Dundee) Endoscopic Psychomotor Tester (ADEPT) in the training box environment has been shown to correlate well with subjective evaluation of operative skill (Francis et al. 2002). ADEPT was developed by the Dundee team specifically for the purpose of assessing technical skill and aptitude for performing laparoscopic surgery. The system's hardware consists of a dual gimbal mechanism that accepts a variety of 5.0-mm standard endoscopic instruments for manipulation in a specifically mapped and enclosed work space. The target object consists of a sprung base plate incorporating various tasks. It is covered by a sprung perforated transparent top plate that has to be moved and held in the correct position by the operator to gain access to the various tasks. Standard video endoscope equipment provides the visual interface between the operator and the target-instrument field. Different task modules can be used, and the level of task difficulty can be adjusted by varying the manipulation, elevation, and azimuth angles. The system's software is designed to (a) prompt the surgeon with the information necessary to perform the task, (b) collect and collate data on performance during execution of specified tasks, and (c) save the data for future analysis. The system was tested and validated in a series of studies (Francis et al. 2001; Hanna et al. 1998); however, these do not appear to have been widely accepted by the surgical community. ICSAD is derived from a generic technology that was applied to minimally invasive surgery but the ADEPT system was specifically designed to assess laparoscopic skills. However, that assessment was abstracted from actual surgery and at no point could ADEPT be immersed in the performance of surgery. For these, and probably many other reasons, ADEPT was never really used as an assessment tool outside the Dundee endoscopic skills laboratory.

Virtual Reality Simulation

It is highly probable that had any of the three assessment systems been developed in the 1980s or earlier, they would have achieved much wider market penetration, acceptance and usage. However, just as these researchers were starting to mature and validate their assessment devices, virtual reality simulation came to the fore. Computer-based simulation has been used for decades in aviation and other professional fields. However, the last 20 years has seen numerous attempts to introduce computer-based simulation into clinical medicine. Surgery, and specifically minimally invasive surgery, has led the way in the development and in the application of this technology in clinical practice. At the beginning of the twenty-first century, use of computer-based simulation for training has expanded into the multidisciplinary fields of catheter-based, image guided intervention, enabling both surgeons and non-surgeons alike to train on new procedures. The widespread introduction and use of computer-based simulation is changing the way that physicians are trained and positively impacts on the treatments patients receive. We believe that this revolution represents a paradigm shift in the way procedural-based medicine will be learned and practiced.

The terms "virtual reality" and "computer-based simulation" are often used interchangeably. Virtual reality, or VR, commonly refers to 'a computer generated representation of an environment that allows sensory interaction, thus giving the impression of actually being present' (Coleman et al. 1994). However, VR is probably best defined by Riva (2003) who suggested that it is a communication interface based on interactive visualization which allows the user to interface, interact with and integrate different types of sensory inputs that simulate important aspects of real-world experience. It allows the user to interact and to experience important aspects of the encounter rather than simply observing. This interaction has important learning implications which will be highlighted in subsequent chapters. Although first proposed as a training strategy for surgery in 1991 by Satava (1993), acceptance of the use of VR for training has been slow due to costs, scepticism within the medical community and the lack of robust scientific evidence to support the efficacy and effectiveness of this training strategy. However, this is rapidly changing.

The first virtual reality surgical simulator in laparoscopic surgery was designed by Satava (1993). He developed it primarily as a training tool to help counteract the difficulties he observed that many of his colleagues were having in acquiring the skills for endoscopic surgery. However, because of the limitations in computer processing capacity, the virtual abdomen was cartoon-like in appearance. Despite this, the simulation was 'realistic' in its anatomical and technical accuracy, allowing trainees the ability to practice skills outside the operating theatre in a computer-based environment. The first VR simulator (or more accurately emulator) to make any headway with the surgical community was the MIST VR system described in Chap. 2. The MIST VR system was designed to develop and to assess minimally invasive surgical skills using advanced computer technology in a format which could be easily operated by both tutor and trainee. The system is comprised of a frame equipped with two standard laparoscopic instruments. This hardware is interfaced with a PC running the MIST VR software. The software creates a virtual environment on the display screen, and is able to track and display the position and movement of the instruments in real time. An accurately scaled operating volume of 10 cm^3 is represented by a three-dimensional cube on the computer screen. The overall image size and the sizes of the target object can be varied for different skill levels. The instrument sensing technology in MIST

VR accomplishes the same measurement as the ICSAD system but is coupled to tasks and measurements that are directly related to MIS performance. Targets appeared randomly within the operating volume according to the task and could be 'grasped' and 'manipulated' (Wilson et al. 1997). In training mode, the MIST VR programme guides the trainee through a series of tasks which progressively become more complex, enabling the development of the hand-eye motor coordination essential for the safe clinical practice of laparoscopic surgery. Each task is based on an essential surgical technique employed in MIS. Performance is *scored* for time, error rate and efficiency of movement for each task, for both hands. Ironically, Imperial College was one of the first teams to complete a preliminary evaluation of MIST VR and their research thrust seemed to emphasize the simulator as an assessment device (Taffinder et al. 1998). The team from Queen's University Belfast also completed an evaluation and their emphasis appeared to emphasize MIST VR as a training device (Gallagher et al. 1999). In 2002 the scientific lead from the Queen's University team, along with a group of surgeons at Yale University, completed the first prospective, randomized, controlled trial of virtual reality training for the operating room (or VR to OR) (Seymour et al. 2002). Gallagher was aware of the potential of MIST VR as an assessment device but knew that it would be easier for the surgical community to accept an evidence-based training device than an assessment device. The Queens University team progressed research on MIST VR as a training device (Gallagher et al. 2000; Jordan et al. 2000, 2001; Pearson et al. 2002) whilst at the same time validating MIST VR assessment metrics (Gallagher et al. 2001, 2003, 2004, 2009; Gallagher and Satava 2002) to the point where (if surgery had chosen) the simulator metrics (time, error and economy of diathermy) had been validated for high stakes assessment. This possibility was never availed of by surgery.

The weakness of the MIST VR system despite its robust scientific validation was that it only assessed performance in one domain and that was MIS. Despite the enthusiasm and undoubted scientific and intellectual contribution of the MIS community to research and thinking about how training should be conducted and assessed, MIS represents only a small portion of surgical practice. However, important lessons can be learned from the MIST VR. The first is that it was developed by a collaborative group including an engineer (Chris Sutton, London, UK), the end user, i.e., a surgeon (Dr. Rory McCloy, Manchester, UK) and an expert in curriculum/metrics development, i.e., a psychologist (Dr. Bob Stone, Manchester, UK). Many simulators are developed by an engineer who has 'consulted' an end user rather than intimately involving them and rarely is a curriculum development and metrics expert involved. Much like a scientific experiment, a simulator is much more difficult to fix at the end of development than at the beginning. Even from a quick overview of MIST VR it was clear from the outset that it was a machine that had been designed as a metric-based training device, built on sound learning theory. It was also very clear that metrics had been developed by the surgeon and the psychologist in a collaborative effort. Psychologists have expertise in a number of domains but one of them is the science of behavior (i.e., sensory, perceptual, cognitive and psychomotor) and all that encapsulates.

How to Develop Metrics from First Principles

There is no magical solution to the issue of metric development, and it is almost certain that good metrics will have to be procedure specific rather than generic. For example, as we have illustrated, while time alone is not a crucial metric for MIS procedure performance, time and the resultant radiation exposure is very critical in the assessment of performance in many image-guided catheter-based procedures where extreme doses of radiation can lead to burns and other dire consequences. The formulation of metrics requires breaking down a task into its essential components (task deconstruction) and then tightly defining what differentiates optimal from suboptimal performance. Unfortunately this aspect of surgical performance (and simulation) has been given all too little attention by the surgeon educators, researchers and the simulation industry. Drawing on the example from the MIS community almost all of the VR simulators use time as a metric. Unfortunately time analyzed as an independent variable is at best a crude and at worst a dangerous metric. For example, in the laparoscopic environment being able to tie an intracorporeal knot quickly gives no indication of the quality of the knot. A poorly tied knot can obviously lead to a multitude of complications. The most valuable metrics that can be provided to a trainee are on errors. The whole point of training is to improve performance, make performance consistent and reduce errors. One of the major values of simulators is that they allow the trainee to make mistakes in a consequence-free environment, before they ever perform that procedure on a patient.

Successful metric development is deceptively simple but crucially depends on the appropriate and clear *identification* of what is to be measured and then carefully *defining* those behaviors in a manner that facilitates their reliable *measurement.*

Metric Identification; Task Analysis

Identifying what it is that you want to measure is often obvious and straightforward, i.e., 'measure surgical performance'. However, the role of what is to be measured should be specified as clearly as possible. For example, you want to measure technical skill during the performance of laparoscopic cholecystectomy. It may also be necessary to identify the context in which you wish to measure the behavior such as surgical trainee learning to perform the procedure or a very experienced consultant surgeon learning to perform the procedure. Very different knowledge sets would be expected from both surgeons and this will impact on the metrics generated to measure their performance. For example, it would be expected that a consultant surgeon was very familiar with the standard operating room setup and the services that they might expect as part of standard operating practices. However, we would also expect that they are less familiar with the operation specific setup of the procedures they are learning. These are just guidelines to help identify behaviors which are to be measured and should not be taken to imply that measurement systems will be different for the same procedure depending on the experience of the surgeon undergoing assessment. They will not.

It is sometimes the case that a behavior which is to be measured is easily identified, e.g., checking that the correct limb on the correct patient is being operated on. However, in many cases, the goal of the program is to develop a set of measurements for a more complex group of behaviors such as those enacted during the laparoscopic cholecystectomy. Analyzing a more complex set of behaviors is facilitated by a process referred to as task analysis. Task analysis is a way of proceeding from the general goal of the program (i.e., measuring surgical performance during a laparoscopic cholecystectomy) to a small number of fairly concrete behaviors. The purpose of task analysis is to identify the specific behaviors required in the performance of a particular surgical procedure and to break down or divide a complex sequence of behaviors into component parts. The initial component of task analysis is to identify the behaviors that are to be measured. This is probably easiest to achieve by observing individuals who are performing the task well and, if possible, observing individual's whose performance of the task is less optimal, e.g., a consultant surgeon and a junior trainee surgeon. The reason we have chosen such extreme comparisons is that this highlights differences in performance parameters and brings to the fore the performance characteristics that are probably most productive to try and measure. What we are seeking to identify is what it is that very experienced surgeons do well and what is it that trainees do badly and that clearly distinguishes the two groups most clearly. It is probably easiest if these performances are video and audio recorded for the task analysis. This means that the same procedure can be viewed repeatedly, thus allowing the task analysis team to develop valuable insights into subtle aspects of procedure performance. It is also valuable if the subject expert, e.g., a consultant surgeon experienced in performing the procedure, is included in the task analysis team. This person should be proficient in performing the procedure but not necessarily an expert. It is more important that they are experienced in training less experienced surgeons to perform the procedure and under ideal circumstances that the video tapes that are being used for the task analysis should be of them performing the procedure or them supervising a trainee performing the procedure. The task analysis group should probably contain more than one such subject expert. Other selection criteria for these individuals might include; (1) they all speak the same language, (2) have relatively good group social skills (not too argumentative, opinionated or shy), (3) are able to genuinely participate in a group discussion and then come to a consensus decision that does not necessarily represent 100% of their opinion. This may sound relatively easy to achieve, but in our experience it is not straightforward. Caution is advised when including very senior or expert members within the group, as their opinions and views may dominate discussion. In our experience this has *always* been counter-productive. Although this is not a therapy group, members will be focusing on procedures which are very familiar to them but they will be looking at the procedure from a perspective which is very novel to them. The product of this group should be performance metrics that represent the views and understanding of surgeons who are experienced in teaching and in the performance of the procedure, not the views of the most senior member of the group or the person who shouts the loudest. An optimal number of procedure experts is about three or five plus the task analysis expert (i.e., the psychologist or behavioral scientist). The task analysis expert must genuinely be comfortable with the process of unambiguous definition of performance characteristics in terms of observable events, as less concretely defined behaviors are almost impossible to measure reliably. They should also be mindful that the outcome of this part of the process is highly predictive of success of the overall project and that the time taken to identify key performance indicators of the operation should be viewed as discrete (unlike psychotherapy). One of the benefits of this process is to help experienced practitioners identify the core (observable) features of safe operative performance rather than operating style or individual preferences that are epiphenomenal to the surgical procedure. Many of the groups that we had taken through this process have found it to be very enlightening and one that has significantly informed their teaching and training style. Another important point of note is that once a group of surgeons have successfully gone through this process (all the way to defining and then actually measuring operative performance) they find it significantly easier to do it the second time. They are more observant when viewing video recordings, parsimonious in their identification of units of performance and where they fit into chains of behavior and then units of assessment. The metric development process usually takes a fraction of the time to complete the second time around, but the group can still be prone to focusing on 'red herrings'.

The behaviors that are identified are a critical feature of the task analysis and it is important that the units of behavior that this group identifies are discrete and observable. This aspect of the task analysis may be difficult because there are no firm rules for dividing behaviors or for establishing the units that constitute meaningful measurable components. Measurement may require smaller or larger units of behavior, depending on the surgical task that is being assessed, over what period of time it is being assessed and the criticality of performance parameters to be measured. Along with the identification of specific performance characteristics to be measured the order or sequence of these behaviors also needs to be specified. This needs to be given due consideration for each surgical procedure being studied as the order in which the procedure progresses may be critical or of relatively minor importance. For example, in laparoscopic cholecystectomy, some surgeons expose the cystic duct and cystic artery, then apply the clips and only then do they dissect the structures. However, other surgeons expose the cystic structures, clip and they dissect each structure separately. Do these differences in surgical practice really affect the outcome of the procedure? Probably not; but it is important that all of these actions are completed during a particular stage of the surgical procedure in a performance unit which is properly sequenced in the operation and should be scored as such. This issue is relatively straightforward, but as the application of metrics to the measurement of surgical performance is relatively new it is highly probable that discussions around similar procedural aspects of surgery will be frequent. These discussions are important as are the decisions arrived at by the task analysis team.

One of the difficult parts of this process for the practising surgeon who performs and trains others for the procedure in question is that their skills have become automated, i.e., their surgical and to some extent also their teaching skills. They perform the tasks well without having to think too much about the fine detail of what it is they are doing. However, if they are asked to review the performance of another surgeon (or even themselves), they are almost always able to indicate what was performed well and what was performed badly. These are the units of behavior that the team should strive to identify. In general, these performance characteristics will include things that the surgeon really should not have done and things that have been done, but possibly they could have been done better. The goal of the task analysis team should be to identify crucial aspects of performance that contribute both to optimal and sub-optimal performance taking account of the tasks that a surgeon does or does not do. This task is made easier by viewing the video recordings in a group setting, verbalizing and discussing what it is that they see that they consider has been done well or was a sub-optimal performance. This helps to generate a shortlist of performance characteristics that might typify good candidates for metric definition. Good candidates for progression into the metric definition process invariably survive the group discussion process and the reason why they are important behaviors in the performance of the surgical procedure have usually also been elucidated as part of the discussion. It is also important at this stage that the performance characteristics that have been identified by the group are translated into concrete and specific behaviors so as to facilitate their definition. Frequently, practising surgeons who train other surgeons have forgotten that they know this information. Many surgeons have described their participation in the task analysis team 'as if they had to take a step back from the performance of the procedure to think about precisely what it is they do or train others to do and why they do it in the way that they do it'. They must then verbalize this process. The person who leads or chairs the entire process often does not have the expertise needed to identify the desired behaviors for task analysis. Indeed, it is an asset that this person is not an expert in the performance of the procedure. However, it is important that they are an expert (usually of a psychologist or a behavioral scientist) in the process of task analysis which lies within the domain. The task of this person is to translate into concrete steps and discrete units of behavior the larger goals that the surgical team have identified. One of the difficulties of a task analysis has to do with the degree of specificity of individual behavior and with the units or amount of behavior that one step should include. For some surgical procedures, many small units of behavior may be grouped into one step, e.g., laparoscopic cholecystectomy grouped into (1) exposure of the cystic structures, (2) clipping and dissection of the cystic duct and artery and (3) dissection of the gallbladder from the liver bed (Ahlberg et al. 2007). For other surgical procedures, e.g., Nissen Fundoplication, many more smaller steps need to be delineated and scored separately (Van Sickle et al. 2008). There are no firm guidelines for delineating the number of steps, but it is likely that the decision will be based on the complexity of the surgical procedure, the operative risk posed by the part of the procedure being assessed and how long it takes to perform that part of the procedure. The effectiveness of metric-based assessment of operative performance depends on identifying specific behaviors so that they can be reliably assessed. The initial task is careful identification and specification of behaviors that are to be measured. The significance of this task should not be underestimated because it is the first step in the process of metric development. The second step is to define the behaviors that have been identified in the task analysis.

Metric Definition

Task analysis identifies the units of behavior that constitute the procedure or part of the surgical procedure to be assessed. Each behavior must then be carefully defined. It is insufficient to describe these behaviors in general terms such as inappropriate, inadvertent, minimal or competent. Definitions of behaviors that make up such general labels may be understood in idiosyncratic terms even among members of the task analysis group. The target behaviors to be measured have to be defined explicitly so that they can actually be observed, measured and agreed upon by individuals doing the assessment. It is insufficient for members of the task analysis team to agree in general terms the definitions of the performance characteristics to be measured. Definitions must be fully and clearly defined and expressed in such a way to minimize vagueness and to facilitate codification. These definitions must also be articulated in such a way that the behaviors can be observed. The definitions should also be as objective as possible so that when the definitions are tested by independent observers the results are reproducible in a reliable fashion.

An initial task of scientific research in general is to identify the construct, domain or focus of interest and then to translate this into measurable operations. Abstract notions such as 'efficiency', 'economy' and 'unnecessary' must be operationalized, that is, made into operational definitions. Operational definitions refer to defining the concept on the basis of the specific operations used for assessment. These definitions will almost certainly be derived from observations of the video recorded surgical procedures and from the personal experience of the procedure experts. Great emphasis should be placed on observation of performance, because overt performance is the most direct and reliable source of information on the surgical performance characteristics to be measured. Operational definitions are essential in the process of objective assessment of surgical skills. However, it should be recognized that operational definitions are limited. In defining an abstract construct such as 'skill' an operational definition does not capture all of the domain of interest. Overall, performance characteristics are simply the observable motor end of a chain of sensory, perceptual and cognitive behaviors, which although not directly observable contribute significantly to skilled performance. An operational definition is best construed as a working definition which ideally reflects central features of the abstract notions such as 'skilled' performance. However, limitations imposed by precise operational definitions are not corrected by the use of vague descriptions of performance characteristics that rely on the implicit knowledge by the observers conducting the assessment.

In general, operational definitions should meet three criteria, i.e., objectivity, clarity and completeness (Kazdin 1994). To be objective, the definitions should refer to observable characteristics of behavior or environmental events. For example, the surgeon wants to use the electrocautery (the observable event is the surgeon asking for electrocautery to be switched to coagulate (or dissect) or an audible hum from the machine working in the background). Another example might be where the surgeon asks for electrocautery to be switched on and proceeds to use it to divide tissues. To be clear, the definition should be so unambiguous that it can be read, repeated and paraphrased by observers. The definition should not require or rely on implicit knowledge or inference from the person conducting the assessment. To be complete, the definition must delineate the boundary conditions so that it is clear when their behavior occurred or did not occur and so it can be scored as such.

Developing a complete definition often creates the greatest difficulty, because decision rules are needed to specify how behavior should be scored. If the range of performance characteristics included in the definition are not described carefully, observers have to infer whether a response occurred or not. In the electrocautery example given above, an operational definition which only included asking the nurse or the assistant to switch on the machine would have been incomplete. The operating surgeon could have communicated what to do to one of them by means of non-verbal gestures. By including the hum of the electrocautery machine in the operational definition this auditory information allows performance to be scored. One of the tips when generating operational definitions is to try and generate situations which occur with reasonable (but low) frequency where the definition would not work and then modify the operational definition so that it covers this potential situation. Operational definitions cannot cover every eventuality but they can give very clear guidance on how these eventualities should be dealt with and scored. Although global and imprecise terms such as ‘inappropriate’, ‘minimal’, ‘obvious’ and ‘competent’ appear attractive in these situations, their lack of clarity and objectivity render them almost useless in this situation. They rely on implicit understandings which cannot be relied on. Generating operational definitions which meet the criteria of objectivity, charity and completeness is no small task. There may even be general agreement in the group about a certain aspect of performance which everyone agrees is important, but may fail to generate an agreed upon operational definition. Although not frequent, this situation does occur. However, without a good working operational definition performance cannot be scored reliably and unless some agreed upon solution is found to this situation the performance characteristics should be excluded from the assessment process. It should also be noted that we never fail to be impressed by the innovation shown by task analysis groups when confronted with this situation.

One example occurred during the task analysis and error definition phase of the Yale VR to OR study (Seymour et al. 2002). During the review of the videotapes it was clear that there were certain instances when the surgeon had both surgical instruments in the patient's abdomen but they were not really doing much with them. Everyone agreed that what was being observed was inefficient use of operating time; however, no clear rule or set of rules emerged that encapsulated all of the observed eventualities. The operational definition that eventually emerged was 'lack of progress'. Immaterial of what the operating surgeon was doing, they were scored as failing to make progress if they had both surgical instruments in the patient's abdomen and achieved absolutely nothing during any 60 s periods of time (which were assessed from other performance characteristics as well). This operational definition encapsulated what other assessments referred to as 'inefficiency' but requires no implicit understanding of what this term means. Indeed, the operational definition of this aspect of performance has been so successful that this has been included in some form in most of the studies objectively assessing surgical performance by direct observation. Specifying behavior and performance characteristics in these terms is a skill and must be learned and practised. What we find particularly attractive about this approach is its objectivity, transparency and replicability.

Metric Assessment

When behavior has been defined in precise terms, assessment can begin. It may be tempting to rely on using the judgment or a general impression rather than an objective assessment to evaluate how an individual has performed during a particular surgical procedure. However, the judgment sometimes does not correspond to the actual objective records of performance. Judgments about performance can be influenced by many factors other than the performance itself. Assessments can be influenced by such factors as attractiveness (Byrne 1961), familiarity (Perloff 2008) or even at what point during the day the assessment is being conducted. Direct observations are designed to reveal more directly than global impressions or ratings of the level, degree or amount of behavior emitted by the person being assessed. Observing behavior has its own obstacles, sources of bias and pitfalls. Despite the efforts that are made in the identification and operational definition of behavior, observations of behavior are not entirely free from human judgment. Typically, observers must record or judge the occurrence or non-occurrence of behaviors in an environment where many other things are ongoing. However, overt behavior is a direct measure of what the person is actually doing or performing and so provides a very useful basis for understanding what that person can actually do under particular circumstances, i.e., can they suture a wound, can they perform a laparoscopic cholecystectomy. There may be arguments about the adequacy of what someone does reflecting what they know. However, in surgery, what they know has been more than adequately assessed for some considerable period. The concern here is being able to assess what they can actually do since knowing how to do something is not the same as actually being able to do it.

Metrics Assessment Strategies

Success or failure of an assessment strategy crucially depends on how well the performance characteristics of interest have been identified and operationally defined. In most objective assessment programs, performance characteristics are assessed on the basis of discrete occurrences of those behaviors or the amount of time that they occurred.

Frequency Measures Assessment Strategy

Frequency counts simply require tallying the number of times a particular behavior occurs during a given period of time, e.g., how many surgical clips did the trainee apply? A frequency measure is particularly useful when the target response is discreet and when it takes a relatively constant amount of time, each time it is performed. A discreet response has a clearly delineated beginning and a clearly delineated end, so that separate instances of it occurring can be counted. The amount of time taken to perform the behavior, i.e., wound clipping, should be relatively constant so that the units counted are approximately equal. Ongoing behaviors such as the use of electrocautery, cleaning a wound whilst suturing or receiving verbal instructions on how to perform or modify performance of the procedure are difficult to record simply by counting because each response may occur for a different amount of time or occurs frequently or sporadically. For example, if a trainee is given instructions for 10 s on one occasion and then for 20 s on another occasion; should this be scored as one or two units on the second occasion? Having chosen to use a frequency assessment strategy means that in this instance, considerable information is lost about the duration of a particular performance characteristic, such as receiving instructions. Frequency assessment is a particularly good strategy when dealing with the discrete units of behavior such as suturing, clipping etc. Frequency measures simply require noting the instances in which the behavior occurred. It is also helpful if the behavior being assessed occurred at a constant period of time. Unfortunately, surgical procedures tend to vary considerably in the amount of time taken to complete them. If a trainee's performance is assessed during a procedure that takes 20 min one day and then they are assessed the next day on an equivalent procedure which takes 30 min, these performances are not directly comparable. However, the rate of response each day can be determined by dividing the frequency with which a behavior occurred by the number of minutes it took to complete each procedure. This measure will give a frequency of response or rate of responding which is comparable for different procedure durations. For example, a trainee is working in the accident and emergency and on Monday they close a scalp wound with four sutures in 10 min. On the Tuesday, they close another scalp wound with seven sutures in 15 min. This means that the rate of response for Monday was 2.5 sutures (i.e., 10/4) per minute and for Tuesday was 2.14 (15/7) per minute.

A frequency-based assessment strategy has several attractive features for use in surgical settings. First, frequency measures are relatively simple to score. Keeping a count of behavior is usually all that is required. Second, frequency measures readily reflect changes over time, and so are particularly useful when assessing the rate of a trainee's learning. Third, frequency measures give a direct measure of the *amount* of performance. Frequency measures are particularly useful when they are being scored automatically, such as in an online learning program or on a virtual reality simulator. In both of these situations, the measures of actual performance are fairly reliable. In Chap. 9, we will discuss how metrics should be applied to e-learning programs and would consider that measures of frequency are probably one of the easiest measures to implement.

Discrete Categories Assessment Strategy

Often it is very useful to classify performance into discrete categories such as correct/incorrect or performed/not performed. Statisticians refer to this type of categorization as a 'dummy variable'. In many ways, discrete categorization is like a frequency measure because it is used for behaviors that have a clear beginning and end and a constant duration. However, there are at least two important differences. The first difference is that with a frequency measure, performances of a particular behavior are tallied and the focus is on a single aspect of performance or behavior. Furthermore, the number of times that the behavior may occur is theoretically unlimited, e.g., the number of times the surgeon may swab a wound clean whilst they are suturing it. Discrete categorization is used to measure whether several different behaviors have occurred or not. There are only a limited number of opportunities to perform the response. For example, discrete gradations might be used to measure how a trainee performed during a simple suturing or closing a wound on a real patient. A checklist could be devised that lists several performance characteristics that are indicative of proficient suturing performance, e.g., choosing the correct suture material, the number of sutures per inch of the wound, sutures spaced equally apart, all knots on the same side of the wound, air knots, wound puckering, etc. The total number of behaviors or steps that have been performed correctly constitute the measure. Discrete categorization is a particularly useful strategy for the assessment of learning. It is also very easy to use because it requires listing a number of behaviors or performance characteristics and checking whether they were performed or not. These scores can be independent, as in the suturing example we have just given or they could be interlinked, such as in the steps of a surgical procedure such as laparoscopic cholecystectomy. Discrete categorization can yield convenient summary scores such as the total number of correct steps in a surgical procedure, or the percentage or proportion of proficient performance characteristics present in suturing performance. Overall, discrete categorization is a very flexible method of observation that allows assessment of all sorts of behaviors irrelevant of whether they are related or independent from each other. Some critics may argue that some units of performance are more critical or more important than others. We agree with this position, but this type of assessment offers a more reliable and replicable assessment strategy working from a clearly defined operational definition, rather than subjective appraisal of the importance or unimportance of a particular unit of behavior. Furthermore, it helps to limit much of the response variability that can occur with frequency assessment strategies, which may disguise important within-subject or between-subject differences.

Interval Recording Assessment Strategy

Performance characteristics are usually measured by observation for a single block of time such as an entire surgical procedure or for a clearly defined part of a surgical procedure. This block of time can be fixed, such as for 10 minute blocks during the suturing and closure of a wound or it could be for part of or an entire surgical procedure. The block of time is then divided into a series of short intervals. During each interval, the target behavior or performance characteristic is scored as having occurred or not having occurred. If a discrete behavior such as the application of electrocautrey occurred during a 15 s interval it is scored as having occurred. If it occurs four times within the same 15 s period it is scored only once. Equally, if electrocautrey is only applied for a brief but perceptible period of time during that 15 s period, it is also scored as having occurred. If the behavior is ongoing with no clear beginning or end, such as in the use of electrocautrey for dissection of the gallbladder from the liver bed, or it occurs for a long period of time, it is scored during each of the intervals in which it has occurred.

Interval scoring of behavior or performance characteristics is facilitated by a scoring sheet on which intervals are represented across time and an example is presented in Table 5.1. In Chap. 6 we will discuss this type of assessment strategy in greater detail. During each eligible interval a '0' or a '1' is recorded to indicate whether the behavior or performance characteristic that is being assessed has occurred or not. In this example, we have scored performance as occurring during each of fourteen, 30 s intervals.

Performance can be recorded for one unit of behavior, or it can be expanded to include multiple units as in the example included here where we have scored three units of behavior. In using an interval scoring system, an observer looks at performance during the interval and when the interval is over, the observer records whether the behavior occurred or not during that interval. If an observer is recording several behaviors that occurred during that interval, a few seconds may be needed to record all of the behaviors observed during that interval. If the observer records a behavior as soon as it occurs, they run the risk of missing other behaviors that occurred in addition to the first behavior that is being scored. This is one of the disadvantages of this type of scoring strategy but it can easily be overcome by video recording performance and by pausing it at the end of each interval to allow for performance scoring. The advantage of time sampling is that it represents observations on performance over a much larger unit of behaviors such as a surgical procedure.

Table 5.1 The number of intervals during which the operating surgeon used electrocautery to dissect tissue, coagulate or when they burned non-target tissue

Unit of behavior	Interval	1	2	3	4	5	6	7	8	9	10	11	12	13	14	Total
1.	Electrocautery dissect	1	1	1	0	0	1	1	1	0	0	0	0	0	0	6
2.	Electrocautery coagulate	0	0	0	1	1	0	0	0	1	1	0	1	1	1	7
3.	Burn non-target tissue	0	1	1	0	0	0	1	0	0	0	0	0	0	0	3

There are a number of features about interval assessment that make it very flexible and easy to use in a wide variety of assessment settings. The first is that interval assessment can be used to record virtually any behavior. It is immaterial whether the behaviors or performance characteristics are discrete, do not vary in duration, are continuous or sporadic, they can be scored as occurring or not occurring during any time period. The second feature of interval assessment that makes it attractive to use is that the results of the assessment are easy to summarize and to communicate. The result is that interval recording can be easily converted into percentages, and then reported to others as behavior occurring as a percentage of the time (intervals) that were assessed. It is probably the easiest and most flexible assessment strategy for new users of this methodology to learn and implement quickly.

Applied Issues in Implementing an Assessment Strategy

Behavior or performance characteristics can usually be assessed in more than one way and no single strategy must be adopted. Also, there are many different measures that can be used to assess behavior or performance characteristics in a given surgical task. The type of assessment strategy used and operational definitions of performance will depend on the behaviors to be assessed and the context in which the assessment is to take place. Live performance assessment in a clinical situation provides less flexibility in the way that the assessment is conducted. However, if it is possible to record performance for subsequent analysis, this gives considerably more leeway to the assessors and facilitates reliability checks. Direct observation of target behavior with live or video recorded performance is the assessment situation that should be the goal. Certain surgical procedures facilitate recording such as laparoscopic or image guided procedures. It is relatively straightforward to capture and record images from these procedures for subsequent analysis. However, image guided procedures represent a minority of surgical practice. Most surgical procedures are still conducted using a traditional open technique. This makes the assessment of traditional open surgical skills in the operating room more challenging, and assessments in settings such as accident and emergency even more challenging due to the sporadic presentation of practical cases. However, these difficulties can be overcome with innovative placement of small imaging devices to capture the surgical performance that is to be assessed. Another possible way of overcoming the assessment problems inherent in these situations is to simulate the scenarios (i.e., accident and emergency or operating room) and to conduct the assessment in the skills laboratory. Anesthetists have been carrying out these types of simulation scenarios for decades; however, they tend to use a less robust assessment methodology (Gaba and DeAnda 1988b)!

Although video recording of operative performance is the assessment strategy of choice because of its usability, check-ability and flexibility, it is not always possible to use this strategy. Some operating rooms may have rules against using these recordings. Some patients and operating room staff may object to being video record and in other situations it may just not be feasible. It is also possible that video recording performance is simply not a feasible option because assessment needs to be conducted there and then with no possibility for subsequent analysis, such as in a high stakes selection assessment (Gallagher et al. 2008). In the assessment of procedural skills in medicine, and particularly in surgery, this is a common occurrence. In this type of situation, there is no alternative other than having performance assessed directly. Assessments are usually completed by placing one or more assessors in a position where they can observe the person being assessed. Occasionally, the assessor may be out of sight behind a one-way mirror in an observation booth adjacent to the operating room or emergency room. If the person being assessed is aware that they are being assessed, this may create a potential problem with this type of assessment. The fact that the person who is being assessed knows they are being assessed may be affected by that fact. This is referred to as a reactivity effect or Hawthorne effect (Landsberger 1968). Assessment is reactive, if the observer's presence alters the behavior of the person being assessed. Several investigators have shown that the presence of an observer may alter behaviors of the person who is being observed (Adair 1984). However, in most cases the effects are temporary, if they occur at all.

This is only one potential source of error. Other potential sources of error originate with the assessor. When observers are first trained to assess behavior, they will probably adhere rigorously to the operational definition. However, over time and after training has finished observers may drift and gradually depart from the original definition. If the criteria that are used for scoring deviate slightly from the original definition, this will influence performance data. To ensure assessors adhere to the original operational definitions periodic retraining, video recording reviews and feedback regarding the accuracy of their scoring during sessions can help minimize assessment drift. Another problem is that assessment bias may originate from expectations that the assessor brings to the assessment situation. They may have certain expectations about how the person being assessed will perform and these expectations may influence the scoring on performance. An added problem is that many of the individuals who are conducting the assessment are more experienced as trainers. Observing performance as a trainer and as an assessor involve two completely different mindsets. What we have frequently observed is that the consultants who are assessing trainees with a training mindset tended to be much more lenient than consultants who are scoring performance with an assessor's mindset. Whilst understandable and commendable, this type of behavior must not be allowed to interfere with an objective assessment programme, particularly if it is for high stakes scenarios such as the continuation of training, selection into higher training or promotion. At the start of a new assessment process, what we tend to do is to remind the consultants that they are conducting an assessment not a training program and that they should score what they see, not what they think the person might be capable of doing on a good day. In general, good operational definitions, careful training of assessors and careful monitoring of assessors performance during the assessment process are usually good protections against biased scoring.

Assessment Reliability

As we have just described, there is always the potential for an unreliable assessment. That is one of the main reasons why it is important for individuals who assess performance to agree on the occurrence or non-occurrence of operationally defined behavior. Inter-observer agreement, inter-rater reliability or reliability of assessment is crucially important. Assessment of performance is only useful when it can be achieved with some consistency. For example, if frequency counts differ greatly depending on who is counting, it will be difficult to know how the person being assessed actually performed. Inconsistent measurement introduces variation into the data that does not accurately represent changes in performance of the person who is being assessed. Large variations or differences between observers is quite worrying and directly impinges on the reliability of the data and the conclusions that can be drawn from them. If these patterns of assessment are present in the data, they need to be elucidated by assessments of the reliability of scoring.

Reliability assessment is also important because it minimizes the opportunity for a bias to creep into the assessment process. Bias may be a result of the assessors definitions or performance drift over time; it could be due to the expectations of the assessor, perhaps because of previous experience with the person being assessed, or it could simply be to do with the time of the day that the performance is being assessed, i.e., a primacy or recency effect (Luchins 1957). One of the easiest ways to check reliability is to have performance assessed by two or more assessors. In this situation it can easily be seen whether the pattern in the data varies as a function of who is doing the assessment or is a genuine reflection of the performance of the person who is being assessed. Agreement between observers provides a simple, efficient and effective check on the consistency of assessments. Reliability checks are also important because they tell us something important about our operational definitions of performance characteristics. Performance may be scored unreliably because the individuals applying the assessment interpret the operational definition differently. This means that the performance characteristic that we wish to assess has not been optimally defined. This important information needs to be known (preferably before assessment proper commences) and once it is known the operational definition can be modified to make it more reliable.

Reliability Assessment: How to Do It

One of the most important aspects in the assessment of performance is to ensure that it is done reliably. At the start of the assessment program we identified in very general terms what it was that we wanted to assess. After viewing video recordings of behaviors or performance characteristics which we wished to assess, we identified a shortlist of reasonable performance measures. We then clearly defined the performance characteristics of the behaviors that we wished to assess. Having agreed on operational definitions the usefulness, reliability and validity of these definitions needs to be assessed before assessment proper begins. It is probably best done by the task analysis group on an ongoing basis particularly for the first procedure from which they have generated metrics. Some surgeons find the process of metric definition very difficult as the process is quite meticulous and some surgeons find the process somewhat pedantic. It is not; it is simply the process of ensuring scientific detail. An assessment process is only as good as the behaviors that have been identified and the definitions have been generated to assess those behaviors.

An easy way to check the reliability of performance definitions is for the group that generated those performance definitions to apply them in the assessment of performance. What we usually do is to get the task analysis group to assess performance on individuals who have been video recorded. We get them to assess video recorded performance independent from their peers. The theory being that this provides the optimal opportunity for reliable performance to occur as it is the individuals doing the scoring who also generated the operational definitions used in the scoring process. Invariably there are disagreements. These occasions are very useful learning events for members of the task analysis team. They very quickly learn the implicit knowledge that each one of them assumes or infers in the definition process. They also realize that if they cannot score the performance reliably the probability that someone reading the definitions for the first time will be able to do so is very low. Indeed, it is at this point that members of the task analysis team embrace the redefinition of the performance characteristic with enthusiasm and with ingenuity or they simply decide to drop the performance characteristic assessment. In many instances dropping the performance characteristic is not really a problem. However, in other instances, the performance characteristic is core to the surgical procedure that failing to generate a reliable and valid operational definition is simply not an option. In Chap. 6 we will describe some very innovative solutions to this problem that some of the teams we have worked with have developed.

Once the definition of performance characteristics have been modified and agreed, training in the application of those assessments is continued with the task analysis group. Toward the latter stages of this training, operational definition changes cease and the emphasis shifts to reliable implementation of those definitions. This training continues with a variety of recordings from different individuals that present with performances that are easy to assess through to performances that are quite difficult to assess. Throughout this entire process the task analysis expert is seeking to identify situations or events when aberrant conditions would lead to a failure in the operational definition to apply, or results that are at odds with what all the other members of the team think. The more detailed the training the less likely this is to occur. Toward the end of this training process the assessors should be subdivided into pairs and their inter-rater reliability checked after each case. Inter-rater reliability (IRR) should always be greater than 80% or IRR $\geq$ 0.8. These training sessions should be conducted as a group (despite the fact that assessment is being conducted in pairs) and all disagreements should be discussed with the group so as to elucidate why the two raters disagreed. Ideally, the two raters should be achieving close to 100% agreement. Toward the end of training reliability assessment of the two raters should become more stringent. The assessors should work independently, without access to one another's scoring sheets and the reliability of their assessments should be checked by an independent person. This independent person who also normally chairs these sessions should be very knowledgeable about how this procedure works. Also, they should not score performance but simply ensure the quality of assessment is maintained and improved where possible.

Inter-rater Reliability Assessment: How It Is Calculated

Inter-observer agreement or inter-rater reliability (IRR) provides an estimate of how consistently behavior or performance is observed and scored. The procedure for estimating inter-rater reliability differs somewhat depending on the assessment method. Agreement for frequency measures requires that two observers simultaneously but independently count the target behaviors during the time set aside for assessment. At the end of the assessment period the frequencies reported by the two assessors are compared to establish if the two assessors recorded the target behavior with equal frequency. A percentage of agreement can be formed to measure the degree with which the two observers agreed in the final counts. To determine the percentage agreement between the two assessors a fraction is formed from the frequency obtained by each observer. Inter-observer agreement or inter-rater reliability is then calculated by dividing the smaller frequency by the larger frequency and multiplying by 100. For example, if during a short surgical procedure one assessor counted the surgeon cleaning the wound with a swab 20 times and the other assessor counted that they cleaned the wound 22 times this would give an inter-rater reliability of 91% (or 20/22 * 100=90.91). Interpretation of this percentage should be cautious. The table indicates that the assessors agreed on the total frequency of the behavior assessed with a 9% margin of error. However, this does not mean that the assessors agreed 91% of the time. Although one of the assessors scored performance as occurring 20 times and the other assessor scored performance as occurring 22 times, there is no way of knowing whether they scored the exact same performance characteristics/behavior. Reliability as assessed here reflects agreement of the total number of behaviors rather than agreement in each specific instance. One of the disadvantages of using a frequency measure in the assessment of behavior is that when the behavior is not operationally defined, a high percentage of agreement for frequency data may still conceal a considerable amount of disagreement, e.g., just like counting apples and oranges and when they are classified as solid

Table 5.2 The number of intervals during which the operating surgeon used electrocautery to dissect tissue, coagulate or when they burned non-target tissue

Units of behaviour	Interval	1		2		3		4		5		6		7		IRR
	Assessor	A	B	A	B	A	B	A	B	A	B	A	B	A	B	
1.	Electrocautery dissect	1	1	1	1	1	1	1	1	0	0	0	1	0	0	0.86
2.	Electrocautery coagulate	0	0	0	1	1	0	0	0	1	1	0	1	1	1	0.57
3.	Burn non-target tissue	1	1	0	0	0	0	0	0	1	1	0	0	0	0	1.00

spherical objects that are fruit and can be eaten. This operational definition fails to include characteristics such as color, taste and texture which considerably limit the interpretation of data generated from observations using this operational definition. Agreement or inter-rater reliability has to achieve an acceptable level before assessment proper can begin. Furthermore, good agreement or high inter-rater reliability should be maintained throughout the assessment process. Although no single criterion for acceptable agreement levels has been set, convention dictates that agreement should be between 80 and 100% (Kazdin 1994).

Calculation of an inter-rater reliability is different for interval methods of assessment. In this type of assessment, inter-rater reliability is calculated on the basis of the proportion of intervals in which the two assessors agreed on the occurrence of assessed behavior. An agreement is scored if both assessors record the occurrence of a particular behavior in the same interval. A disagreement is scored when one of the assessors scores a behavior as occurring in an interval and the other does not. Table 5.2 shows the data from two assessors of one subject's performance on three units of behavior, i.e., electrocautery dissection, electrocautery coagulation and burning non-target tissue. Both assessors agreed that the subject used electrocautery to dissect tissues in intervals 1, 2, 3 and 4. They also agreed that they did not use it during intervals 5 and 7 but disagreed on whether they used it or not during interval 6. IRR is calculated for this behavior by dividing the number of intervals (7 intervals) into the number of agreements (6) and multiply by 100, i.e., $6 \div 7 = 0.86 * 100 = 86\%$. This means that the assessors agreed on performance assessment for 86% of the intervals or IRR = 0.86. There were three intervals when the assessors disagreed on the electrocautery coagulation behavior $4 \div 7 = 0.57 * 100 = 57\%$. This result indicates that the two assessors only agreed on performance assessment for just over 50% of the intervals, which is just slightly better than by chance. If this occurred in a real situation, it would be investigated

Table 5.3 The number of intervals during which the operating surgeon used was assessed as burning non-target tissue by assessors 'A' and 'B'

Interval	1		2		3		4		5		6		7		8		9		10	
Rater	A	B	A	B	A	B	A	B	A	B	A	B	A	B	A	B	A	B	A	B
Burn-non target tissue	1	1	1	1	0	0	1	0	1	0	1	0	1	0	1	0	1	1	1	1

11		12		13		14		15		16		17		18		19		20		21		22		23	
A	B	A	B	A	B	A	B	A	B	A	B	A	B	A	B	A	B	A	B	A	B	A	B	A	B
0	0	0	0	0	0	0	0	0	0	0	0	0	0	0	0	0	0	0	0	0	0	0	0	0	0

21		22		23		24		25		26		27		28		29		30		31		32		33	
A	B	A	B	A	B	A	B	A	B	A	B	A	B	A	B	A	B	A	B	A	B	A	B	A	B
0	0	0	0	0	0	0	0	0	0	0	0	0	0	0	0	0	0	0	0	0	0	0	0	0	0

immediately and an explanation and remedy sought. Both assessors agreed 100% of the intervals on their assessment of burning non-target tissue, which is the ideal (but uncommon) situation. Some researchers may be tempted to take the mean IRR for the three behaviors that were assessed and claim that overall the ≥ IRR 0.8 (actual mean = 0.81) which statistically is correct but methodologically incorrect as it misrepresents how reliable the assessment actually was. We shall discuss this issue in greater detail in Chap. 7.

We can see in Table. 5.3 the assessment data of a subject who was operating using electrocautery. These data show the assessment of their performance by the rater 'A' and rater 'B' for burning non-target tissue with the electrocautery instrument. Most of the instrument usage occurred during the first 10 assessment intervals. The assessors agreed that from interval 11 to interval 33 there was no observed usage of the instrument. However, during the first 10 intervals both assessors agree on four intervals that they did burn non-target tissue (intervals 1, 2, 9 and 10) and that there was no burning during interval 3. They disagreed on an assessment of performance for intervals 4, 5, 6, 7 and 8. The data summary indicates that there were 33 assessed intervals and the assessors disagreed on their assessment for 5 of these. This may indicate that their inter-rater reliability would be, 28 ÷ 33 = IRR 0.85 (or 85% agreement). This would appear satisfactory; however, it is misleading.

This inter-rater reliability is determined by dividing the number of intervals in which both observers marked the behavior as occurring (i.e., agreeing) by the number of agreements *plus* the number of intervals in which one observer scored the behavior as occurring and the other did not (i.e., disagreements). In this example, both assessors agreed that the behavior occurred in four intervals (intervals 1, 2, 9 and 10) but they disagreed on its occurrence in five intervals (intervals 4, 5, 6, 7 and 8). Therefore, the inter-rater reliability formula for these data is $4 \div 9 = 0.44$ (i.e., 44%) which is a much less impressive level of agreement. Although the assessors recorded behavior for 33 intervals, not all of the intervals were used to calculate inter-rater reliability. An interval is counted only if at least one of the assessors records the behavior as occurring. In situations like this, intervals where neither assessor recorded the behavior as occurring are excluded. If these intervals were to be included they would have to be considered as agreements as both observers agreed that the behavior being assessed did not occur. If these intervals were included as agreements, this would grossly inflate the reliability estimates beyond the levels obtained when occurrences alone are counted as agreements. To avoid this situation convention dictates that we restrict counting agreements to response occurrence intervals only. The rule of thumb that we have always used is to only include behavior in the assessment definition process which occurs with 'reasonable' frequency.

This approach to the assessment of inter-rater reliability may seem somewhat strict. The main concern is whether agreement should be restricted to intervals for which either assessor recorded an occurrence of the behavior or should we also include intervals for which both observers agreed on the non-occurrence of the behavior. This is an important issue because the estimate of inter-rater reliability depends on the frequency of the behavior being assessed and on whether occurrence and/or non-occurrence agreements are included in the formulae. If the person being assessed performs that target behavior relatively frequently or relatively infrequently, the assessing surgeons are unlikely to have a high proportion of agreements on occurrences or non-occurrence respectively. Both of these scenarios will have a significant impact on reliability estimates. Kazdin (1994) has discussed this problem and suggested additional formulas for a possible ways of using both occurrence and non-occurrence intervals.

The calculation of inter-rater reliability is no small matter as failure to reach a satisfactory level on a continuous basis during the assessment of performance indicates that there is a problem with the assessment process. Assessments should be transparent, objective and fair. Failure of two assessors to reach a satisfactory level of agreement i.e., 80% or greater on a regular basis, may be due to a problem with operational definition of the behaviors being assessed or of training the individuals to use the assessment. Whatever the source of the problem it needs to be resolved urgently. That is one of the main reasons why we recommend that inter-rater reliability assessments are conducted after each person's assessment has been completed. This means that problems can be identified very quickly and an immediate solution sought. In Chap. 6 we will work through a number of examples of this assessment methodology being implemented in a variety of settings. We will also explain how we have combined the assessment strategies for one assessment program. In Chap. 7 we will return to the issue of assessment reliability and how it is calculated and reported.

Summary

Surgery has always believed in the value of objective assessment of surgical skills. Unfortunately up until the 1990s, operating time was used as a surrogate measure of skill. From that time surgery has pioneered a number of methodologies that purport to objectively assess surgical skills. One of these, OSATS, relies on generic descriptions of performance characteristics, which are rated on a 1–5 point Likert scale. Unfortunately OSATS uses descriptions of performance characteristics that have no uniform and global understanding of their meaning and instead relies on an implicit understanding which is assumed to be shared between surgeons. We suspect that this may lead to problems, e.g., achieving a satisfactory level of inter-rater reliability. OSATS also fails the fundamental test of transparency because it relies on implicit knowledge of the assessor. Other assessment devices such as ICSAD may be able to objectively track and quantify psychomotor performance; however, this information is only useful when it is coupled with contextual information which still requires the objective assessment of surgical skills. ADEPT was devised as a pure assessment device of surgical skills and was never intended as an assessment of clinical skills in vivo. It has never been widely adopted. Simulation, whether it be virtual reality or physical models, still requires the contextual information to define whether the surgical performance that has been recorded is right or wrong. This requires a group of subject experts to perform a task analysis on the surgical skills that are to be assessed. They must then identify the observable features of optimal and sub-optimal performance and then generate an operational definition of what these are so that they are scoreable in an objective, transparent and fair manner. To ensure that this is the case, the group of experts should score video recorded performance to establish the reliability of the assessment process they have devised. Only when they are able to achieve acceptable levels of inter-rater reliability of assessed performance greater than 80% should the assessment process be implemented *in vivo*. Objective assessment of surgical skills be reliable but it should also be transparently seen to should be so.

References

Adair JG. The Hawthorne effect: a reconsideration of the methodological artifact. *J Appl Psychol*. 1984;69(2):334-345.

Ahlberg G, Enochsson L, Gallagher AG, et al. Proficiency-based virtual reality training significantly reduces the error rate for residents during their first 10 laparoscopic cholecystectomies. *Am J Surg*. 2007;193(6):797-804.

Byrne D. Interpersonal attraction and attitude similarity. *J Abnorm Soc Psychol*. 1961;62(3):713-715.

Catania A. *Learning*. Englewood Cliffs: Prentice-Hall; 1984.

Coleman J, Nduka CC, Darzi A. Virtual reality and laparoscopic surgery. *Br J Surg*. 1994;81(12):1709-1711.

Darzi A, Smith S, Taffinder N. Assessing operative skill. *BMJ*. 1999;318(7188):887.

Francis NK, Hanna GB, Cuschieri A. Reliability of the Dundee Endoscopic Psychomotor Tester (DEPT) for dominant hand performance. *Surg Endosc*. 2001;15(7):673-676.

Francis NK, Hanna GB, Cuschieri A. The performance of master surgeons on the Advanced Dundee Endoscopic Psychomotor Tester: contrast validity study. *Arch Surg*. 2002;137(7):841.

Gallagher AG, Satava RM. Virtual reality as a metric for the assessment of laparoscopic psychomotor skills. Learning curves and reliability measures. *Surg Endosc*. 2002;16(12):1746-1752.

Gallagher AG, McClure N, McGuigan J, Crothers I, Browning J. Virtual reality training in laparoscopic surgery: a preliminary assessment of minimally invasive surgical trainer virtual reality (MIST VR). *Endoscopy*. 1999;31(4):310-313.

Gallagher AG, Hughes C, Reinhardt-Rutland AH, McGuigan J, McClure N. A case-control comparison of traditional and virtual-reality training in laparoscopic psychomotor performance. *Minim Invasive Ther Allied Technol*. 2000;9(5):347-352.

Gallagher AG, Richie K, McClure N, McGuigan J. Objective psychomotor skills assessment of experienced, junior, and novice laparoscopists with virtual reality. *World J Surg*. 2001;25(11):1478-1483.

Gallagher AG, Smith CD, Bowers SP, et al. Psychomotor skills assessment in practicing surgeons experienced in performing advanced laparoscopic procedures. *J Am Coll Surg*. 2003;197(3): 479-488.

Gallagher AG, Lederman AB, McGlade K, Satava RM, Smith CD. Discriminative validity of the minimally invasive surgical trainer in virtual reality (MIST-VR) using criteria levels based on expert performance. *Surg Endosc*. 2004;18(4):660-665.

Gallagher AG, Neary P, Gillen P, et al. Novel method for assessment and selection of trainees for higher surgical training in general surgery. *Aust N Z J Surg*. 2008;78(4):282-290.

Gallagher AG, Leonard G, Traynor OJ. Role and feasibility of psychomotor and dexterity testing in selection for surgical training. *Aust N Z J Surg*. 2009;79(3):108-113.

Ghazisaedy M, Adamczyk D, Sandin DJ, Kenyon RV, DeFanti TA. *Ultrasonic calibration of a magnetic tracker in a virtual realityspace. Proceedings of the IEEE Virtual Reality Annual International Symposium (VRAIS 95)*, Research Triangle Park, NC, March 1995.

Gordon R. *Great Medical Disasters*. London: House of Stratus Ltd.; 2001.

Hance J, Aggarwal R, Stanbridge R, et al. Objective assessment of technical skills in cardiac surgery. *Eur J Cardiothorac Surg*. 2005;28(1):157-162.

Hanna GB, Drew T, Clinch P, Hunter B, Cuschieri A. Computer-controlled endoscopic performance assessment system. *Surg Endosc*. 1998;12(7):997-1000.

Jordan JA, Gallagher AG, McGuigan J, McClure N. Randomly alternating image presentation during laparoscopic training leads to faster automation to the "fulcrum effect". *Endoscopy*. 2000;32(4):317-321.

Jordan JA, Gallagher AG, McGuigan J, McClure N. Virtual reality training leads to faster adaptation to the novel psychomotor restrictions encountered by laparoscopic surgeons. *Surg Endosc*. 2001;15(10):1080-1084.

Kazdin AE. *Behavior Modification in Applied Settings*. Pacific Grove: Brooks/Cole Publishing Co.; 1994.

Kohn LT, Corrigan JM, Donaldson MS. *To Err Is Human: Building a Safer Health System*. Washington: National Academy Press; 2000:196-197.

Landsberger HA. *Hawthorne Revisited*. New York: Cornell University Press; 1968.

Larsen CR, Grantcharov T, Aggarwal R, et al. Objective assessment of gynecologic laparoscopic skills using the LapSimGyn virtual reality simulator. *Surg Endosc*. 2006;20(9):1460-1466.

Luchins AS. Primacy-recency in impression formation. In: Hovland CI, ed. *The Order of Presentation in Persuasion*. New Haven: Yale University Press; 1957:33-61.

Martin JA, Regehr G, Reznick R, et al. Objective structured assessment of technical skill (OSATS) for surgical residents. *Br J Surg*. 1997;84(2):273-278.

Meyer K, Applewhite HL, Biocca FA. A survey of position trackers. *Presence: Teleoperators and Virtual Environments*. 1992;1(2):173-200.

Nixon MA, McCallum BC, Fright WR, Price NB. The effects of metals and interfering fields on electromagnetic trackers. *Presence*. 1998;7(2):204-218.

Pearson AM, Gallagher AG, Rosser JC, Satava RM. Evaluation of structured and quantitative training methods for teaching intracorporeal knot tying. *Surg Endosc*. 2002;16(1):130-137.

Perloff RM. *The Dynamics of Persuasion*. New York: Lawrence Erlbaum Associates; 2008.

Raab FH, Blood EB, Steiner TO, Jones HR. Magnetic position and orientation tracking system. *IEEE Trans Aerosp Electron Sys*. 1979;AES-15(5):709-718.

Reber AS, Reber ES. *The Penguin Dictionary of Psychology*. London: Penguin Books; 1985.

Regenbogen SE, Greenberg CC, Studdert DM, Lipsitz SR, Zinner MJ, Gawande AA. Patterns of technical error among surgical malpractice claims: an analysis of strategies to prevent injury to surgical patients. *Ann Surg*. 2007;246(5):705.

Riva G. Applications of virtual environments in medicine. *Methods Inf Med*. 2003;42(5): 524-534.

Satava RM. Virtual reality surgical simulator. The first steps. *Surg Endosc*. 1993;7(3):203-205.

Senate of Surgery. *Response to the General Medical Council Determination on the Bristol Case: Senate Paper 5*. London: The Senate of Surgery of Great Britain and Ireland; 1998.

Seymour NE, Gallagher AG, Roman SA, et al. Virtual reality training improves operating room performance: results of a randomized, double-blinded study. *Ann Surg*. 2002;236(4):458-463; discussion 463-454.

Smith SG, Torkington J, Brown TJ, Taffinder NJ, Darzi A. Motion analysis: a tool for assessing laparoscopic dexterity in the performance of a laboratory-based laparoscopic cholecystectomy. *Surg Endosc*. 2002;16:640-645.

Spencer F. Teaching and measuring surgical techniques: the technical evaluation of competence. *Bull Am Coll Surg*. 1978;63:9-12.

Taffinder N, Sutton C, Fishwick R, McManus I, Darzi A. Validation of virtual reality to teach and assess psychomotor skills in laparoscopic surgery: results from randomised controlled studies using the MIST VR laparoscopic simulator. *Stud Health Technol Inform*. 1998;50:124-130.

Van Sickle K, Ritter EM, Baghai M, et al. Prospective, randomized, double-blind trial of curriculum-based training for intracorporeal suturing and knot tying. *J Am Coll Surg*. 2008;207(4): 560-568.

Wilson MS, Middlebrook A, Sutton C, Stone R, McCloy RF. MIST VR: a virtual reality trainer for laparoscopic surgery assesses performance. *Ann R Coll Surg Engl*. 1997;79(6):403-404.

Chapter 6
Metric-Based Simulation Training

Computer-based simulation has several advantages when compared with conventional methods for surgical training. One major advantage is that the same experience or sequence of events can be replicated repeatedly. This repetition allows the trainee to learn from mistakes in a safe environment. Another benefit which is probably of equal if not more omportance is the objective feedback a trainee can receive. Since everything a trainee "does" on a computer-based simulator is essentially data, all actions can be tracked. In addition to crude measures such as performance time, detailed data such as instrument path length, speed of instrument movement, and the exact location in space of any instrument at any point in time is recorded. While these data alone are meaningless, it can be used by subject matter experts to create a set of very robust and objective performance metrics. A simulator without metrics is really no better than an expensive video game. While the main function of metrics is to provide the trainee with objective and proximate feedback on their performance, they also allow the trainer to objectively assess the progress of the trainee throughout the training process. This allows the trainer to provide formative feedback to aid the trainee in acquiring skill. While providing this formative feedback is currently the most valuable function of objective assessment with simulation, inevitably, simulators will be used for summative assessment. This testing will then be used for processes such as selection and credentialing in the future much like knowledge testing is used now. In order for simulators to be applied to such high-stakes assessment, this will require a much more rigorous set of metrics and currently is still in the experimental phase. When this does come to the fore it is certain the metrics for that simulator must be shown to meet the same psychometric standards of validation as any other psychometric test (Gallagher, Ritter, and Satava 2003).

In Chap 5 we described the formulation of metrics which require breaking down a task into its essential components and then tightly defining what differentiates optimal from suboptimal performance. Unfortunately this aspect of simulation has been given all too little attention by the simulation industry. Drawing on the example from the MIS community, almost all of the VR simulators use execution time as a metric. Unfortunately time analyzed as an independent variable is at best crude

A.G. Gallagher and G.C. O'Sullivan, *Fundamentals of Surgical Simulation*, Improving Medical Outcome - Zero Tolerance,
DOI 10.1007/978-0-85729-763-1_6,

and at worst a dangerous metric. If performance is considered as a function of time and quality, the relationship can be represented by the following equation:

$$\text{Performance} \sim \frac{\text{Quality}}{\text{Time}}$$

Thus performance is directly proportional to quality and inversely proportional to time. With this relationship, if quality is held constant and time decreases, then performance is improved. Conversely, if a large increase in quality is gained from a minimal increase in time, performance is still improved despite the longer execution time. While this is obviously an oversimplified relationship, it serves to illustrate the importance that if time is to be used as a metric, some metrics to assess quality must also be included. For example, in the MIS environment, being able to tie an intracorporeal knot quickly gives no indication of the quality of the knot. A poorly tied knot can obviously lead to a multitude of complications. There are only a few reports in the literature that use objective quality analysis due to the difficulty in acquiring this type of information, but this type of information is greatly facilitated in the computer-based environment.

The most valuable metrics that a simulation can provide is identification of errors. The whole point of training is to improve performance, make performance consistent and to reduce errors. Simulation designers must take great care to create error metrics that both train safe behavior as well as not allow unsafe behavior. As mentioned previously one of the major benefits of simulation is that trainees are allowed to make mistakes in a consequence-free environment, before they ever perform that procedure on a patient. However, if a simulator allows a trainee to perform an unsafe manoeuvre without identifying it as an error, dangerous behaviors can be trained, possibly becoming difficult to untrain later. Thus, omitting important error metrics and allowing unsafe behavior must be avoided, and this requires close collaboration with procedure content experts who are also familiar with simulation. The end result of a good simulator with well-designed metrics is a training system where trainees can learn both what TO do and what NOT to do when operating on patients. In the didactic part of the curriculum, the student must be taught exactly what the error is and then should be tested to insure that they are able to identify when they make an error, before starting on the simulator. The errors must be quantified so as to be completely unambiguous. Without robust metrics the simulator is at best an expensive video game and at worst an adverse outcome waiting to happen.

Development of Metrics

LC Metrics: Identification

Surgical training should achieve a number of goals. Obviously it should bring about an improvement in performance. However, it should also lead to more consistent performance and specifically related to surgery it should also lead to a reduction in errors. On the first occasion that metrics were developed for study the researchers

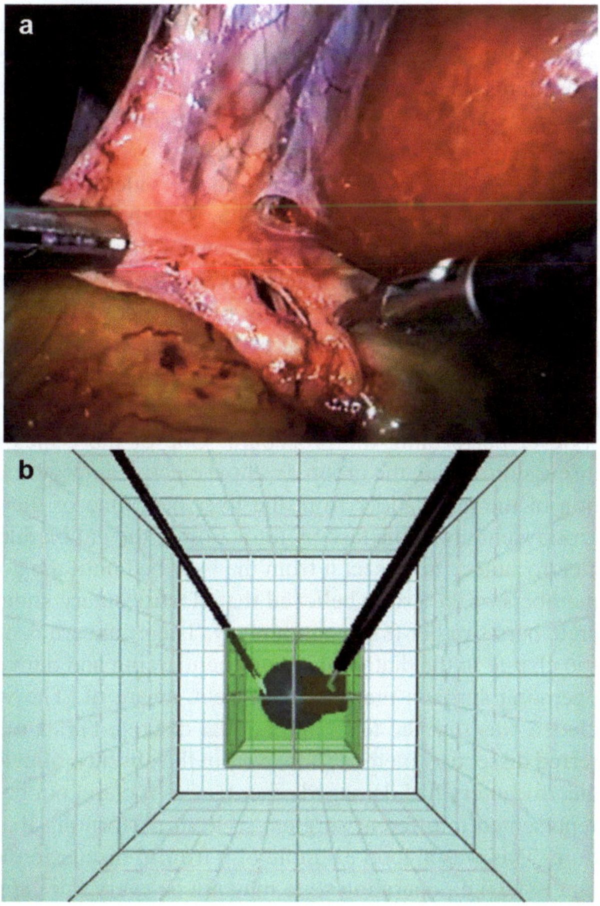

Fig. 6.1 (**a**, **b**) Surgical diathermy of the gallbladder from the liver bed during a LC and task 6 on the MIST VR trainer used in the first VR to OR clinical trial. MIST VR screen appearance on "Manipulate and Diathermy" task. The sphere, which must be precisely positioned within a virtual cube, presents a target for the L-hook electrosurgery instrument. Objects may be positioned anywhere within the defined operating space

were specifically interested in errors not least because of how central this theme should be to medical education and training (Seymour et al. 2002). The specific procedure that they were interested in was laparoscopic cholecystectomy (LC) because of how commonly it is practiced. The researchers wanted to measure how much transfer of training there was from training in a virtual environment to the real world. They focused on LC and in particular one part of the LC that is approached with a reasonably common methodology by most surgeons, i.e., diathermy of the gallbladder from the liver bed. Another advantage of choosing this part of the procedure is that it has a clear beginning and an end (removal of the gallbladder). This is one of the important pre-requisites for the implementation of a metric-based program. This part of the procedure also involves sophisticated two-handed coordination of surgical instruments, retraction of the gallbladder and the application of diathermy to the correct tissue plane. The researchers also chose this part of the operation because it bears striking resemblance to task 6 (Manipulate and diathermy) on the MIST VR system and therefore an appropriate simulation task already existed which could be used to train the required technical skills to perform the procedure (Fig. 6.1a, b).

All LC that were performed by the VR to OR investigating team were video recorded for subsequent analysis. The video recordings consisted of LC surgical procedures that they themselves had performed or were performed by a surgeon in training whom they were proctoring/mentoring. There then followed a period of unfettered viewing of these tapes by the group. The group were asked to identify what surgical behavior they saw on the video recordings that represented optimal performance and what behavior they saw that represented less than optimal performance. During subsequent discussions of these observations they were also asked to recount performance characteristics that they had previously observed during an LC which were not observed in any of the recordings that were being reviewed. All potential measures of surgical performance were then collated and discussed extensively. The discussion centered around issues such as whether an observed performance characteristic was an error or not and whether it just represented a different style of performing the procedure. One of the issues that generated considerable discussion among the group was how electrocautery should be applied for the dissection of the gallbladder from the liver bed. One of the very senior surgeons in the group went about the task by retraction of the gallbladder and then using continuous electrocautery to dissect it from the liver bed until the goal had been achieved. Other members of the group believed that electrocautery should have been applied in discrete bursts rather than continuously. Their concern centered on the risk of the electric charge in the diathermy instrument arcing and damaging other tissues which the operating surgeon may not have been aware of. The way that this issue was concluded was that the team agreed that discrete bursts of electrocautery was the preferred dissection method; however, in the absence of evidence that continuous use of electrocautery had damaged other tissues it could not be scored as an error. It simply represented a different surgical style of performing that part of the surgical procedure. This was a good example of a fruitful discussion which centered on an important issue, i.e., operating style may not be every ones approach of choice but it is not necessarily wrong either and only the outcome of that approach should be scored as an error or not, depending on what actually happens, not what might happen. The latter issue will be returned to in the discussion of 'attending takeover' metric definition. As the definition of metrics currently stands the researchers were primarily interested in scoring the outcome of performance and did not focus on operating style; however, the possibility of this happening in the future cannot be precluded. It is probable that as the focus on surgical outcomes moves away from the operating procedure and their outcomes to specific intra-operative techniques it is highly probable that many surgical procedures may move to standard operating procedures (SOPs) just as in other high-skills industries. This would necessitate a move away from 'how I do it' type of practice to 'this is the way it should be done from best practice principles'. Indeed, it is also highly probable that the techniques for SOPs may be worked out on high-fidelity virtual reality simulations rather than on patients and not simply focus on patient outcomes but also on time taken to perform the procedure, costs of instrumentation and disposables used during the performance of the procedure. These questions will almost certainly impact on who or how many surgeons can be trained during surgical procedures since it is now well established that training a junior surgeon during a operation has considerable time implications for the completion of the case (Wilson et al. 2010).

LC Metrics: Operational Definition Development Issues

From the list of performance characteristics a number of potential measures were put forward as prime candidates to be included in our measurement protocol. These were gallbladder injury, liver injury, dissection on the incorrect tissue plane, burning non-target tissue with the electrocautery instrument and tearing or ripping through tissues rather than burning through them. Although other surgical events were discussed, it was concluded that they occurred so infrequently that it would not be reasonable to include them as events in the study. Discussion did centre around a number of other issues, one of which concerned performance etiquette with the electrocautery instrument. As indicated in our previous discussion about how the electrocautery instrument should be used to dissect the gallbladder from the liver bed the concern was primarily about safety. This issue emerged again when viewing a number of other video recordings when it was observed that some of the surgeons were using the electrocautery instrument without being able to clearly visualize what they were doing. After some discussion it was concluded that observers could not tell whether the electrocautery instrument had a charge running through it are not, but it was safer to assume that it had unless there was convincing evidence to the contrary. It was at this point that the investigators included 'instrument out of view' as a metric error.

Defining Operating Efficiency

There was also considerable discussion around the issue of operating efficiency. The team were aware of the consensus among many in the surgical community that efficiency of operating was probably a good indicator of the skill of the surgeon. However, they were uncomfortable with how efficiency had been operationalized in other assessment protocols such as OSATS (Martin et al. 1997). In the OSATS Likert-scale descriptions, they had one assessment variable which purported to measure 'time and motion'. The anchoring descriptors included 'many unnecessary moves', 'efficient time and motion but some unnecessary moves' and 'economy of movement and maximum efficiency'. The problem that the team had with this whole issue was that they agreed with the concept, but disagreed with how it had been operationalized. They found it difficult to conceptualize how a consensus could be reached on what might be classified as 'unnecessary'. For example, how frequently had the operating surgeons to do something before it was classified as unnecessary and could the observers (and by implication the assessors) be sure that the surgeon was performing an action that for them was goal directed but for the observer the goal was unclear. Another difficulty that the team had was how to operationally define concepts such as 'efficient time and motion'. They could certainly have developed quantitative ratios to operationally define this concept; however, this would almost certainly have been meaningless to the general population of surgeons who would have been conducting the assessment. It would also have been quantitatively meaningless unless it was known what the population mean and standard deviation time and motion performance characteristics were for performing those precise manoeuvres during a laparoscopic cholecystectomy. Lastly, the team was concerned that although they as a group knew what they meant when they talked about economy of movement; they were not sure that they could communicate these ideas in such a way that they could be as well understood and reliably identified by someone hearing about the concept for the first time. This is an important issue as replicability is a cornerstone of the scientific method.

In the computerized environment, concepts such as economy can be operationally defined and these definitions can be applied to measure surgical performance. For example, MIST VR has the facility to measure *Economy of movement* by each surgical instrument for each hand, separately. This metric is relatively straightforward to generate as the computer can easily measure the optimal distance the instrument needed to travel from its start to the target, as well as the actual distance travelled, and therefore any excess distance travelled is a measure of economy of movement. However, whether that metric is meaningful or a reliable measure is a different but important matter. Despite the fact that computer tracked performance on MIST VR can be applied consistently using precisely the same assessment formulae for different individuals, there can still be assessment problems. For example, Gallagher et al. (2001) and Gallagher and Satava (2002) investigated the psychometric properties of MIST VR assessment metrics. In both studies it was found that the MIST VR metrics (time, errors, economy of (instrument) movement and economy of diathermy) distinguished between experts. It was also found that the internal reliability of these metrics was high (range 0.9–0.98). These are fundamental benchmarks in the appraisal of any psychometric assessment device. However, only the measurements of time to perform the task, the number of errors enacted and economy of diathermy demonstrated a sufficiently high test–retest reliability measure. The test–retest reliability measures for economy of movement were 0.5–0.7. These parameters indicate that the performance characteristic called economy of movement was not being sufficiently and reliably assessed between assessment trials. The majority of surgeons would probably agree that they can recognize a surgeon who is using laparoscopic instruments inefficiently. While this shared wisdom may be the starting point for attempts to measure an important aspect of surgical performance, inability to provide an operational definition which can be scored reliably renders this performance metric of limited usefulness. Metrics, whether they are scored by a computer or by an individual, must reach the same psychometric benchmarks of reliability and validity. It is unclear why these metrics were found to be unreliably associated with MIST VR performance but the fact is that this was found and reported in the scientific literature meant that this metric could not be used in the VR to OR clinical trial. An important lesson that should probably be taken from this example is that if a computer cannot score a well-defined performance characteristic reliably it is highly probable that this same task will pose even greater difficulties for human scorers.

The VR to OR team were all aware of the scientific findings and the importance of published research on the economy of movement as discussed above. These findings were not just from the data generated by virtual reality simulators, but also from assessment devices such as ICSAD (Smith et al. 2002) which we have discussed in Chap 5. It had been shown in a number of studies using ICSAD that experienced surgeons showed more efficient movements than their less senior colleagues (Datta et al. 2002). The problem for the VR to OR team was that they could not use a device such as ICSAD in the operating room because of its unreliability close to metal which would conduct the signal, but more importantly, because it would also be too intrusive. Despite extensive discussions and numerous definitions of what economy of the instrument usage or economy of instrument movement meant no satisfactory definition could be reached. By satisfactory we mean that the definitions that were generated by the VR to OR team would need to work easily when applied to common surgical events during a LC. However, what the team found was that the definitions simply did not encapsulate what they wanted to measure despite the fact that the entire team agreed that in many of the video recordings there were good examples of inefficient performance. There was some discussion about the 'purposefulness' of this period of inactivity by the operating surgeon. At this point it was decided by the group that no measure would be used that would involve any inferences about behavior that were not directly observable.

The stalemate was broken when the team started to describe what it was they saw that indicated to them that the operating surgeon was behaving in an inefficient manner. These types of comments included, "he stood there and did nothing" and "I'm not sure what she was doing during that time but I didn't see much sign of activity". Out of this discussion came performance characteristics that were scorable . The performance characteristic of the metric that was identified was 'lack of progress'. By this it was meant that the surgeon had both surgical instruments inside the patient's abdomen but was making no progress toward completion of the surgical procedure. They might have had the instruments in the patient's abdomen but not in contact with tissues; they might have been grasping tissues with one instrument and touching or prodding tissues with the other instrument but did not appear to be doing anything that would get them closer to dissection of the gallbladder from the liver bed. Furthermore, 'lack of progress' was only scored if they achieved absolutely nothing within a 60 s period of time. This was a very liberal criterion, which meant that if they performed any correct surgical act, no matter how small (e.g., one very brief burst of electrocautery on tissues that they were trying to dissect) within the 60 s period this metric error was not scored. Despite this liberal definition, data from the clinical trial showed that this metric distinguished between trainee surgeons who were performing the LC better than those who were not.

A number of lessons were learned by the VR to OR team during this exercise. Probably the most important lesson that was learned was that some operational characteristics which appear to be easy to identify and agree upon are much more elusive when trying to specify an operational definition of how they should be scored. There is a fundamental difference between describing and defining a behavior or performance characteristic. In general parlance describing behaviors may be satisfactory to communicate ideas and concepts; however, on their own they are inadequate for the reliable assessment of that behavior. Generating the language or characterizing an aspect of the behavior that is to be assessed is a skill that continues to develop over a career of practice. Some performance characteristics are more difficult to operationally define than others and some are not adequately definable. In the example we have discussed here the concept of 'economy' or 'efficiency' was one such category that was very difficult to adequately define. Even when the operational definition had been generated the researchers were not at all confident that it would be adequate to encapsulate what it was they were trying to measure. However, with perseverance and ingenuity an operational definition was eventually arrived at that proved extremely valuable. Indeed, this definition of clinical performance has been so successful in characterizing operative clinical performance that it has been used in a wide variety of other clinical studies (Ahlberg et al. 2007; Van Sickle et al. 2008b).

Attending/Consultant Surgeon Takeover

Another problem that the team had to confront related to the issue of purposefulness of some aspect of performance or some behavior that the trainee surgeon was just about to enact, but was stopped by the supervising surgeon. In behavioral science, measurement aspects of human performance such as purposefulness cannot be directly assessed and are usually inferred from something that the person does. Furthermore, although the purpose or the intention of a person's behavior may be inferred, these inferences are frequently colored by the outcome of the behavior. Take for example the behavior of an entrepreneur who implements a new business program for the sole purpose to make money but ends up affecting the environment in the process. If he implements his business plan and in the process he ends up helping the environment, then people generally say he *unintentionally* helped the environment; if he implements his business plan and in the process he ends up harming the environment, then people generally say he *intentionally* harmed the environment. The important point is that in both cases his only goal was to make money (Knobe 2003). To simplify matters, it is probably best just to score what actually happened rather than what might have happened and for what reasons.

From the unfettered viewing of LC and video recorded procedures a large number of potential metrics were identified by the team. However, one of the problems with these metrics was that they occurred with such infrequency that they were difficult to include in a metric scoring system. A common theme which runs through many of these events was that they were behaviors which might have caused injury to the patient had the trainee been allowed to continue. Frequently what happened was that the trainee started to perform some aspect of the surgical procedure in such a way that it posed a risk to the patient, but they were not allowed to complete what they were doing by the supervising surgeon because they also recognized the potential consequences of the trainee surgeon's actions. Sometimes, what was observed was that the trainees did not even get to perform the potentially dangerous behavior before the supervising surgeon stopped them. This made generating an operational definition of the trainees performance characteristics very difficult for two reasons. The first was that the types of actions were so variable from poor instrument coordination to inability to recognize anatomical landmarks or be able to proceed to the next step in the surgical procedure. The second was that the trainee was frequently not allowed by the supervising surgeon to perform certain actions. In essence, this would have meant that the team would have had to generate a definition for something that did not happen. The problem was eventually solved when the focus of measurement shifted from the behavior of the trainee to the trainer. A consistent aspect of what the team wanted to measure was that the trainee was behaving in a way that caused concern to the supervising surgeon and so they intervened to assist in their performance or to take over the operation and perform that part of the surgical procedure themselves. 'Attending a takeover' as a metric error had a number of advantages. The first is that it indicated that things were not going as planned during the surgical procedure. It also indicated that the supervising surgeon was concerned enough that they felt they had to intervene or takeover performing the procedure. They could have done this for a wide variety of reasons which included safety of the patient. It may also have been to assist the trainee with a particularly difficult aspect of a case or it might have been to stop the trainee doing something which the supervising surgeon believed would have exposed the patient to increased risk. As assessors of the trainees' performance the team could not reliably infer the motivations of the supervising surgeon. However, what they could reliably score was that the supervising surgeon felt concerned enough that they assisted or took over the rest of the operation. If it was unclear why the supervising surgeon took over operating, they were asked after the procedure to give explicit reasons.

There was also some discussion about which point in the procedure assessment of performance should begin. Different surgeons had different operating styles and ways that they approached the procedure. However, it was quickly agreed that scoring of the procedure should commence on first contact of diathermy with tissue. This definition allowed surgeons to get a comfortable grip on the gallbladder so that it could be retracted thus allowing for dissection of connective tissue to the liver. Likewise the procedure would be considered. The complete scoring criteria/metric errors and the agreed operational definitions are given in Table 6.1.

The procedure started when diathermy made first contact with the tissue and was complete when the last attachment was divided. These start and endpoints were chosen because they were common to all laparoscopic procedures.

Another point of note about the metrics is that the VR to OR team tried to anticipate where anomalies might occur in the application of the metrics and then include further clarification to the metric definition to deal with the anticipated ambiguity.

Table 6.1 The metric errors and their operational definitions which were used to assess surgical performance for the VR to OR (Seymour et al. 2002)

Metric errors/criteria of injury assessment	Operational definition
Procedure **START**	First contact of diathermy with tissue
Procedure **END**	Last attachment is divided
Failure to progress	No progress made in excising the gallbladder for an entire minute of the dissection. Dealing with the consequences of a predefined error represents lack of progress if no progress is made in excising the gallbladder during this period
Gallbladder injury	There is gallbladder wall perforation with or without leakage of bile. Injury may be incurred with either hand
Liver injury	Necessitates capsule penetration and may have bleeding
Burn nontarget tissue	Any application of electrocautery to non-target tissue with the exception of the final part of the fundic dissection where some current transmission may occur
Tearing tissue	Uncontrolled tearing of tissue with the dissecting or retracting instrument
Incorrect plane of dissection	The dissection is conducted outside the recognized plane between the gallbladder and the liver (i.e. in the sub-mucosal plane on the gallbladder, or sub-capsular plane on the liver)
Instrument out of view	The dissecting instrument is placed outside the field of view of the telescope such that its tip is unviewable and can potentially be in contact with tissue. No error will be attributed to an incident of a dissecting instrument out of view as the result of a sudden telescope movement
Attending takeover	The supervising attending surgeon takes the dissecting instrument (right hand), or retracting instrument (left hand) from the resident and performs a component of the procedure

For example, in FAILURE TO PROGRESS the team wondered what would happen if a trainee enacted some kind of error which interfered with the normal flow of the procedure. The conclusion was that if the trainee was dealing with the consequences of something that was a direct consequence of what they did and thus were unable to make progress with gallbladder dissection they should be scored as unable to make progress. In contrast, if an error (e.g., diathermy instrument out of view) was enacted by the trainee whilst the person operating the camera made a sudden movement with the telescope which meant that viewing was lost by the operator, no error would be scored for that period. What the team attempted to do in developing operational definitions of the performance characteristics they were going to measure was to provide definitions that best characterized what it was they were scoring.

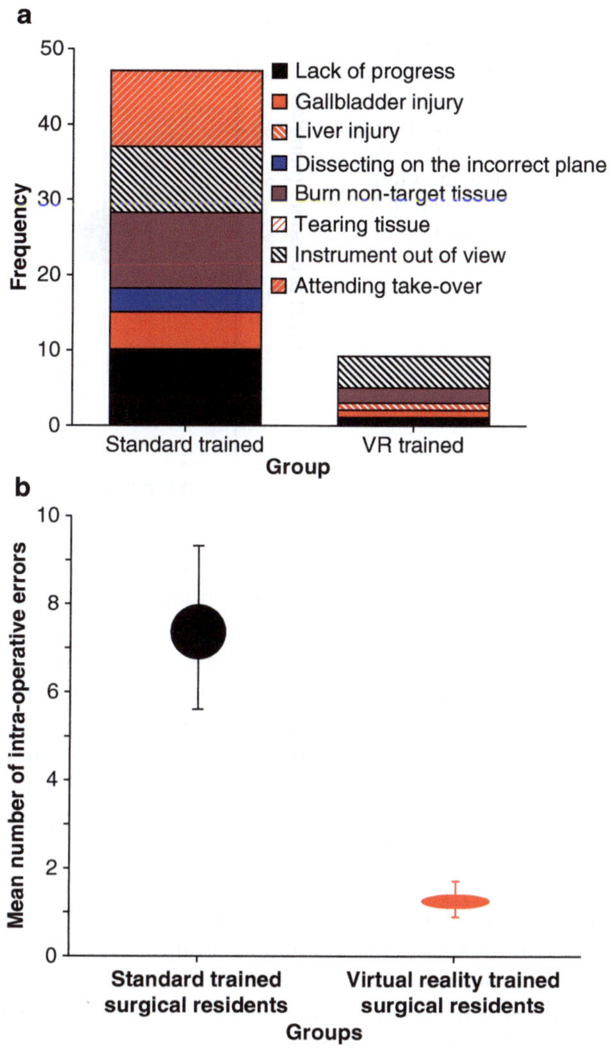

Fig. 6.2 (**a**) The frequency of the different intra-operative errors made by the standard trained and the virtual reality trained group during the dissection of the gallbladder from the liver bed during in the VR to OR study (data sourced from Seymour et al. 2002). (**b**) Mean and standard deviation number of intra-operative errors made by the standard trained and the virtual reality trained group during the dissection of the gallbladder from the liver bed during in the VR to OR study (Data sourced from Seymour et al. 2002)

Figure 6.2a shows the frequency of occurrence of eight different types of intra-operative errors defined and scored by the team. For the errors that were enacted the standard training group were making more of each type. Neither group enacted an error of tearing tissues. Only the standard training group made errors in the liver injury and dissection in the incorrect plane error categories. All attending takeover errors were enacted by trainees in the standard training group. Figure 6.2b shows the mean and standard deviation number of errors and enacted by other standard and virtual reality training group. The virtual reality trained group made significantly fewer objectively assessed intra-operative errors. Indeed, it was found that the virtual reality training group made six times fewer objectively assessed intra-operative

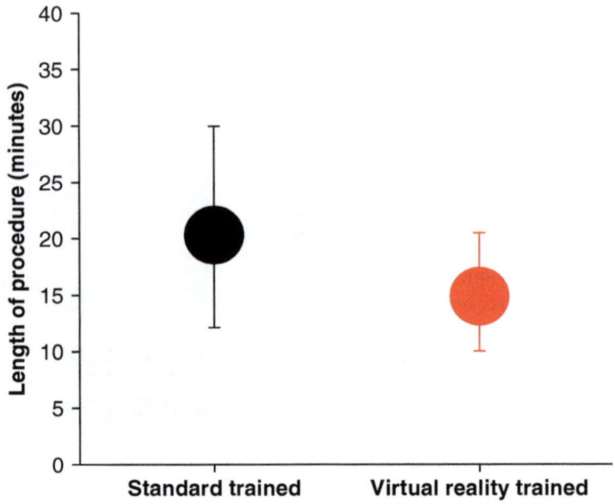

Fig. 6.3 Mean and standard deviation number of minutes the standard trained and the virtual reality trained group took to perform the dissection of the gallbladder from the liver bed during the VR to OR study (Data sourced from Seymour et al. 2002)

errors. This was the first clinical trial to show that virtual reality trained surgeons performed significantly better than traditionally trained surgeons (Seymour et al. 2002).

The amount of time taken to perform the procedure was also assessed. As pointed out earlier, time on its own is a crude performance metric. However, if quality is held constant and time decreases, then performance is improved. Thus when time is assessed along with these performance metrics we should have a good overall characterization of surgical performance. The mean number of minutes (and standard deviations) taken to perform the dissection of the gallbladder from the liver bed are shown in Fig. 6.3. As can be seen the surgeons in the VR trained group performed the task considerably faster than the standard trained group, i.e., 29% faster. These data coupled with those on intra-operative errors indicate very clearly that the performance quality of the VR trained group is very clear in comparison to the standard trained group who took longer to perform the procedure and made more errors. It should also be noted that the inter-rater reliability for the assessment of all of the surgeons' operative performance during video reviews was $91 \pm 4\%$ (range 84–100%). At no point did it drop below 80%. The issue of inter-rater reliability will be discussed in more detail in Chap. 7 as it is an important measure of how well the operational definitions are working and also the level of agreement between surgeons who were scoring performance.

Although the results from the VR to OR were generally well received by the surgical community, there were some critics who pointed out that the results only represented a small part of the surgical procedure, i.e., dissection of the gall bladder from the liver bed. The results did show proof of concept, but as the surgical community pointed out more evidence was needed to show the value of virtual reality simulation as a training tool. It was at this point that metrics were developed for the rest of the laparoscopic cholecystectomy surgical procedure. Metrics for the dissection portion of the procedure already existed, were published and good lessons had been learned about the development process involved in metric identification and metric definition. Good lessons had also been learned about training surgeons how to reliably identify intra-operative errors.

The metrics for the rest of the LC procedure were developed in the same way that the metrics had been developed for the dissection of the gall bladder portion of the procedure. There was an unfettered review of videotaped LC surgical procedures which had been performed by very experienced and less experienced laparoscopic surgeons. A shortlist of metric errors was drawn up whilst looking at the specific parts of the operation where intra-operative errors had not yet been identified, i.e., the exposure portion and the clipping and dissection portion (Table 6.2). Metric errors which had been identified in the previous study (Seymour et al. 2002) and were applicable to these as portions of the surgical procedure were used again. These metric errors include gallbladder injury, instrument out of view and attending takeover. Metric errors specific to the exposure portion of the procedure included incorrect angle of gallbladder retraction, dropped gallbladder retraction and cystic duct injury. Intra-operative errors specific to the clipping and dissection portion of the procedure concentrated on the application of the clips and included performance characteristics such as dropping a clip, clips placed too close or too far apart, trying to cut clips with the scissors. Other scissor errors included cutting non-target tissue and dividing tissues too close to the clips. The metric errors were scored on an interval scoring schedule the same as shown in Table 5.2, Chap. 5.

Figure 6.4 shows the mean and standard deviation number of errors enacted by the two groups during LC procedures 1, 5 and 10. The results showed that the virtual reality training group made significantly fewer objectively assessed intra-operative errors in all three of the cases that were assessed. They also showed that not only did the virtual reality trained group perform better than the standard trained group, i.e., they made less errors and also performed at this level consistently as indicated by the smaller standard deviation bars. They also had an absence of a learning curve across the three procedures. In contrast, the standard trained group showed considerable intra-group performance variability and their mean performance during procedure five was worse than during procedure one. Furthermore, inter-rater reliability (IRR) throughout the assessment of intra-operative performance was high, i.e., 0.98 (98% agreement between raters).

A Modified Interval Scoring System for Advanced Laparoscopic Surgery

During the development of metrics for the exposure, clipping and dissection elements of the LC, it became clear that the interval scoring methods that have been developed for the dissection of the gallbladder from the liver bed would not be optimal for scoring the clipping and dissection elements of the procedure. This was because this part of the procedure was very brief. Consequently, we modified the interval scoring schedule and instead of having intervals that were based on a fixed

Table 6.2 Operative error definitions for the exposure, clipping and dissection portion of the LC surgical procedure

Exposure errors	
Exposure starts:	Once fundus is stable
Exposure ends:	When clip appears
1.	Lack of progress: Absolutely no progress is made for an entire minute. Each minute spent dealing with the consequences of a predefined error represents lack of progress and should be evaluated as such
2.	Burn non-target tissue: Any application of electrocautery to non-target tissue
3.	Nontarget structure injury: There is a perforation or tear of a non-target structure (i.e. liver, bowel, common duct) with or without associated bleeding or bile leakage. Injury in this instance does not include electrocautery along the surface, as this would be classified as burning non-target tissue
4.	Instrument out of view: A dissecting instrument with cautery capability is placed outside the field of view of the telescope such that the tip is unviewable. An instrument will be considered to have cautery capabilities at the moment that cautery is applied to tissue and at all times thereafter until the instrument is changed. Hook instruments are an exception in that they are considered to always have cautery capabilities. No error will be attributed to an incident of an instrument out of view as the result of a sudden telescope movement
5.	Attending takeover: The supervising attending surgeon takes the dissecting instrument or retracting instrument from the resident and performs a component of the procedure. The error occurs throughout the entire period the attending has control and each interval during this period will be evaluated as such. The error ends once the resident resumes control of the instrument(s)
6.	Gallbladder injury: There is a gallbladder wall perforation with or without leakage of bile
7.	Cystic duct injury: There is a perforation or tear of the cystic duct indicated by leakage of bile
8.	Inappropriate dissection: Dissection is conducted such that either (1) tearing of tissue occurs during dissection within the triangle of Calot, or (2) the plane of dissection within the triangle extends to include areas along the common bile duct
9.	Incorrect angle of gallbladder retraction: Retraction of gallbladder is provided such that dissection proceeds within an inadequately distracted or "closed" Triangle of Calot prior to fenestration of triangle window
10.	Dropped retraction: Retracted tissue is suddenly dropped. Errors are counted only if re-grasping and retraction along a similar angle are subsequently required
Clipping and tissue division errors	
Clipping starts:	The appearance of the clip
Clipping ends:	Once clip is placed

Table 6.2 (continued)

General errors (applies to both clipping and transection)	
1.	Attending takeover: For definition see number 5, exposure
Clipping application errors	
2.	Clip overlap: Clip placed on previously placed clip
3.	Clip spacing error: Less than 1 mm spacing between distal porta and proximal gallbladder clips
4.	Poor clip orientation: Clip placed >10° from perpendicular as oriented to cystic duct or cystic artery after clip applier is removed
5.	Partial closure: Partial closure of cystic artery or duct (clip does not completely cross structure)
6.	Poor application: Clip is applied such that it is (1) incompletely closed, (2) scissored or (3) requires re-grasp manipulation
7.	Poor visualization: Clip applied without visualization of the tip of the clip applier
8.	Non-target tissue clipped: Clip applied to non-target tissue caught in closed tip outside cystic duct or cystic artery
9.	Clip drop: Clip comes out of clip applier prior to application. Application occurs once any part of the structure being clipped is within the jaws of the clip applier
Tissue division errors	
10.	Inappropriate division: Cut less than 1 mm to nearest porta side clip
11.	Clip cutting: Scissors closure on clip
12.	Nontarget injury: Cut non-target tissue

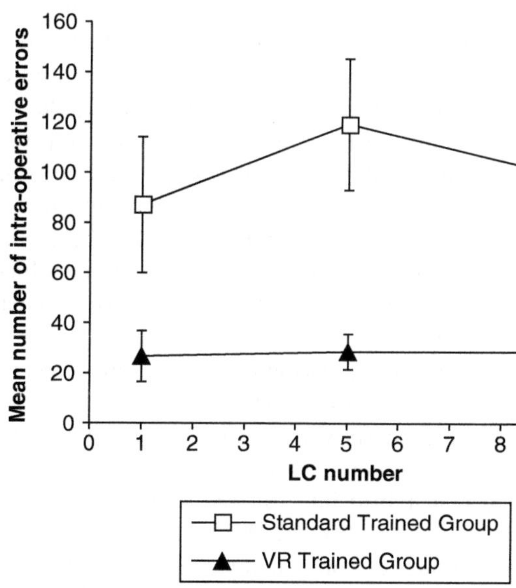

Fig. 6.4 Mean and standard deviation number of intra-operative errors made by the standard trained and the virtual reality trained group for the entire LC during trainees 1st, 5th, and 10th procedures in the VR to OR study (Ahlberg et al. 2007)

period of time, i.e., 60 s, we developed an event-driven scoring schedule. This schedule is best explained by describing how the metrics for an advanced laparoscopic procedure were developed and applied to the assessment of intra-operative performance.

Nissen fundoplication is considered an advanced laparoscopic surgical procedure. Technical skills, such as intracorporeal suturing and knot tying, are fundamental to becoming proficient in advanced laparoscopic procedures and is a procedure that surgical trainees are not allowed to attempt until the senior years of their training. In a study investigating training methods for intracorporeal suturing, Van Sickle et al. (2008) used a similar training and assessment methodology as the Seymour et al. (2002) and Ahlberg et al. (2007) studies. Trainee surgeons in a traditional training group and simulation training group performed the fundall suturing portion of a laparoscopic Nissen fundoplication. A standardized three-suture fundoplication was performed with the first and most cephalad suture being placed by the attending/consultant surgeon. The remaining two sutures were replaced by the trainees. The first trainee placed a suture which consisted of a fundal-esophageal-fundal bite followed by the tying of a slipknot. On the second trainee placed suture, the esophageal bite was omitted. The trainee surgeon's performance in placing the sutures and tying the knots was video recorded for subsequent analysis. The intra-operative errors were generated and operationally defined using the same method as described for the LC.

In the development of metrics for the Nissen fundoplication, it became clear during the viewing phase of video recorded intra-operative performance that a strictly timed interval schedule would not be optimal for scoring. Preliminary discussions about the modified interval scoring method centered around reducing the interval from 60 to 30 s or possibly 15 s. However, no satisfactory agreement could be reached on optimal timing for assessment intervals. An alternative strategy was suggested, which meant that intervals could be defined by intra-operative events rather than time. The advantage of this approach is that each step in the suturing procedure is discreet and all steps must be completed by all subjects. The steps in the suturing procedure were defined in the same way as the errors were defined and are shown in Appendix III. Furthermore, it was also decided that rather than scoring intra-operative errors just once during each interval that there should be a frequency count instead. The scoring matrix that resulted from this is shown in Table 6.3.

The scoring matrix shows the stages/steps in the performance of the suture on the vertical axis and the intra-operative errors on the horizontal axis. For the second suture the scoring matrix was the same except there was no 'esophageal bite' step. Metric errors were scored as frequently as they occurred. What the researchers developed was a hybrid interval-frequency scoring method which has been validated (Van Sickle et al. 2008a). As can be seen from Table 6.3, four out of the ten metric errors could be scored at any stage during the suturing procedure. Six of the ten metric errors could only be scored at specific steps of the suturing procedure.

Table 6.3 The matrix for scoring intra-operative performance for the first suture performed by the Nissen Fundoplication surgical trainees (Van Sickle et al. 2008b)

Suturing errors score sheet Suture # __________

	Missed Grasp	Tear/ Injured Tissue	Instrument Not assist	Excess Manipulation	Incom/ Repeat bite	Needle out of view	Missed Loop	Tail Looped	Fail to Sq knot	Scissors Touch tissue
Insert/ Orient										
Fundal bite 1										
Esophageal bite										
Fundal bite 2										
First throw										
Second throw										
Slip knot										
Cinching										
Squaring										
Third throw										
Cutting										
Total										

For example, when the needle was inserted and during the orienting process the trainee had not yet got to the stage where they were driving the needle through the fundus of the stomach so this error could not be scored. However, they could miss the grasping of the needle, they could tear or injure tissue with the needle and they could handle the needle inefficiently (which was operationally defined as grasping the suture or the needle more than two times during a step). Also, during the first two throws when the surgeon was starting to tie the knot they were not making a bite

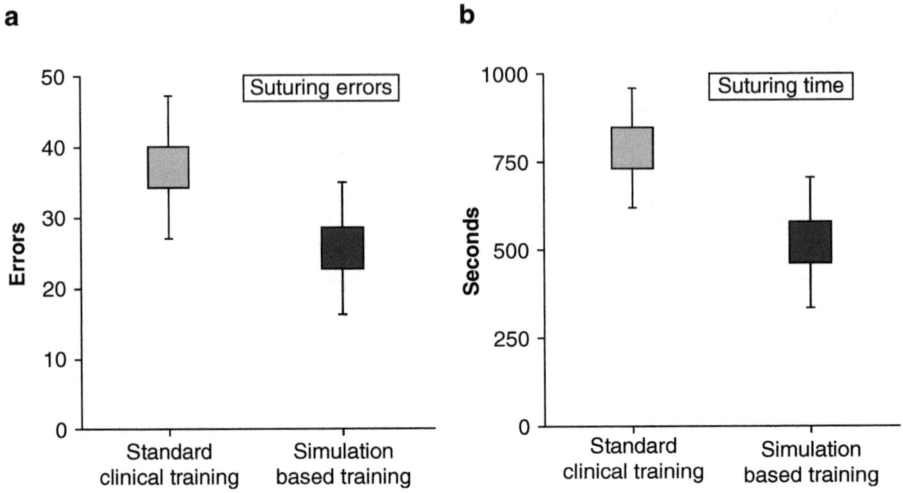

Fig. 6.5 (**a**) Suturing total errors, simulation-based laparoscopic suturing curriculum (*dark gray bar*) versus standard clinical training (*light gray bar*); *p* 0.01; unpaired t-test. (**b**) Suturing total time, simulation-based laparoscopic suturing curriculum (*dark gray bar*) versus standard clinical training (*light gray bar*); *p* 0.004; unpaired *t*-test

at tissue, nor had they tied the knot so they could not square it and they were not using scissors; this meant that none of these metric errors can be scored during this step.

Figure 6.5a, b shows the mean and standard deviation number of errors made by the simulation and standard trained groups and the time they took to perform both sutures. The simulation curriculum trained group made significantly fewer intra-operative errors and performed the procedure significantly faster. Interobserver agreement between the rating surgeon investigators was calculated by dividing the number of agreements between the raters by the sum of the number of agreements and disagreements, and IRR > 0.8.

This study demonstrates a number of important points about the assessment methodology. The first is that the methodology is flexible enough to be applied to a wide variety of clinical situations, from basic laparoscopic surgical skills as demonstrated in LC to more advanced laparoscopic skills such as in Nissen fundoplication. In the latter surgical procedure, the researchers modified the interval methodology from traditional time-based intervals to event-based intervals. However, the operational definitions for both the intra-operative errors and the steps in the operative procedure were produced from the same methodology as described in Chap. 5. In another validation study (Van Sickle et al. 2008b), this modified assessment method demonstrated construct validity between expert and less experienced laparoscopic surgeons performing the sutures for Nissen fundoplication. It also demonstrated high inter-rater reliability which is a fundamental requisite for an assessment process which aspires to be used for high-stakes assessment. We will discuss this issue in more detail in Chap. 7.

In Vivo Metric-Based Assessment

The ideal situation for research and assessment purposes is to be able to video record performance for subsequent analysis. However, this is not always possible such as in the assessment of technical skills for career advancement. In Ireland, Gallagher et al. (2008) have reported on an assessment system they used to help select surgeons into the higher surgical training program. The researchers argued that a fundamental aspect of a selection system for career advancement is that it should be objective, transparent and fair. However, the selection system should also assess individuals on performance characteristics that were related to the job or training they were about to undertake. As surgeons applying for entry to a surgical training program for higher surgical skills, technical skills were a fundamental aspect of what they would be required to do. They designed a multiskill, multitask surgical assessment programme which was used to help select candidates into the higher surgical training programme. The assessment programme consisted of all shortlisted candidates being assessed on their surgical technical skills on 10 separate skills stations. These were basic surgical skills that the applicants would have been expected to have been taught and encountered during the first two years of their basic surgical skills training program and as such the tasks were not new to the applicants. All candidates completed all 10 skill stations which took between 20 and 30 min depending on the station. Each skills station was staffed by a consultant surgeon who was experienced in the training and teaching of surgical trainees. The consultant surgeon scored performance by the candidates using procedure-specific marking criteria which had been agreed in advance by a separate group of surgical trainers.

One of the tasks consisted of the excision of a sebaceous cyst and then suturing the wound closed with interrupted sutures and is shown in Fig 6.4. Candidates had 20 min to complete the task and the task-specific marking criteria are shown in Table 6.4.

Metrics were developed in the same way that we have previously described. However, the difference on this occasion was that great emphasis was placed on ensuring that the scoring criteria was as transparent as possible since performance was not being video recorded for later analysis. The researchers were also mindful of the issue of how usable the scoring criteria that they generated would have to be. In practice, this meant that the first opportunity they had to train the consultant surgeons performing the assessment on the assessment methods was on the morning of the assessment itself. The task analysis and operational definitions had been completed and agreed on by a smaller group of surgeons who were very similar in profile (i.e., clinical experience, teaching experience and training experience) to the surgeons who were conducting the assessment on the day. Table 6.4 shows just one example of the assessments that were used (Carroll et al. 2009; Gallagher et al. 2008, 2009). The assessment was not simply about whether the surgeon could perform the procedure or not but how well they performed the procedure. Other aspects of the procedure that directly related to technical performance were also

Table 6.4 Procedure specific marking criteria for excision of subcutaneous lesion

1. Anatomy	
Name any two different anatomical locations of Lipoma	Yes □ No □
Name a syndrome associated with Lipoma (i.e., Dercums disease)	Yes □ No □
2. Medication	
Candidate was able to name a local anesthetic	Yes □ No □
Candidate was able to name the dose	Yes □ No □
Candidate was able to name the dose with adrenaline	Yes □ No □
Candidate was able to name the side effects of local anesthetic (i.e., fitting and arrhythmias)	Yes □ No □
3. Incision	
<4 cm in length	Yes □ No □
Linear incision rather than an ellipse	Yes □ No □
4. Excision/exposure	
Candidate was able to name three instruments chosen and used to perform the procedure (not a scalpel)	
Instrument 1	Yes □ No □
Instrument 2	Yes □ No □
Instrument 3	Yes □ No □
5. Closure	
Candidate used interrupted suture to close incision	Yes □ No □
No evidence of candidate tearing/injuring tissue (i.e., scraping sound from tissue model)	Yes □ No □
Correct number of throws	Yes □ No □
No evidence of tail loop (i.e., rabbit ear(s))	Yes □ No □
Knot squared	Yes □ No □

assessed. These included the assessment of whether the candidates knew the appropriate anatomy, the medication that could be used for the procedure and the correct dosage; the type of incision that they made, the instruments used to perform the procedure and how well they closed the incision. On the morning of the assessment the surgeons were instructed and shown examples of how to score the tasks and were specifically instructed that they were to score with an 'assessor' rather than a 'trainer' mindset. They were also instructed to score what they observed that the candidate did while performing the procedure, not what they thought the candidate might be capable of on a 'good' day.

Under these circumstances it is very difficult to assess performance characteristics such as 'economy' and 'efficiency' in the same way that can be assessed on a video recording. However, efforts were made to score the aesthetics of their performance, which almost certainly is a surrogate of performance efficiency. Suturing technique was assessed, but so also was how they sutured, e.g., were they tearing or injuring tissue as they sutured; how neat were their knots? The assessment criteria could have been expanded to include factors such as whether the cyst bulb was removed intact or not and possibly whether there was puckering of the wound. However, even as reported here the operationalized assessment criteria for excision of subcutaneous lesions were able to distinguish between candidates performance on this very basic surgical task. On average, candidates who were selected for higher surgical training performed the task 10% better than those who were not.

Metric Development; Lessons Learned

Thinking about and generating operational definitions for performance characteristics that are to be trained and assessed is a very different way of thinking about education and training in surgery. Ironically, practicing surgeons who regularly teach and train junior surgeons have this information at their fingertips. However, rarely do they actually think about and recount precisely what it is that they are trying to achieve in the education and training of their junior colleagues. Involvement in a team whose job is to formulate metrics for the assessment of surgical performance forces surgeon educators to define precisely what is that they are trying to train and to describe in detail how performing some aspect of a surgical procedure one way means that it is performed well rather than wrongly. Most practicing surgeons recognize the value of this type of strategy, whilst at the same time finding it very difficult. The difficulty for many surgeons is that many subtle details are included in their operative practice and have been automated, which ensures they perform the procedure well. As discussed in Chaps. 2 and 3 procedural memory is our memory for how to do things. Procedural memories are automatically retrieved and utilized for the execution of the step-by-step procedures involved in both cognitive and motor skills; from riding a bicycle to performing a commonly practiced surgical procedure. These skills are emitted without the need for conscious control or attention. Procedural memory is a type of long-term memory. This is the final phase in Fitts (Fitts and Peterson 1964) model of skill acquisition and it involves perfecting skill acquisition so that skills can be practiced with minimal conscious or cognitive effort. The positive consequences of automation are that it frees up cognitive resources to attend to other aspects of the operation. The disadvantage of automation is that the actual step-by-step detail of the technique is lost to many of the practitioners and they are unable to explain in words what it is they do and how they do it. With effort, most surgeon trainers can master the skill of recounting in detail precisely what it is that they do and the important detail of how they do it a particular way and why. Most proficiency surgeons are aware of the different ways or styles of performing some aspect of a surgical procedure and they have chosen the way that they do it for particular reasons, i.e., it makes performance easier, more efficient, or makes a later stage in the procedure easier to perform. To be a productive member of the task analysis team they should readily (genuinely) recognize that theirs is only one style and for training purposes and successful metric development they may have to concede that their way may be uncommon or indeed inferior to another approach that they had not considered.

The Imperative of Metrics

Metrics lie at the core of what simulation is (or at least should be). To develop metrics it is necessary first of all to understand the detail of performing a surgical procedure. It is necessary to know the steps and the order in which they are performed in the procedure and then be able to describe in detail, how best the steps can be accomplished. It is in the level of detail that metrics are derived. These are also the types of detail simulations should be developed from. Simulations should primarily be about training individuals using the steps by which a procedure should be performed and how best to achieve these steps. Crucially, the performance characteristics enacted by the trainee in achieving these steps must be assessable. That is why metrics must be at the core of simulation development. Unfortunately, many simulations seem to be developed to look like the procedure and metrics are only an afterthought. These types of simulations, no matter how good they look, are nothing more than video games.

The type of performance characteristics that we have detailed here, how they are identified and operationally defined should be the building blocks for efficient and effective simulation. This changes the goal of simulation development from 'we needed to build a simulation that looks like the actual surgical procedure' to 'we need to build a simulation that trains and assesses the performance characteristics that will best generalize to the actual surgical procedure'. The ideal situation would be to build a simulation that looked like the actual surgical procedure and was an effective trainer. However, the latter aspect of this scenario is the most important part of the simulation. This also explains why MIST VR is to date the most effective virtual reality trainer in surgery yet the tasks look nothing like the real surgical tasks. The developers concentrated on simulating tasks that would train the appropriate two-handed psychomotor coordination necessary for the safe performance of a laparoscopic cholecystectomy. They also ensured that these performance characteristics were easily assessable using valid and reliable metrics (Gallagher et al. 2001; Gallagher and Satava 2002). The result was that this was the first virtual reality simulator to show in a prospective, randomized, blinded clinical trial that training on it to defined performance criteria significantly improved intra-operative performance on a real patient (Seymour et al. 2002).

Identification of the important performance characteristics that are the requisites of good surgery is a crucial and fundamental part of the metric development process. It is important that surgeons chosen as part of the task analysis team are very familiar with the procedure they are about to analyze. They do not have to be expert in the performance of the procedure, but they do have to be safe practitioners and good teachers and trainers. The process of choosing suitable surgeons may sound easier than it actually is. Some surgeons are simply so experienced in the performance of the procedure that their skills have automated to the extent that the details of how they perform the procedure are not consciously analyzable by them. Other surgeons are comfortable in performing the procedure in a certain way but have difficulty understanding or appreciating a different way. The amount that these two types of surgeons could contribute to the task analysis is probably limited. Another

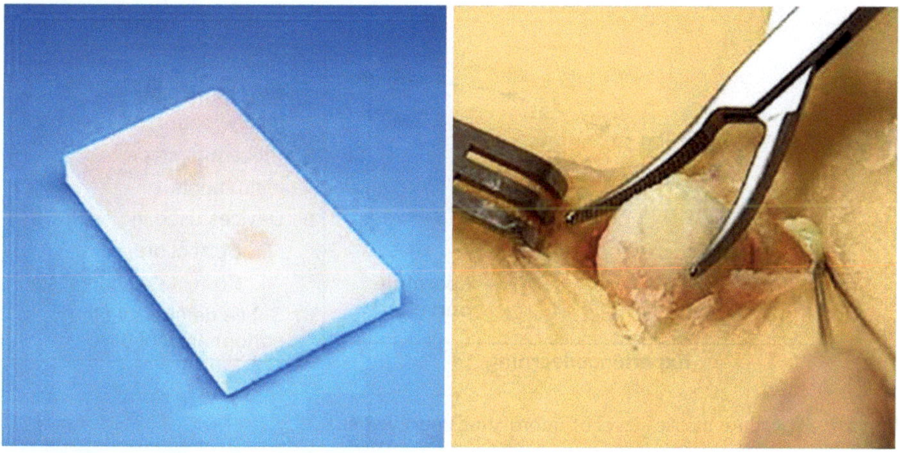

Fig. 6.6 Open surgical skills assessment task which consist of the excision of a sebaceous cyst and then suturing the wound closed. The metrics developed for the *in vivo* task would be applied to this silicone model for training and assessment

group of surgeons who should be given serious consideration to be included in the task analysis team are very senior trainee surgeons. What we have found is that very senior trainees (SpRs or Fellows) are skilled enough to know how to perform the procedure optimally but have not automated to the extent where they are unaware of the detail of their performance. The other advantage of having this group is that they can act as 'expert novices'. By this we mean they are experienced enough to remember what aspects of performing the procedure they found most difficult to grasp or practice, what aspects of training they found most helpful in overcoming these difficulties and what it was about their own or a peer's performance that indicated the problem had been resolved. The task could be as simple as the excision of a sebaceous cyst which is easily simulated using a silicone model (Fig. 6.6).

Metric Information

Metrics are important because they convey information about the performance characteristics of the person doing the procedure. With the average practicing surgeon this is not a factor that is at the forefront of consideration. We simply know that they are experienced in performing the procedure and their outcomes are good. However, the detail of how they actually achieve this is important information that can guide how best we train and assess surgeons in training to ensure that they are on the same performance trajectory. Figure 6.7 shows a hypothetical performance learning curve and numbered points along the curve. The first point, number 1, gives the most basic information about performance, i.e., time on task. This information conveys little or nothing about detail of performance or whether the procedure was performed the right way or the wrong way or how well it was performed.

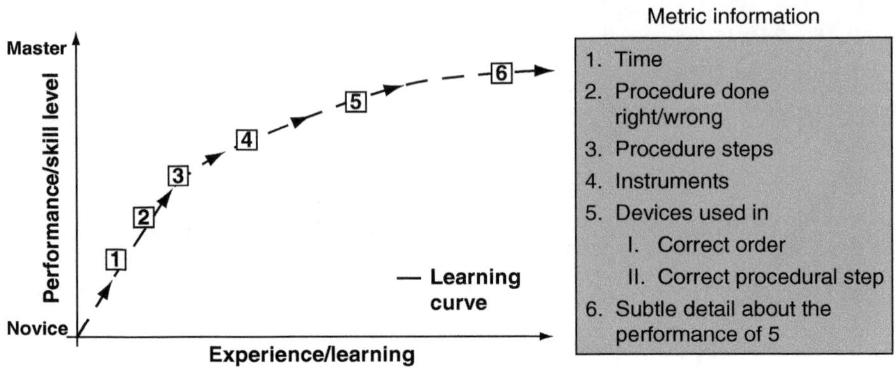

Fig. 6.7 Procedure metrics level of information conveyed

Point 2 on the learning curve gives us information about time on task and whether it was done right or wrong. Information conveyed in point 3 includes all the prior information and whether the correct procedural steps were followed are not. In point 4 this information is supplemented with knowledge on the instruments used to perform the procedure and is added to again in point 5 about the correct instrument being used during the correct step. Point 6 subsumes all prior information and also conveys detail on subtle aspects of device and procedural step interaction that informs us of how well the procedure was done. Each level of metric information subsumes the prior level of metric information and adds something new as well. This is the level of information that metrics should aim to achieve during their development. Efficient and effective simulation training has at its core information feedback to the learner. In Chap. 4 we explained that feedback on performance is one of the most important sources of information that can directly affect learning procedural skills. Computerized simulation models make it easier to provide quantitative feedback on performance when compared with silicon models or animal tissue models. However, for this feedback to be useful it requires appropriate and inappropriate performance characteristics to have been operationally defined in a way that is unambiguously quantifiable. Therefore, the function of the simulation model is not simply to look and feel like whatever procedure is trying to be simulated. Rather, it is a vehicle for providing feedback on gross and subtle aspects of task performance on the simulated model, to the learner. In this configuration the simulation context and face validity take secondary importance to the metrics and are simply the vehicle for collecting metric information on performance.

Summary

Metric-based assessment is a fundamental aspect of effective simulation for training surgical skills. Identification and operational definition of important performance characteristics which are crucial to efficient and effective surgery are the cornerstones of good metrics. Operational definitions are not as easy to develop as it might appear. However, they are essential for the objective, fair and transparent assessment of performance. Performance metrics are derived from the experience and observations of surgeons experienced in performing the procedure. Operational definitions should convey in words what many surgeons experience as implicit knowledge. The problem with implicit knowledge is that it makes for ambiguous assessment criteria. Unambiguous, explicit and quantitative feedback provides the best information on which to improve performance. The task analysis in which performance characteristics to be trained and assessed are identified should provide the core information for the simulation development. Simulations should be a vehicle for the delivery of metric-based performance feedback rather than something that approximates the look and feel of performing the procedure on a patient.

Appendix: Emory VR to OR Lap. Chole. Procedure-Related Definitions for Master Study

Exposure

Exposure Starts: Once fundus is stable
Exposure Ends: When clip appears

Exposure Errors

Lack of Progress – Absolutely no progress is made for an entire minute. Each minute spent dealing with the consequences of a predefined error represents lack of progress and should be evaluated as such.

Burn Non-target tissue – Any application of electrocautery to nontarget tissue.

Non-target structure injury – There is a perforation or tear of a non-target structure (i.e. liver, bowel, common duct) with or without associated bleeding or bile leakage. Injury in this instance does not include electrocautery along the surface, as this would be classified as burning non-target tissue.

Instrument out of view – A dissecting instrument with cautery capability is placed outside the field of view of the telescope such that the tip is unviewable. An instrument will be considered to have cautery capabilities at the moment that cautery is applied to tissue and at all times thereafter until the instrument is changed. Hook instruments are an exception in that they are considered to always have cautery capabilities. No error will be attributed to an incident of an instrument out of view as the result of a sudden telescope movement.

Attending takeover – The supervising attending surgeon takes the dissecting instrument or retracting instrument from the resident and performs a component of the procedure. The error occurs throughout the entire period the attending has control and each interval during this period will evaluated as such. The error ends once the resident resumes control of the instrument(s).

Gallbladder injury – There is gallbladder wall perforation with or without leakage of bile.

Cystic duct injury – There is a perforation or tear of the cystic duct indicated by leakage of bile.

Cystic artery injury – There is a perforation or tear of the cystic artery indicated by hemorrhage. Scoring continues until the hemorrhage is arrested. If a clip is applied, it is applied safely and appropriately, otherwise it is considered an error for the interval it was placed.

Inappropriate dissection – Dissection is conducted such that either (1) tearing of tissue occurs during dissection within the triangle of Calot, or (2) the plane of dissection within the triangle extends to include areas along the common bile duct.

Incorrect angle of gallbladder retraction – Retraction of gallbladder is provided such that dissection proceeds within an inadequately distracted, or "closed" Triangle of Calot prior to fenestration of triangle window.

Dropped retraction – Retracted tissue is suddenly dropped. Errors are counted only if re-grasping and retraction along a similar angle are subsequently required.

Clipping/Tissue Division

Note:

1. *Given that total clipping time may take less that 1 min, scoring intervals for this segment will be event driven. Each clip placement will be considered a separate event. Additionally the transection of the cystic artery and the cystic duct will be considered separate events.*
2. *If the cystic artery, or cystic duct are not exposed together prior to clipping and tissue division of each respective structure, the clip/tissue division evaluation will proceed for the exposed structure, followed by a continuation of the exposure evaluation until the unexposed structure is prepared (i.e. if the cystic artery is clipped prior to cystic duct exposure, the cystic artery clipping and division will be evaluated until transection of tissue occurs, then the exposure evaluation will continue until a clip designated for the cystic duct appears).*

Clipping Start: The appearance of the clip

Clipping End: Once clip is placed

Tissue Division Start: The appearance of shears

Tissue Division End: Transection of tissue

General Errors (applies to both clipping and transection)

Attending takeover – The supervising attending surgeon takes the dissecting instrument or retracting instrument from the resident and performs a component of the procedure. The error occurs throughout the entire period the attending has control and each interval during this period will evaluated as such. The error ends once the resident resumes control of the instrument(s).

Clipping Application Errors

Clip overlap – Clip placed on previously placed clip.

Clip spacing error – Less than 1 mm spacing between distal porta and proximal gallbladder clips.

Poor clip orientation – Clip placed $>10°$ from perpendicular as oriented to cystic duct or cystic artery after clip applier is removed.

Partial closure – Partial closure of cystic artery or duct (clip does not completely cross structure).

Poor Application – Clip is applied such that it is (1) incompletely closed, (2) scissored or (3) requires re-grasp manipulation.

Poor visualization – Clip applied without visualization of the tip of the clip applier.

Non-target tissue clipped – Clip applied to non-target tissue caught in closed tip outside cystic duct or cystic artery.

Clip drop – Clip comes out of clip applier prior to application. Application occurs once any part of the structure being clipped is within the jaws of the clip applier.

Tissue Division Errors

Inappropriate division – Cut less than 1 mm to nearest porta side clip.

Clip cutting – Scissors closure on clip.

Nontarget injury – Cut nontarget tissue.

Dissection

Dissection Start: Appearance of hook cautery instrument

Dissection End: Gallbladder is free from liver bed

Dissection Errors

Lack of Progress – No progress is made for an entire minute of the dissection. Each minute spent dealing with the consequences of a predefined error represents lack of progress and should be evaluated as such.

Burn Nontarget tissue – Any application of electrocautery to nontarget tissue with the exception of the final part of the fundic dissection where some current transmission may occur.

Instrument out of view – The dissecting instrument is placed outside the field of view of the telescope such that the tip is unviewable. No error will be attributed to an incident of an instrument out of view as the result of a sudden telescope movement.

Attending takeover – The supervising attending surgeon takes the dissecting instrument or retracting instrument from the resident and performs a component of the procedure. The error occurs throughout the entire period the attending has control and each interval during this period will evaluated as such. The error ends once the resident resumes control of the instrument(s).

Gallbladder injury – There is gallbladder wall perforation with or without leakage of bile.

Liver injury – There is liver capsule and parenchyma penetration, or capsule stripping with or without associated bleeding.

Incorrect plane of dissection – The dissection is conducted outside the recognized plane between the gallbladder and the liver (i.e. in the submucosal plane on the gallbladder, or subcapsular plane on the liver).

Tearing tissue – Uncontrolled tearing of tissue with the dissecting or retracting instrument.

References

Ahlberg G, Enochsson L, Gallagher AG, et al. Proficiency-based virtual reality training significantly reduces the error rate for residents during their first 10 laparoscopic cholecystectomies. *Am J Surg*. 2007;193(6):797-804.

Carroll SM, Kennedy AM, Traynor O, Gallagher AG. Objective assessment of surgical performance and its impact on a national selection programme of candidates for higher surgical training in plastic surgery. *J Plast Reconstr Aesthet Surg*. 2009;62(12):1543-1549.

Datta V, Chang A, Mackay S, Darzi A. The relationship between motion analysis and surgical technical assessments. *Am J Surg*. 2002;184(1):70-73.

Fitts PM, Peterson JR. Information capacity of discrete motor responses. *J Exp Psychol*. 1964;67(2):103-112.

Gallagher AG, Ritter EM, Satava RM. Fundamental principles of validation, and reliability: rigorous science for the assessment of surgical education and training. *Surg Endosc*. 2003;17(10): 1525-1529.

Gallagher AG, Satava RM. Virtual reality as a metric for the assessment of laparoscopic psychomotor skills. Learning curves and reliability measures. *Surg Endosc*. 2002;16(12):1746-1752.

Gallagher AG, Richie K, McClure N, McGuigan J. Objective psychomotor skills assessment of experienced, junior, and novice laparoscopists with virtual reality. *World J Surg*. 2001;25(11): 1478-1483.

Gallagher AG, Neary P, Gillen P, et al. Novel method for assessment and selection of trainees for higher surgical training in general surgery. *ANZ J Surg*. 2008;78(4):282-290.

Gallagher AG, Leonard G, Traynor OJ. Role and feasibility of psychomotor and dexterity testing in selection for surgical training. *Aust N Z J Surg*. 2009;79(3):108-113.

Knobe J. Intentional action and side effects in ordinary language. *Analysis*. 2003;63(3):190.

Martin JA, Regehr G, Reznick R, et al. Objective structured assessment of technical skill (OSATS) for surgical residents. *Br J Surg*. 1997;84(2):273-278.

Seymour NE, Gallagher AG, Roman SA, et al. Virtual reality training improves operating room performance: results of a randomized, double-blinded study. *Ann Surg*. 2002;236(4):458-463. discussion 463-454.

Smith SG, Torkington J, Brown TJ, Taffinder NJ, Darzi A. Motion analysis. *Surg Endosc*. 2002;16(4):640-645.

Van Sickle K, Baghai M, Huang IP, Goldenberg A, Smith CD, Ritter EM. Construct validity of an objective assessment method for laparoscopic intracorporeal suturing and knot tying. *Am J Surg*. 2008a;196(1):74-80.

Van Sickle KR, Ritter EM, Baghai M, et al. Prospective, randomized, double-blind trial of curriculum-based training for intracorporeal suturing and knot tying. *J Am Coll Surg*. 2008;207(4): 560-568.

Wilson T, Sahu A, Johnson DS, Turner PG. The effect of trainee involvement on procedure and list times: a statistical analysis with discussion of current issues affecting orthopaedic training in UK. *Surgeon*. 2010;8(1):15-19.

Chapter 7
Validation of Metrics Coupled to Simulation Training

In the previous chapters we identified very specific human factor reasons why medical procedures such as image guided surgery are difficult to learn and practice. They make unique perceptual, cognitive and psychomotor demands on the trainee and practitioner. The same research that has allowed us to identify these difficulties also provides us with potential solutions. One of the most important ways individuals learn is through "knowledge of results" of what they do and how their actions (or inaction) impacts where intended. The natural world provides human beings with ecologically valid information on their knowledge of results. However, this feedback information can be delivered at times when it is not contiguous to the behavior of the individual. In other words, an individual can do something which has negative consequences in the real world but they may not see the consequences of their behavior until much later. They fail to establish a relationship between their behavior and the negative results or outcomes and consequently, they almost certainly fail to modify their behavior.

In Chap. 5 one of the metric errors that we discussed was "instrument out of view". Why would we identify this apparently benign behavior as a source of potential error? One of the major reasons is that the operating surgeon needs to be able to visualize the working end of all their operating instruments, at all times throughout the procedure (whether the procedure is a traditional open or an image guided). This is particularly true when they have an electrocautery attached to one of the operating instruments. When electrocautery is attached to a surgical instrument, it can be used for coagulation or dissection. Furthermore, as the instrument is usually being used in an enclosed, moist, space, the electrical charge from the instrument can arc and damage other tissues. This can occur even in optimal conditions. However, if the surgeon cannot see the working end of the instrument, the possibility of observing this potentially dangerous event is eliminated. Consequently, if the patient develops a fever and other possible abdominal symptoms post-operatively because of an inadvertent electrocautery injury to tissues such as the bowel, the surgeon is unlikely to form the link between their unobserved behavior and post-operative complications. If these events occur on a frequent enough basis, the link will eventually be established. The real-world consequences of this type of

A.G. Gallagher and G.C. O'Sullivan, *Fundamentals of Surgical Simulation*, Improving Medical Outcome - Zero Tolerance,
DOI 10.1007/978-0-85729-763-1_7,

learning are that a number of patients will suffer post-operative complications before the surgeon learns the contiguous relationship between the post-operative complications and their failure to monitor electrocautery instruments during surgery. Contrast this situation with the surgeon who has experienced a fatality from major intrathoracic bleeding after an endoscopic thoracic sympathectomy for palmar hyperhidrosis following an intra-procedural surgical mishap (Ojimba and Cameron 2004); the contiguity between surgery and the mortality will serve as a very powerful learning aid.

The fact that we know (from decades of quantitative psychological research) that this is how individuals learn, i.e., knowledge of results, means that we can use this information to design more efficient and effective learning strategies. Rather than allowing the consequences of events to occur as they would in the natural order of things we can impose order on the contiguity of the events. The same consequences that occur in the natural world and control learning can be organized in such a way to ensure more effective and efficient learning. In the previous chapter, we described a way to identify potential relationships such as the one we have just described. We also proposed that these operationally defined units of behavior can be used as metrics for training purposes. Metrics are simply a set of measurements that help to quantify performance and give some indication whether or not goals have been or are being met. The enterprise under discussion here is the training of skills. It should be clear from Chaps. 5 and 6 how crucial metrics are for training and for the assessment of skills. We also believe that skills, training, assessment and metrics are integrally linked.

Metrics are an essential and vital part of any good training programme, whether that training programme is online, physical models, cadavers or virtual reality. Metrics are important for the trainee because they allow them to observe what they are/are not doing right and what they are/are not doing well and to modify their performance accordingly. They can enable the trainee to know how they are performing in comparison to their peers and how much their performance needs to improve to be on a par with more experienced colleagues. The same metrics can also be used to inform the trainer about how an individual or cohorts of trainees are learning. It allows trainers to identify in a timely manner which individuals are struggling with the training programme and affords the opportunity to set in motion a remediation or support program. Taken a step further, it also allows the trainer to identify when a trainee is exhibiting the skills and at the performance and consistency level that would indicate proficiency and thus are probably ready to progress to more advanced surgical procedures, level of responsibility in the operating room or possibly in their career. In previous studies it has been demonstrated that metric-based training to proficiency improvements intra-operative performance (Ahlberg et al. 2007; Seymour et al. 2002; Van Sickle et al. 2008). In these studies the proficiency-based training groups made significantly fewer objectively assessed intra-operative errors than the traditionally trained groups. This means that the performance of the surgeon in the operating room which has been shaped and optimized by metric-based simulation training has, in all probability, implications for patient safety. These metrics can have implications for the trainee surgeon in terms of when they get to do more advanced surgical cases or possibly, when they do or do not advance in their career. The implication of both of these conclusions is that we must make every effort to ensure that the metrics we use for training and assessment do what they are supposed to do; that they are reliable and valid. It is these metrics that will guide decision-making about the effectiveness of training and even when training can be considered complete. In the next chapter we shall discuss the concept of proficiency and how at the start of the twenty-first century this concept has been embraced by surgery and other procedural-based medical disciplines. However, it is important to note that the concept of proficiency is meaningless unless it has been appropriately defined and that this definition actually derives from something meaningful in the real world. The operationalized definition of proficiency that we support is one that is quantitatively defined and benchmarked (Champion and Gallagher 2003; Gallagher and Cates 2004b; Gallagher et al. 2005). The implementation of a proficiency-based progression training program which is robust, objective, transparent and provides fair validation evidence on the chosen metrics is of primary importance. This evidence is critical for the demonstration of the value of the chosen metrics, but it is also an important step in demonstrating the value of the methodology and metrics to the medical community; In order for it to be accepted the medical community have to have confidence in the outcome. Consequently, this venture requires meticulous validation efforts by the surgical community. Medical disciplines such as surgery have not always achieved this level of rigor. For example, the quality of surgical research was roundly criticized by the Lancet in the 1990s (Horton 1996). In this unprecedented attack the editor published a paper which called into question the quality of much surgical research. In his editorial "Surgical Research or Comic Opera?" Horton expressed grave reservations about the utility, validity and usefulness of much surgical research. Although the editorial received the predictable indignant response from the surgical community, Horton did make some valid points about the scientific quality of surgical research.

About the same time as the Lancet article, surgery was in the throes of embracing a new approach to performing surgery, i.e., MIS. By the mid-1990s it was clear that a higher rate of complications was associated with the learning curve of the surgeon (Centres 1991; Moore and Bennett 1995; Wherry et al. 1994) and there was an urgent search for new approaches to the training of surgeons which would help them overcome the unique human-factor problems associated with learning laparoscopic surgery. In the surgical training centers around the world that had developed training programs, there was a rush to publish validation evidence purporting to show that their laparoscopic training program worked (Geis et al. 1994; Melvin et al. 1996; Rosser et al. 1998). One of the new approaches was virtual reality training (Gallagher et al. 1999; Sutton et al. 1997; Taffinder et al. 1998). The surgical community greeted (and to some extent still do) VR simulation training in surgery with considerable scepticism and made explicit requests for evidence that simulation was a valid tool. In 2002, the first prospective, randomized, blinded, controlled, clinical validation trial of VR to OR was reported in the surgical literature (Seymour et al. 2002). It was followed two years later by a similar study (Grantcharov et al. 2004).

Both studies used a similar experimental design and concluded that virtual reality training improved intra-operative performance. The Seymour et al. (2002) study was particularly interesting because it was the first time that simulator metrics had been used to quantitatively define proficiency. Rather than requiring trainees for a number of trials (as in the Grantcharov et al. 2004 study), they continued to train until they could consistently reach the proficiency benchmark.

Validation will assume an increasingly important role in the future, particularly if surgery moves to high-stakes assessment of surgical skills. On the basis of assessment with validated tests, trainee surgeons may or may not be allowed to continue in their surgical training. Similarly, senior surgeons may "choose" to continue or stop practicing surgery on the basis of the results of the tests of technical skill. Therefore, the issue of validation and the scientific integrity of these studies must be beyond reproach. Perhaps because of the necessity to design new training methodologies in response to the introduction of minimally invasive surgery, endoscopic surgeons have some of the "best" developed understanding of the issues relating to validation of any of the surgical specialties. However, these issues will almost certainly confront other clinical specialties such as interventional cardiology, interventional radiology, urology etc.

Scientific validation is a common activity in industry and in academic disciplines such as psychology. In industry, verification and validation is the process of checking that a product, service, or system meets specifications and it fulfills the intended purpose. These are critical components of a *quality management system* such as *ISO 9000*. Verification is a quality control process that is used to evaluate whether or not a product, service, or system complies with regulations, specifications, or conditions imposed at the start of a development phase. Validation is the quality assurance process of establishing evidence that provides a high degree of assurance that a product, service or system accomplishes its intended requirements. It is sometimes said that validation can be expressed by the query "Are you building the right thing?" and verification by "Are you building it right?"

The scientific validation activity in psychology can be traced back to work undertaken more than a century ago. Two of the pioneers were Charles Edward Spearman (1863–1945) and James McKeen Cattell (1860–1944). Both men had studied under *Wilhelm Wundt* at the University of Leipzig and Spearman brought the methods to England (University College London) and Cattell to the USA (initially at *University of Pennsylvania* and latterly at Columbia University in New York). Both men are famous for their psychometric contributions to the study of intelligence. Among Spearman's achievements was the discovery of the general factor ("g") in human intelligence as well as the development of statistical tests. Cattell was the first Professor of Psychology in the United States at the *University of Pennsylvania* and long-time editor and publisher of scientific journals and publications, most notably in the journal *Science*. He established one of the most successful "mental testing" corporations anywhere in the world called "The Psychological Corporation". Its education testing unit was re-branded as Harcourt Brace Educational Measurement in 1995 and then shortened in 1999 to Harcourt Educational Measurement.

The growth and variety of tests (good and bad) developed rapidly during the twentieth century largely in the USA. In 1974, in response to concerns about test development and usage in a wide variety of settings the American Psychological Association (APA), the American Educational Research Association and the National Council on Measurement in Education developed standards for judging and assessing tests. These are referred to as the *Standards* (APA 1999). This publication does not lay down rules about test quality, but rather gives guidelines on a number of issues relating to administration, interpretation, ethical issues, appropriate norms, etc. However, it also provides rigorous, well-proven "guidance" on validation, reliability and error measurement of tests. Some key concepts relating to APA standards are defined below.

> *Validity*: [*def*: generally the property of being true, correct and in conformity with reality]. This meaning, common in ordinary parlance, is typically not intended in the technical literature. In logic, the property of an argument or conclusion is that it is deemed to be valid because it conforms to proper logical principles. The assumption here is that the reasoning itself must be correct. An argument may have validity in the sense that it follows logical reasoning, but does not correspond with reality and thus is not "valid" – but the fault will be with the principal assumptions and not with the reasoning process. In testing, the fundamental property of any measuring instrument, device or test is that it "… measures what it purports to measure". Therefore validity is not a simple notion, but rather it is comprised of a number of "first principles". The result is that within the testing literature, a number of validation benchmarks have been developed to assess the validity of a test or testing instruments. These are *Face*, *Content*, *Construct*, *Concurrent*, *Discriminate* and *Predictive* Validity and each of these are defined and described below (Reber and Reber 1985).

> *Face Validity:* [*def*: a type of validity that is assessed by having experts reviews the contents of a test to see if it seems appropriate]. Simply stated, an evaluation to determine whether the test will measure what it is supposed to. It is a very subjective type of validation and is usually only used during the initial phases of test construction.

Unfortunately, most surgeons tend to evaluate a simulator on the basis of face validity. One of the goals that we would like this book to accomplish is to empower the reader to evaluate a simulator on a more substantive basis rather than just how "pretty" it looks alone. This matter goes beyond the issue of price as some very expensive simulators, particularly endovascular simulators, look like they provide very high fidelity simulations. Surgeons may be taken in by the fact that the simulator is immersed in an environment that looks like a real operating room or cath. Lab. and indeed to perform the procedure on the simulator using the same devices as they would in a patient. However, if the devices do not behave the same in the simulator as they would inside a real patient, questions should immediately be asked about the fidelity of the procedural simulation. Additionally, the simulator should provide proximate feedback to the trainee and trainer on performance. These feedback metrics should consist of more than measurements of the amount of time to perform the procedure, devices used during the procedure and whether the procedure was completed or not. Ideally, the device should give formative and summative feedback which informs the trainee about aspects of their performance that needs to be improved. Formative feedback should be given proximal to performance as this has been shown repeatedly to be one of the most efficient mechanisms of learning. Proximal feedback informs the trainee about what they did wrong (or nearly did wrong) at the time they did it and with which instrument. Usually the trainee will be aware of this, during or shortly after, but if they don't, it is a good idea if the simulator has the facility to inform the trainee of precisely what it is they did wrong.

One of the best examples of how surgery got face validity appraisal wrong is the MIST VR simulator reviewed briefly in Chap. 2. When this virtual reality simulator (or more accurately, emulator) was introduced into the market in the late 1990s, it was widely dismissed by the surgical community. It was probably dismissed because at that time it looked and behaved nothing like the stereotypical image that most of the surgical community had about surgical simulation. The preconceptions that the surgical community had about simulation derived from information on simulation in the aviation industry. MIST VR did not attempt to simulate the look and feel of realistic tissues. It also had only a limited number of instruments that trainees could use during the procedure and the simulations of these instruments looked almost cartoon-like. The reasons why MIST VR looked like it did at that time were sound; desktop computing simply did not have the processing capacity at that time to render volumetric tissues in real time. What the developers went for instead was training the appropriate hand-eye coordination to perform one of the gold standard laparoscopic surgical procedures, i.e., laparoscopic cholecystectomy. Despite being dismissed by the surgical community, MIST VR remains the best validated surgical simulator in medicine today. This validation includes the demonstration that training on MIST VR to a quantitatively defined level of proficiency improved intraoperative performance (Gallagher et al. 1999, 2004; Gallagher and Satava 2002; Seymour et al. 2002; Winder et al. 2004).

> *Content Validity:* [*def*: an estimate of the validity of a testing instrument based on a detailed examination of the contents of the test items]. The evaluation is carried out by reviewing each item to determine whether it is appropriate to the test and by assessing the overall cohesiveness of the test items, such as whether the test contains the steps and skills that are used in a procedure. Establishing content validity is also a largely subjective operation and relies on the judgments of experts concerning the relevance of the materials used.

Content validity requires more rigorous assessments than face validity. Content validity should assess whether the information being trained or taught as part of the simulation is appropriate and correct. For example, it would be entirely inappropriate to construct a simulation that trains junior surgeons to perform a common surgical procedure using an uncommon method. The simulation should provide a reference procedure, which should be performed in a way that is widely agreed among the surgical community. This may change as more advanced and more complicated simulations come to the market. But most simulations that are currently available have been devised for surgeons and physicians in training. Medicine as a whole has done a particularly good job in developing consensus around the content of national courses that are to be delivered for training purposes. This has usually been done by national professional bodies, and has been mostly concerned with published information, either in book form or online. The contents of simulations that are currently on the market have been devised largely by collaborations between a company that has developed the simulation and the surgeons or physicians that have been most appropriate to advise on the development of the simulation project and possibly a medical device manufacturer. We believe that this is probably an unsatisfactory state of affairs and professional bodies should become more involved in helping to shape how simulations look, feel, behave and perform. National professional bodies are probably concerned that if they dictate what simulations should look like, they will be responsible for paying for it, in part at least. This almost certainly is what will happen, as it is a logical development of simulation training that is owned (in part at least) by the national professional bodies that are responsible for training and credentialing. Currently there is a free for all, and it has been more by accident rather than design that no major medical adverse events have been associated with a simulator. However, this is an event that is waiting to happen. All it will take for this scenario to happen is the development of a bad simulation for the use or delivery of a new medical device that trains inappropriate or dangerous behavior. On the face of it (to non simulation subject experts), the simulator looks like it will train the appropriate behavior and is therefore approved for training purposes. This same simulator is then used as part of an FDA or CE agreed educational and training package for a clinical trial involving a new surgical device or instrument. A cohort of subjects are trained on the simulator, they acquire bad habits or dangerous behaviors which they then replicate in the operating room or catheterization laboratory which results in a number of adverse clinical events before the trial can be stopped.

We have considerable sympathy for the simulation device manufacturers and developers, because once national professional bodies become involved in the regulation and development of simulation, progress will almost certainly be slowed. However, what the companies may wish to do is to charge the national professional societies for their development time and not just for project milestones. This may have the effect of encouraging the national societies to be more expeditious in project development. We are not sure over what time frame these developments will happen. What we are certain of is that the current setup is probably not acceptable. Currently, the development of content for a new simulation is guided by a group of procedure enthusiasts (surgical/medical), device experts and the simulation company. This group may or may not have expertise in curriculum development and learning theory and practice, but it almost certainly will not have expertise in the development and use of metrics. Whilst it is important how the simulator looks and feels it is essential that it has appropriate metrics. A really nice simulator without metrics is nothing more than a fancy video game!

Whilst there are no hard and fast rules as to the optimal composition of the team which should be responsible for the development of simulation content, there are a number of individuals who are essential. Essential members of the team are the simulation developers, who will know what expertise they possess as a group and the constraints and capabilities of the technology. The next *group* of essential members of this team are the physicians/surgeons. These individuals need to be very experienced (not necessarily expert) in using the device or performing the procedure for which they are developing the simulation. There is no required ideal number, only it should be more than one and less than a "committee" (probably between three and five is about right). The next essential member of this team is a behavioral scientist, who understands human factors as they apply to medical procedures, behavior definition and metric construction. This group should also contain expertise on curriculum design and validation. An essential component of this working group is that they have an excellent and open working relationship. The process of optimal simulation development is probably best guided by the expression "do what you can when you can". This will definitely mean compromise by almost every member of the group in terms of what and how they want to achieve. However, what must not be compromised is allowing something to seep into the development which might compromise patient safety. This group should be careful not to get delayed or sidetracked by issues that are not solvable in the near future. For example, physicians may insist that the simulator delivers veridical haptic feedback whilst the developers realize that this engineering simply is not possible. A good compromise might be that information about haptic forces is delivered via another sensory modality such as a visually or an auditory stimulus. A simulator does not have to be perfect in every detail to be more effective, efficient and safer than what is currently available for training purposes. If it meets none of these criteria at the outset, the project is doomed to failure.

> *Construct Validity:* [*def*: a set of procedures for evaluating a testing instrument based on the degree to which the test items identify the quality, ability or trait it was designed to measure]. As more traits or performance qualities are identified, construct validity must be updated. A common example is the ability of an assessment tool to differentiate experts and novices performing a given task.

Construct validity is probably best summarized by the question "are we measuring or assessing what we think we're measuring?" Construct validity is a type of validation that is based on the accumulation of evidence from numerous studies using the instrument or device being evaluated. A single study may be conducted with the goal of assessing the construct validity of a simulator. However, this demonstration alone is insufficient to conclude that construct validity of the device has been unequivocally demonstrated. If the results of this study are reliable and valid, it is simply a matter of time before they are replicated. Construct validity studies are some of the first studies to be completed with a simulation device to demonstrate that the performance of novices and experts or individuals' very experienced in performing the procedure on real patients can be distinguished by their performance. This evidence may be as crude as the finding that novices simply could not complete the procedure, or complete it safely to the more sophisticated metric distinctions between the quality of performance by the experts and novices. The former information is of interest, but probably not of much assistance for designing an optimal training curriculum. The latter, of metric-based distinctions between performances, is what should guide training. As discussed in Chap. 4, an essential component of efficient and effective training is feedback.

One of the very attractive features of simulation technology is that it affords the opportunity to provide this type of feedback in a form that is controllable by the trainer through the simulation platform. This feedback mirrors and augments what the trainee would get in the real world but allows for it to be compressed into meaningful learning chunks. It thus facilitates in a very powerful way the efficiency and effectiveness of learning complex procedural skills for the practice of medicine in an environment that is risk free for patients. Construct validity information can also be very useful in the operational definition of proficiency. Proficiency-based progression in skills training is still a relatively new concept in surgical training. As we shall see in Chap. 8 proficiency definition benchmarks are important to get right, because if this definition is too stringent the trainee will never reach the proficiency level. If the level is set too low, trainees will struggle to demonstrate transfer of training to clinical results, or predictive validity. That is why proficiency definitions are established on a small number of performance metrics that are highly predictive of performance. For example, in the original VR to OR study using MIST VR, only two performance metrics were used in the definition of proficiency, i.e., error and diathermy scores (Seymour et al. 2002). Although a number of construct validation studies have been conducted on the MIST VR metrics, only two of the possible six performance metrics were used in the operational definition of proficiency. Instrument errors and economy of diathermy were used because the researchers were attempting to train safe, effective and efficient use of two surgical instruments to dissect the gallbladder from the liver bed. Furthermore, construct validation studies had shown that both of these metrics were very powerful predictors of level of skill (Gallagher et al. 2001; Gallagher and Satava 2002; Winder et al. 2004). These metrics distinguished between surgeons of different levels of laparoscopic experience not only in terms of overall performance, but also in terms of performance consistency. The results of these studies showed that more experienced surgeons performed better consistently in comparison to less experienced and novice laparoscopic surgeons. This type of information based on quantitative data is invaluable in constructing the definition of proficiency.

Concurrent Validity: [*def*: an evaluation in which the relationship between the test scores and the scores on another instrument purporting to measure the same construct are related]. This would be used when introducing a new assessment tool to replace a pre-existing "gold standard" assessment tool.

Concurrent Validity can be said to have been demonstrated if there is a high concordance between two tests that purport to measure the same thing. For example, we would expect a surgeon who is very experienced in laparoscopic procedures to perform well on a laparoscopic virtual reality simulator. We would assume that laparoscopic surgery and virtual reality simulations of laparoscopic surgery elicit the same human factors in the performance of the tasks. One of the problems that many simulations encounter is the discordance between observed, objectively assessed performance on the simulator and the reported performance of surgeons in the operating room. When this situation has occurred the surgeon has invariably blamed the simulator. However, we are not sure that this is a valid conclusion. In a study conducted at the American College of Surgeons Clinical Congress in 2003,

210 experienced laparoscopic surgeons participated. All of the surgeons were required to complete a very simple virtual reality task and an almost identical task in a box trainer. Both types of tasks were repeated twice. Test subjects were allowed two trials on each task because the researchers were not particularly interested in the learning curve on each task. What they were interested in was the correlation between two almost identical tasks, one real-world task and the other a virtual task. The surprise finding from this study was that of the 210 experienced, practicing laparoscopic surgeons assessed, 15 of them could complete none of the tasks. It was also found that between 2% and 12% of the surgeons performed more than two standard deviations from the mean. Some of the surgeon's performance was *20* standard deviations from the mean (Gallagher and Smith 2003). Overall, 10% of the surgeons tested performed the task significantly worse than the group's average performance.

These results initially shocked the researchers as they had difficulty accounting for the proportion of surgeons who had performed so poorly. However, on reflection, the surgeons' performance had been assessed with a well-validated simulator (i.e., MIST VR) and a simple laparoscopic task which they had the opportunity to practice. The simulator outcomes were difficult to dismiss because it had just been shown in a prospective, randomized, blinded clinical trial to improve performance in the operating room. It is difficult to say whether the surgeons who performed badly on the assessment at the American College of Surgeons meeting also performed badly in the operating room. What we can say is that we have made similar observations to the ACS study. In studies that we have been involved in, some apparently well-respected surgeons performed poorly on the simulator. In the aviation industry this would not really be an issue. Their attitude is very simple, i.e., they would accept the results from the simulation. In surgery the opposite is true. A number of years ago, one of us (AGG) was trying to convince a group of Swedish surgeons visiting Atlanta, Georgia, about the contrast between subjective appraisal and objective assessment of surgical performance. In an informal demonstration each surgeon was asked to tie their best surgical knot using an open surgical setup. All of the knots tied by the surgeons were objectively assessed using a methodology that has already been validated for the assessment of laparoscopic knot quality (Van Sickle et al. 2005). All of the surgeons reported that they were confident that they had tied very good surgical knots which would not slip. Each surgeon observed as their knot was assessed with the tensiometer. Despite having deliberately tied surgical knots that would not slip, 25% of them did. They admitted that they found these results indisputable. Studies on the concurrent validity of simulations are extremely rare; however, we believe that they will become much more common as soon as the objective assessment of technical skills becomes a widespread exercise. We will discuss these points further in Chaps. 11 and 12.

Discriminate Validity: [*def*: an evaluation that reflects the extent to which the scores generated by the assessment tool actually correlate with factors with which they should. This is a much more sophisticated analysis which requires that those factors which should correlate highly actually do, as well as those factors which should correlate poorly do so. An example of this would be an assessment tool that could differentiate ability levels within a group with similar experience, such as discriminating abilities of all the surgical trainees in post-graduate year 1 (PGY1).

As medicine and medical procedures come to rely more and more on image guided technology tests, that can discriminate between the types of individuals capable of learning these methods must be identified. This type of testing will become more important in helping to guide graduating medical students about which type of procedural medicine their skills and aptitudes may be best suited. This type of testing is common in high-risk, high-skill industries such as aviation. Image guided interventions make greater perceptual, cognitive and psychomotor demands than more traditional approaches to interventions. These perceptual, cognitive and psychomotor abilities are not equally distributed across the population, even among a population as highly selected as medical students. As we have discussed in Chaps. 3 and 4, the greater the ability, aptitude or skill of the individual in a particular domain (e.g., spatial ability) the lower the cognitive effort required to perform well on the task. These findings have profound implications for the selection of individuals for training in image guided procedures such as laparoscopic surgery, interventional cardiology, interventional radiology and anesthetics. Peripheral or regional anesthesia will become the anesthetic method of choice for most medical procedures. This type of procedure requires very different technical skills of the anesthetist. This means that in many cases, the anesthetist will have to navigate a cannulae or catheter and wire to a particular nerve, under image guidance and maintain anesthesia on that nerve throughout the procedure. Not all individuals who are accepted into medical school will be capable of learning to perform image guided procedures. Medicine needs to be able to identify who these individuals are and guide them toward medical careers that their skills are better suited to. Some preliminary work has been done in this area. For example, it has been found that psychometric tests to assess the ability of the individual to reconstruct 3-D from 2-D information correlate very well with performance on a number of laparoscopic surgical tasks (Gallagher et al. 2003b). It has also been found that performance on psychometric tests that assess perceptual and visual-spatial ability predict the duration of training (e.g., number of training trials) required on a flexible endoscopy virtual-reality simulator to reach proficiency (Ritter et al. 2006). It is unlikely that disciplines such as surgery will have to develop from first principles bespoke human factor psychometric tests which will help them to discriminate between those they should select into training in areas such as minimally invasive surgery. However, caution is advised in choosing the tests, and where possible, it should be data driven.

Predictive Validity: [*def*: the extent to which the scores on a test are predictive of actual performance]. An assessment tool used to measure surgical skills will have predictive validity if it selects who will and who will not perform actual surgical tasks well (Reber and Reber 1985).

While all of these validation strategies have merit, construct and predictive validity are the most likely to provide clinically meaningful and useful data in the short term. The other validities focus upon the assessment of the training or test rather than upon clinical outcomes. All of the validation strategies are important in the construction of a test for high-stakes assessment; however, currently there is no mandated requirement for such a test. There is definitely a distinct need for improved training strategies in all types of surgery, and particularly for MIS. These skills have proved much harder to train and teach than was originally expected, and the performance of advanced MIS currently requires most surgeons in training to undergo additional training. The most important question to ask is "does this device or training strategy train or assess the skills it is supposed to"? This question may be partially answered in the skills laboratory, but can only be conclusively answered in the operating room (OR). New training strategies should be conclusively shown to improve performance in the OR (i.e. establishing predictive validity based upon clinical performance) before they are widely implemented.

It is still not accepted by most medical practitioners that simulation training improves clinical performance and that the efficacy of simulation training remains unproven. In one systematic review of the literature on simulation training, the authors concluded that computer simulation generally showed better results than no training at all (and than physical trainer/model training in one RCT), but was not convincingly superior to standard training (such as surgical drills) or video simulation, particularly when assessed by operative performance (Sutherland et al. 2006). It should be noted that when the reviewers described the control group as "no training", strictly speaking, that was inaccurate. All of the subjects included in the clinical validation studies were enrolled on a surgical training programme at the time of the assessment tests. This means that the simulation trained group's performance was compared to the performance of trainees in the traditional training programme. Calling the control group a "no training" condition is misleading. The other point about this comparison is that the simulation training group need not necessarily have performed better to be judged a success. All that the researchers had to demonstrate was that simulation training was at least equivalent to traditional training. In fact, simulation training has been shown to significantly improve intra-operative performance (Ahlberg et al. 2007; Grantcharov et al. 2004; Seymour et al. 2002). Researchers investigating the predictive validity of simulation training for improved intra-operative performance should be mindful of what they are trying to demonstrate. The goal of their research efforts should be to demonstrate that the training programme they have devised is at least equivalent to traditional training methods.

When simulation is better accepted by the medical community other kinds of predictive validity will be used. One of these has already been instigated by the FDA. In 2004, the FDA was being asked by a number of medical devices companies to approve a new treatment for the prevention of stroke, i.e., carotid artery stenting with embolic protection. There was good clinical evidence that this treatment was superior at preventing strokes in high-risk patients than the traditional surgical treatment of endarterectomy (Yadav et al. 2004). A number of different clinical groups wanted to perform the treatment using these new devices but each possessed a different skill set. The interventional cardiologists had extensive catheter and wire skills but limited experience in the carotid vessels; vascular surgeons had extensive experience operating in the carotid arteries, but variable catheter and wire skills.

Other groups who sought to do the procedure were interventional radiologists, interventional neuro-radiologists and neurosurgeons. In a landmark decision, the FDA concluded that all of these groups of physicians could perform the procedure as long as they demonstrated proficiency on a high fidelity, full procedural, full physics, virtual reality simulator (Gallagher and Cates 2004a). This decision meant that it was the individual physician's performance on the simulator that predicted whether they were allowed to perform the procedure on a patient or not. This kind of evidence-based decision making, as it relates to the skilled performance of medical practitioners, by governmental organizations will become more common. We also believe that performance on simulators will become an integral part of the credentialing process.

High fidelity, full physics, virtual reality simulators currently have the capability of simulating patient specific anatomy which allows the physician to practice the procedure on the simulator before carrying it out on the real patient (Cates et al. 2007). The potential of this facility for validating new interventional devices and new procedures is enormous. In the very near future we will see this facility used in the development of a relatively new treatment for acute ischemic stroke due to the acute large vessel intracranial occlusion, i.e., endovascular mechanical thrombectomy. Training in the procedural skills for every area of medicine exposes the patient to some risk. However, all intracranial interventions expose the patient to extremely high risk of adverse events, even by fully trained highly skilled interventionalists. Endovascular mechanical thrombectomy is probably one of the highest risk of procedures that can be performed and there are no training models other than cadavers and the real (very ill) patient. Virtual reality simulation on a full physics platform provides the opportunity for the physician to get high fidelity real-time training for procedures such as endovascular mechanical thrombectomy. This means that they can go into the operating room or Cath. Lab. very well prepared. This facility could potentially serve another purpose, helping the physician decide whether or not they should do the procedure on the patient. In a clinical trial of an endovascular mechanical thrombectomy device, it has been shown that the mortality rate was 34% (Smith et al. 2008). In ideal circumstances, the patient would be admitted to hospital and scanned to confirm that they had had a stroke due to a large vessel intracranial occlusion. The data from the CT scan could then be downloaded to the simulator and formatted and volumetric rendered so as to allow the operating physician the opportunity to rehearse the procedure in the simulator whilst waiting on the patient to be prepared and transported to the angiography suite. If they were unable to complete the most challenging aspects of the procedure with a high probability of safety on the simulator, they almost certainly would not attempt the procedure on the real patient. In this way the simulator becomes a tool for predicting the likelihood of success of the procedure and thus aids decision-making about whether or not to operate.

The types of validation studies that have been conducted on simulation models are fairly basic. The range and number of validation studies will expand enormously as leaders in the surgical and medical communities become more comfortable and assured about the potential, strengths and limitations of simulation technologies. However, these validation studies must also demonstrate that the derived data are reliable.

Reliability: [*def*: a generic term to cover all aspects of the dependability of a measurement device or test]. The essential notion is consistency, or the extent to which the assessment tool yields the same results when used repeatedly under similar conditions. Specific methods have been devised to establish the reliability of any assessment tool. Two common methods are the *split-half* method and the *test–retest* method. For the split-half method, test items from a single test occasion are split and then the internal consistency of the assessed items is calculated using a range of statistical methods. The test–retest method determines the reliability of a test by administering it on two or more occasions. Both methods are used to generate a reliability coefficient, which is a quantitative expression of the reliability of the tests and ranges between 0 and 1. A good reliability coefficient has been approximated as values ≥ 0.8. Although lower values (i.e., ≤ 0.7) have been reported they are generally frowned on in the behavioral sciences. Other useful measures of reliability such as "alpha", "coefficient alpha", "Cronbach's alpha" or "internal consistency" are relatively easily generated with statistical software packages. Reliability of a test is simply a statistic that can be calculated from *any* set of data. A widely used rule of thumb is that a test should not be used if it has an alpha value <0.7 (see below) and it should not be used for important decisions about an individual unless the alpha value >0.9.

Interpretation of Reliability Coefficients

While validation seems to be reasonably understood by the surgical community, issues pertaining to reliability interpretation appear to be less well understood. This issue is important because a person who does not understand what test reliability means may let their general evaluation data from a test or training device be influenced too strongly about statements of its reliability. The word "reliably" as used in our common speech carries favorable connotations, for example, a reliable (*good*) man, a reliable (*upstanding*) firm, a reliable (*worthwhile*) product. Researchers and clinicians are also likely to conclude that a reliable test is *ipso facto* a good test for any purpose they have in mind. Such erroneous conclusions can have serious implications as measuring something reliably tells us very little. To interpret reliability we need to know more about what the test actually does measure especially the outcome of validation efforts.

Another problem with describing the reliability of a test is that it is frequently interpreted as the amount of agreement between two measures (e.g., two testing occasions or two raters). It is not. Correlation coefficients are often confused with reliability coefficients; however, correlation coefficients are no more than measures of *association*. Association simply infers that there is some relationship between observations; agreement implies a sameness or equal value. Therefore, citing a correlation coefficient as a quantitative measure of agreement is at best misleading and at worst inaccurate. There are a number of reasons for this. The first is that a correlation turns out to be higher if there is a great deal of range or spread in the scores of the group on which it is based than it does if the members of the group score closer

Table 7.1 Hypothetical (data set 1) from two raters on a 5-point Likert scale on the performance of 12 residents

Residents name	Rater 1	Rater 2	Rater 1 deviations from mean	Rater 2 deviations from mean	Product of deviations	Absolute agreement between raters
R1	5	4	1.30	1.30	1.69	No
R2	4	3	0.30	0.30	0.09	No
R3	3	2	−0.70	−0.70	0.49	No
R4	2	1	−1.70	−1.70	2.89	No
R5	4	3	0.30	0.30	0.09	No
R6	5	4	1.30	1.30	1.69	No
R7	4	3	0.30	0.30	0.09	No
R8	3	2	−0.70	−0.70	0.49	No
R9	2	1	−1.70	−1.70	2.89	No
R10	5	4	1.30	1.30	1.69	No
R11	4	3	0.30	0.30	0.09	No
R12	3	2	−0.70	−0.70	0.49	No
Mean	3.67	2.67			1.06	
SD	1.07	1.07			1.07	

together. Thus when interpreting reliability of a test or device one should ensure that the two groups of scores have about the same amount of variability.

A second reason is that a correlation coefficient will always be greater than the reliability coefficient. This may be partly overcome by looking at the r^2 of the correlation, which gives the percentage of variance shared by the two variables in question. For example, a correlation of $r=0.8$ accounts for 64% of the variance for the two variables. However, this again gives no indication of the amount of agreement. Another approach is to look at the concordance between the two variables. *Concordance* in general terms means agreement, harmony or the degree, which a pair shares. In statistical terms, concordance coefficient, usually abbreviated W, is an index of the divergence of the observed agreement in rankings from the maximum possible agreement. This statistic is also known as *Kendall's coefficient of concordance*. The coefficient of concordance, W, expresses the degree of agreement or association on a scale from 1 showing complete agreement and 0 indicates no agreement. Consider the following hypothetical example for the data presented in Table 7.1.

The first three columns show names of 12 residents and the scores of two independent raters. The raters are rating the resident's performance on a 5-point Likert-scale. The means and standard deviations for each rater are also given. From the data it can be seen that both ratings are very similar and consistent, i.e., Rater 1 always rates performance 1-point better than Rater 2. This consistency is reflected in the correlation between the two scores, $r=1.0$. However, although both ratings are consistent they have not "absolutely agreed" on the scores of a single resident but this is not reflected in the correlation coefficient. Nor is this lack of absolute agreement reflected in the observed internal consistency coefficient alpha (or α) where $\alpha=1.0$. The coefficient of concordance for the same data gives a more accurate picture where $W=0.195$. From this simple example it can be seen how statistical correlation may be mistaken for estimates of agreement. However, it is possible to derive a reliability coefficient called the *standard error of measurement* (s.e.m.) from knowledge of the internal consistency (alpha) of the test and the standard deviations of the test scores (Cooper 2002).

Columns four and five give the deviations from the mean score for Rater 1 and 2 and column six gives the product of these deviations, the mean and standard deviations of these deviations. Thus the formula for the standard error is

$\text{s.e.m.} = \text{sd} * \sqrt{1-\alpha}$	$= \text{s.e.m.} = 1.07 * \sqrt{1-1}$
	$= \text{s.e.m.} = 1.07 * 0 = 0$
	$\text{s.e.m.} = 0$

The larger the s.e.m. the more reliable the data and vice versa. This calculation gives a more accurate reflection of data in terms of absolute agreement. In the example data that we cite it could be argued that absolute agreement may not be that important because generally the two raters are on the same pole of the scale; however, this may not always be the case. This is one of the major difficulties of using Likert-type scales. Another problem with Likert sales of more than two points is the difficulty in training raters to agree >80% (IRR of $r=0.80$) of the time which is the accepted quality benchmark for inter-rater reliability assessment.

The behavioral approach to the assessment of two raters reliability takes a much more rigorous approach and as a statistical method is very straightforward and systematic. It is also well developed and validated in a wide variety of settings and easily applicable to almost any assessment situation. This approach simply asks if the raters agreed or disagreed on the occurrence/non-occurrence of an event. These events are usually scored from unambiguous event definitions (Chap. 5) and the metric used to assess the statistical quality of that methodology is known as inter-rater reliability (IRR). Although it may look similar to a correlation coefficient and is scored from 0 (*no agreement*) between raters to 1 (*total agreement*) between raters, it is a very unforgiving metric. Inter-rater reliability means the degree or proportion of times to which two or more independent observers agree in their ratings of a test subject's behavior. It is normally calculated:

$$\frac{\text{Observation event agreements}}{\text{Total number of observations}}$$

Using the formulae cited above the IRR between the two raters in Table 7.1 is 0 (i.e., agreements (0)/total observations (12)=0). The two raters have not agreed on one score for any of the 12 observations! Even though R1 consistently scored one point higher than R2 on every measurement (the association or correlation coefficient=1), there was absolutely no agreement (reliability coefficient=0) between the two raters. Inter-rater reliability demands agreement, not association. To demonstrate IRR, some agreement is introduced into the dataset (Table 7.2).

Table 7.2 Hypothetical (data set 2) from two raters on a 5-point Likert scale on the performance of 12 residents

Residents name	Rater 1	Rater 2	Rater 1 deviations from mean	Rater 2 deviations from mean	Product of deviations	Absolute agreement between raters
R1	5	*5*	1.33	2.08	2.77	Yes
R2	4	*4*	0.33	1.08	0.36	Yes
R3	3	*3*	−0.67	0.08	−0.05	Yes
R4	2	1	−1.67	−1.92	3.21	No
R5	4	3	0.33	0.08	0.03	No
R6	5	4	1.33	1.08	1.44	No
R7	4	3	0.33	0.08	0.03	No
R8	3	2	−0.67	−0.92	0.62	No
R9	2	1	−1.67	−1.92	3.21	No
R10	5	4	1.33	1.08	1.44	No
R11	4	3	0.33	0.08	0.03	No
R12	3	2	−0.67	−0.92	0.62	No
Mean	3.67	2.92			1.14	
SD	1.07	1.24			1.27	

Table 7.2 presents essentially the same set of data as Table 7.1, except the first three residents scores for Rater 2 have been replaced so that the scores agree with those of Rater 1. The same calculations as in the previous example are re-computed and found that for this data set $r=0.934$, $\alpha=0.965$ and $W=0.1024$. Thus the s.e.m. can be calculated

s.e.m. = sd * $\sqrt{1-\alpha}$	= s.e.m. = 1.27 * $\sqrt{1-0.965}$
	= s.e.m. = 1.27 * 0.035 = 0.237
	s.e.m. = 0.237

The IRR for the behavioral method is fairly similar to the s.e.m. method (i.e., agreements (3)/total observations (12) = 0.25). So we can see that as agreement between raters improves so do the s.e.m and IRR.

How Reliable Is the Reliability Assessment?

This problem with interpretation of IRR has been commented on before (Gallagher et al. 2003a; Kennedy et al. 2008). Likert-type scales such as Objective Structured Assessment of Technical Skills (OSATS) (Martin et al. 1997) have frequently been reported as a superior method of assessment methods in comparison to check-list scales. We do not think that the matter is that simple and we are aware of a number of significant problems with Likert scales.

Consider the following hypothetical example for the data presented in Table 7.3. In the table are the hypothetical data from seven trainees who have been assessed by

Table 7.3 Hypothetical scores from seven trainees who have been assessed by two examiners "A" and "B" on the OSATS traditional 5-point Likert scale (1–5)

	Example 1		Example 2		Example 3		Example 4		Example 5		Example 6		Example 7	
OSATS Assessment variable	"A"	"B"	"A"	"B"	"A"	"B"	"A"	"B"	"A"	"B"	"A"	"B"	"A"	"B"
Respect for tissue	5	5	5	5	5	5	5	5	*5*	*4*	*5*	*1*	*2*	*4*
Time and motion	5	5	5	5	5	5	5	5	*5*	*4*	*5*	*1*	*2*	*3*
Instrument handling	4	4	4	4	4	4	4	4	*4*	*3*	*4*	*2*	*3*	*5*
Knowledge of instruments	4	4	4	4	4	4	4	4	*4*	*3*	*4*	*2*	*3*	*5*
Use of assistants	4	4	4	4	4	4	4	4	*4*	*3*	*1*	*4*	*4*	*2*
Flow of operation and forward planning	3	3	3	3	3	3	*3*	*2*	*3*	*2*	*1*	*4*	*3*	*2*
Knowledge of specific procedure	5	5	5	5	5	5	*5*	*4*	*5*	*4*	*2*	*5*	*5*	*3*
Quality of the final product	4	4	*5*	*4*	*5*	*2*	*5*	*4*	*5*	*4*	*2*	*5*	*5*	*3*
Σ	34	34	35	34	35	32	35	32	35	27	24	24	27	27
Mean	4.25	4.25	4.38	4.25	4.38	4	4.38	4.00	4.38	3.38	3	3	3.38	3.38
SD	0.71	0.71	0.74	0.71	0.74	1.1	0.74	0.93	0.74	0.74	1.7	1.7	1.19	1.19
Corr.	$r=1.0$		$r=0.88$		$r=0.36$		$r=0.83$		$r=1.0$		$r=-0.9$		$r=-0.32$	
IRR	IRR=100%		IRR=88%		IRR=88%		IRR=62%		IRR=0%		IRR=0%		IRR=0%	

two examiners “A” and “B” on the traditional 5-point Likert scale (1–5). We have included an eighth measurement category (i.e., “Quality of the final product”) to the global rating scale which validation evidence has been reported on by the group at Imperial (Hance et al. 2005).

Traditionally the vast majority of users of OSATS report a correlation coefficient or an Alpha coefficient as their measure of inter-rater reliability. The problems with this approach which we have outlined above are also demonstrated in Table 7.3. Example 1 represents the ideal where the two raters “A” and “B” agree consistently on their rating of the examinee across all eight assessment criteria. This provides a reliability coefficient of $r=1.0$ as assessed by Pearson Product Moment Correlation Coefficient, $r=1$ for Cranach’s Alpha. These data also provide an Inter-rater Reliability of 1.0 or 100% agreement as assessed by the more traditional method (Martin et al. 1993).

Using the formulae cited above, the IRR between the two raters in Example 1, Table 7.3 is 1! (i.e., agreements (8)/total observations (8) = 1) indicating total agreement between the examiners. In Example 2 there is very good agreement between the examiners with only one point difference on the last assessment variable. This agreement is reflected in the total scores from the two examiners, the correlation between their score ($r=0.88$) and their IRR = 0.88 (or 88% agreement). In Example 3 there is also only one disagreement between the examiners but the difference on this variable is 3 points. In contrast to Example 2 this difference has a very large effect on correlation estimates of reliability ($r=0.36$) but only a modest impact on the more traditional method of estimating reliability, i.e., IRR = 0.88 (88% agreement). Although the difference between the total scores for examiners “A” and “B” is the same for Example 4 as it is for Example 5 (35 vs. 32), rather than disagreeing on just one assessment variable by 3 points they disagree on three variables by 1 point each. In contrast to Example 3 this has very little impact on the reliability correlation coefficient ($r=0.83$) but a much larger impact on the more traditional measure (IRR = 0.62, (62% agreement)).

Example 5 presents a very different picture. Although the examiners did not agree on one single assessment variable score, as reflected in total scores a correlation estimate of reliability indicates the contrary ($r=1.0$) whilst the more traditional estimate gives a more accurate picture, i.e., IRR = 0. In Examples 6 and 7, despite not agreeing on a single score for either of the two subjects the total score for both examiners is the same. In Example 6 the correlation estimate of reliability is a high negative correlation ($r=-0.9$) and a low negative correlation for Example 7 ($r=-0.32$) despite the fact that the total scores for the subject in Example 7 are higher than in Example 6. The more traditional measure of reliability is zero for both assessments (IRR = 0). The important thing to note about Examples 6 and 7 is that the total score of examiners “A” and “B” is the same (Example 6, $\Sigma=24$ and Example 7, $\Sigma=27$) but these scores were derived by entirely different performances on the eight assessment variables.

The assessment of reliability within-subject is a difficult task, as the seven examples we have just given clearly demonstrate. However, a further problem seems to be associated with the use of data generated from Likert-type assessment scales

Table 7.4 Hypothetical scores from one anesthesia trainee who has been assessed by two examiners "A" and "B" on the 6-point Likert scale DOPS scale (where 1 and 2 = below expectations, 3 = borderline, 4 = meets expectations and 5 and 6 = above expectations)

Direct Observation of Procedural Skill (DOPS) anesthesia	Example 8	
	Resident 1	Resident 1
Assessment variable	Assessor "A"	Assessor "B"
Demonstrates understanding of indications, relevant anatomy, technique of procedure	*4*	*5*
Obtains informed consent	5	4
Demonstrates appropriate pre-procedure preparation	2	6
Demonstrates situation awareness	5	5
Aseptic technique	*6*	*3*
Technical ability	*6*	*2*
Seeks help where appropriate	*6*	*6*
Post procedure management	*6*	*6*
Communication skills	*3*	*6*
Consideration for patient	*4*	*5*
Overall performance	*6*	*5*
Σ	53	53
Mean	4.82	4.82
SD	1.40	1.33
Corr.	$r = -0.5$	
IRR	0.27 (27% agreement)	

http://www.bartsandthelondon.nhs.uk/docs/DOPs.pdf

such as OSATS. The data from the seven examples in Table 7.3 will serve to demonstrate the problem. There was a wide range of agreements by examiners "A" and "B" from zero to 100%. However, what some researchers appear to be doing is using the total score from examiners "A" and "B" for each subject as their dependant variables for the assessment of reliability rather that their true estimate of reliability (Bann et al. 2003; Khan et al. 2007). The true estimate of inter-rater reliability for the seven examples is the mean of the reliability estimates which gives a value of 0.41 for estimates based on a correlation coefficient and 0.48 based on an IRR estimate. What some researchers appear to be doing in their assessment of inter-rater reliability is calculating reliability based on the total score for each subject by examiners "A" and "B". The reliability coefficient based on correlating the scores of examiner "A" with examiner "B" for the seven subjects is 0.781 and 0.871 for Cranach's Alpha. This gives a very misleading impression about how reliably the assessors were in applying the scale to the seven hypothetical assessment candidates.

Compounding potential problems with reliability estimation that we have already identified in Table 7.3 are further potential problems which are demonstrated in Table 7.4. In Example 8 a trainee/resident is being assessed by examiners "A" and "B". Despite only agreeing on three assessment areas both examiners efforts have come up with the same total score, i.e., 53. This means that the trainees, mean score = 4.82 would locate them on the DOPS scale as "Meets expectations" (borderline "Above expectations"). However, both examiners arrived at this score by very different paths. This is important because examiner "A" has rated the trainee as "Borderline" or "Below expectations" for Aseptic technique and Technical ability, both of which are of particular importance for the practice of medicine. No indication of this disagreement by the examiners is reflected in the total score but is reflected in the measures of reliability.

Inter-Rater Reliability Assessment; Group or Individual Level of Reliability?

Larsen et al. (2006, 2008, 2009) using a modified version of the OSATS Likert scale have come up with a novel way of calculating IRR. They assessed the performance of laparoscopic surgical gynecologists who were assigned to novice ($n = 8$; <10 procedures), intermediate ($n = 7$; 20–50 procedures) and expert ($n = 6$; >200 procedures) groups. Each of the surgeons performed a laparoscopic salpingectomy which was video recorded and subsequently assessed by two independent observers expert in laparoscopic gynecological surgery (i.e., had performed >2000 laparoscopic gynecological procedures). The video-taped surgical procedures were assessed on the traditional 5-point OSATS Likert scale (score range min. 5 to max. 35). They were also assessed on five other items which were also scored on an OSATS like Likert scale with the exact same score range. One of the items (item 10) was subsequently dropped from the analysis due to unavoidable procedural performance differences between surgeons, i.e., some of them simply did not do step 10 in their normal clinical practice. The authors then applied the formulae that we have given above (agreements/total number of observations) to assess IRR, with one modification. The calculation of IRR is meant to be done at the individual level, but Larsen et al. (2008) calculated it at the group level. For example, they had eight novices who were assessed on nine different OSATS-like assessment items, total number of observations = 72 and there were 14 disagreements. This gives an IRR = 0.806 (i.e., $72 - 14 \div 72 = 0.806$) which is above the acceptable 0.8 level. This seems on the surface to be a perfectly acceptable method of calculating IRR. However, IRR is meant to be calculated at the individual level for a number of very good reasons. These are probably best construed as objectivity, transparency and fairness checks for the *individuals* being assessed. The data presented by Larsen et al. are for the overall IRR of the group and they give no indication of individual IRR levels. However, from the data they have supplied we can draw a number of inferences. For example, if there were 14 disagreements in 72 observations of eight candidates that means that there were on average 1.75 disagreements per candidate. However, at the analysis level of the individual, a disagreement either happened or it did not. This means that it is impossible to have 0.75 of a disagreement. In reality this would mean there were two disagreements for this individual which would mean for that individual that their IRR was <0.8 (i.e., $9 - 2 \div 9 = 0.78$) and if there was more than two disagreements for any one candidate this would mean that IRR would fall well below the accepted level (e.g., $9 - 3 \div 9 = 0.67$). It is highly likely that there were no disagreements between assessors but it is also highly likely that there were more than two disagreements between assessors for some subjects. Although it is important that the overall IRR is >0.8, it is even more important that this applies at the level of the individual assessment because if all individual assessment reach >0.8 IRR this guarantees the group result will reach this level, but not vice versa.

We are at a loss to explain why experienced researchers continue to try and invent a new way of assessing IRR when a parsimonious, tried and tested method already exists. The method proposed here, i.e., agreements/total number of observations, has been used effectively and efficiently in a number of other studies which have assessed procedural skills (Ahlberg et al. 2007; Seymour et al. 2002; Van Sickle et al. 2008). The method is easy to use and one of its major advantages is that it can be used in vivo to assess the reliability of ongoing assessments. This means that any IRR anomalies can be picked up as soon as they happen and can be investigated by the independent arbitrator of the assessment and disagreements clarified and corrected where necessary. This is an important quality assurance measure for organizations conducting an assessment for high stakes such as career progression. If there is a problem with the reliability of the assessment, it can be fixed on the day of the assessment. Discrepancies in IRR >20% can in our experience occur for a number of very straightforward reasons which include genuine disagreement between assessors on their scoring of performance; misunderstanding between raters as to precisely what it is they are supposed to score, i.e., using personal criteria rather than the operationalized definitions given by the assessment body; task failure which was taken account of differently by the two assessors and scoring performance with the wrong "mind-set". One of the challenges we continually face is convincing consultants that when they are scoring performance they must think like assessors and not trainers and score only what they see and not how they "think" the person would perform on a good day.

However, the greatest problem we see in the objective assessment of surgical performance is asking experienced surgeons to score performance that has not been well operationally defined or where there is ambiguity in the scale that they are using. This is one of the reasons that we are not strong supporters of Likert-type scales. For example, in the original OSATS scale we are not convinced that there is a uniform and global understanding and implicit definition between surgeons of what "competent use of instruments" or "efficient motion" means. Most surgeons probably have a fair idea what these concepts mean but for reliable assessments these generalizations are not acceptable. Performance to be assessed must be unambiguously defined so as to make it easy for the assessor to decide when it occurred or did not occur. Furthermore, this type of approach makes it considerably easier to establish reliable assessment behavior. This approach may take the "art" out of performance assessment and make it more scientific but it facilitates reliable assessment and minimizes the potential for legal challenges to performance assessment. As performance assessment for career progression or continuance becomes more common, we envisage that legal challenges to these assessments may become a regular occurrence. Our concern is that some of the popular assessment methods reported in the research literature do not fare well on close scrutiny.

It is for these reasons that studies purporting to assess the reliability of an assessment of procedural skills should…

(a) Conduct an inter-rater reliability assessment on each subject assessed
(b) Conduct inter-rater reliability assessments (where possible) on the day and preferable immediately after testing has been completed
(c) Only use data from subjects that reach the international standard for inter-rater reliability, i.e., IRR > 0.8
(d) Investigate IRR levels that fall below this benchmark and where possible remediate immediately
(e) Report the mean or median and standard deviation or interquartile range of IRR measures
(f) Report how many or what proportion of subjects were excluded because they failed to meet the acceptable IRR criteria.

Assessment of doctors' skills is an onerous task that must reach the current international standards. This means that not only must an assessment be valid and reliable as an overall assessment scheme, but it must also demonstrate already defined levels of inter-rater reliability at the level of the individual. Testing must be seen to be objective, and fair but also transparent. In the quest for assessment strategies of surgical performance, it is important that individuals who observe performance agree on the occurrence/non-occurrence of key behaviors. This is essential to ensure that evaluation of the desired behaviors remains consistent and is not subject to development of a single observer's bias over time. The main reasons for this are (1) assessment will only be useful if it can be achieved with some consistency, (2) if a single observer is recording performance their data may simply reflect a change in that observered definition over time, i.e., they may become biased or less stringent over time. This will become apparent very quickly with a second observer and with continuous checks on the IRR coefficient. (3) Agreement between observers is important because it tells us something about how we have defined the behavior of interest. The first step in good science is to unambiguously and parsimoniously define what is to be measured. Ultimately the ability to accurately and reliably measure performance will result in objectively proven training strategies to produce the desired level of performance.

Why should the reliability of assessment for procedural skills be treated differently from pencil and paper tests? In the former, tests are administered under the *exact* same testing conditions for everyone being tested. There are right and wrong answers on paper and pencil tests with the answers clearly specified in advance and validated with a team of experts. Indeed, procedures have been so well worked out that in some cases tests can even be scored by a computer. These standardized procedures have been set in place to minimize the extent to which subjectivity can seep into the assessment process. However, potential sources of bias in the assessment process are still not taken for granted by psychometricians who are continuously vigilant for it and systematically check for its presence. Assessment of performance such as technical skills is more prone to bias seepage than the standardized test format because of the sheer potential variability in the process. Whether the performance of an individual is being assessed in the skills laboratory or in a clinical situation, there are enormous potential sources of variation from the anatomy that a patient presents, task variability of synthetic models, time of the day that the candidate is being assessed, candidate order (e.g., primacy vs recency effect), attribution bias by the examiner (because of prior knowledge or experience of the exam candidates) and reporting bias by the examiner. The potential for bias to creep into the assessment process is enormous and that is why it is essential that every effort is made and is seen to be made to control for these sources of bias and error. It is also essential that when bias or error does occur it is picked up on at the earliest possible occasion preferably during testing where something can be done about it. If during high-stakes assessment bias or error is not discovered until after assessment has been completed, very little can be done about it other than report that it has occurred. Using correlations or coefficient alpha or other statistical methods to assess IRR will only give an overall assessment of reliability. Furthermore, this information is only available AFTER all candidates have been assessed and requires at least some statistical knowledge and access to the appropriate software. Assessment of IRR as we have suggested here, i.e., agreements/total number of observations, can be conducted by any examiner and ensures accurate information on IRR as soon as assessment has been completed on each candidate. Furthermore, if IRR for each candidate is >80% this ensures the overall "group" results will have IRR >80%. However, ensuring group IRR of >80% does not ensure the same at the level of the individual as we have demonstrated in the examples we have given in Tables 7.1–7.3.

Summary

The expansion and implementation of metric-based simulation education and training will require robust validation evidence to convince a sceptical medical community that this is a better way to prepare surgeons and other physicians for operating on patients. Validation methods have been well worked out in disciplines such as psychology and education for the best part of a century and with internationally agreed standards since the mid-1970s. The vast majority of validation studies on simulation technology have been on construct and predictive validity. As confidence and experience grows with simulation technology the range and number of validation studies will grow. These developments must be coupled with reliable assessment tools that are objective, fair and transparent. The development of robust and reliable behavioral assessment tools is relatively new to surgery and other medical disciplines but not to science and education. The concept of test or assessment reliability has been well thought out with unambiguous clarity as to what is acceptable and what is not.

In psychology and behavioral science, performance assessment inter-rater reliability, inter-rater agreement, or concordance is the degree of agreement among raters of performance. It gives a score of how much homogeneity, or consensus, there is in the ratings given by judges. It is useful in refining the tools given to human judges, for determining if a particular measurement scale or instrument is appropriate for measuring a particular variable. If various raters do not agree with an acceptable level of consistency (i.e., >80%), either the scale is defective or the raters need to be better trained or indeed retrained. On encountering studies that claim to report on validation and reliability efforts of training and assessment strategies the surgical community is advised to interpret some of these claims with caution. Some may be precisely what they claim to be, but others will not. As surgical education moves from the dogma of the past to the evidence-based world of the future, we must not discount the well-established behavioral science principles of experimental design, validation, and reliable assessment that will help us improve training and ultimately patient care.

References

Ahlberg G, Enochsson L, Gallagher AG, et al. Proficiency-based virtual reality training significantly reduces the error rate for residents during their first 10 laparoscopic cholecystectomies. *Am J Surg*. 2007;193(6):797-804.

APA. (1999). NCME (American Educational Research Association, American Psychological Association, & National Council on Measurement in Education). *Standards for educational and psychological tests*.

Bann S, Kwok KF, Lo CY, Darzi A, Wong J. Objective assessment of technical skills of surgical trainees in Hong Kong. *Br J Surg*. 2003;90(10):1294-1299.

Cates CU, Patel AD, Nicholson WJ. Use of virtual reality simulation for mission rehearsal for carotid stenting. *J Am Med Assoc*. 2007;297(3):265.

Centres R. Cholecystectomy practice transformed. *Lancet*. 1991;338(8770):789-790.

Champion HR, Gallagher AG. Surgical simulation - a 'good idea whose time has come'. *Br J Surg*. 2003;90(7):767-768.

Cooper C. *Individual Differences*. London: Arnold; 2002.

Gallagher AG, Cates CU. Approval of virtual reality training for carotid stenting: what this means for procedural-based medicine. *J Am Med Assoc*. 2004a;292(24):3024-3026.

Gallagher AG, Cates CU. Virtual reality training for the operating room and cardiac catheterisation laboratory. *Lancet*. 2004b;364(9444):1538-1540.

Gallagher AG, Satava RM. Virtual reality as a metric for the assessment of laparoscopic psychomotor skills. Learning curves and reliability measures. *Surg Endosc*. 2002;16(12):1746-1752.

Gallagher AG, Smith CD. From the operating room of the present to the operating room of the future. Human-factors lessons learned from the minimally invasive surgery revolution. *Semin Laparosc Surg*. 2003;10(3):127-139.

Gallagher AG, McClure N, McGuigan J, Crothers I, Browning J. Virtual reality training in laparoscopic surgery: a preliminary assessment of minimally invasive surgical trainer virtual reality (MIST VR). *Endoscopy*. 1999;31(4):310-313.

Gallagher AG, Richie K, McClure N, McGuigan J. Objective psychomotor skills assessment of experienced, junior, and novice laparoscopists with virtual reality. *World J Surg*. 2001;25(11): 1478-1483.

Gallagher AG, Ritter EM, Satava RM. Fundamental principles of validation, and reliability: rigorous science for the assessment of surgical education and training. *Surg Endosc*. 2003a;17(10): 1525-1529.

Gallagher AG, Cowie R, Crothers I, Jordan-Black JA, Satava RM. PicSOr: an objective test of perceptual skill that predicts laparoscopic technical skill in three initial studies of laparoscopic performance. *Surg Endosc*. 2003b;17(9):1468-1471.

Gallagher AG, Lederman AB, McGlade K, Satava RM, Smith CD. Discriminative validity of the minimally invasive surgical trainer in virtual reality (MIST-VR) using criteria levels based on expert performance. *Surg Endosc*. 2004;18(4):660-665.

Gallagher AG, Ritter EM, Champion H, et al. Virtual reality simulation for the operating room: proficiency-based training as a paradigm shift in surgical skills training. *Ann Surg*. 2005;241(2): 364-372.

Geis WP, Coletta AV, Verdeja JC, Plasencia G, Ojogho O, Jacobs M. Sequential psychomotor skills development in laparoscopic colon surgery. *Arch Surg*. 1994;129(2):206.

Grantcharov TP, Kristiansen VB, Bendix J, Bardram L, Rosenberg J, Funch-Jensen P. Randomized clinical trial of virtual reality simulation for laparoscopic skills training. *Br J Surg*. 2004;91(2):146-150.

Hance J, Aggarwal R, Stanbridge R, et al. Objective assessment of technical skills in cardiac surgery. *Eur J Cardiothorac Surg*. 2005;28(1):157-162.

Horton R. Surgical research or comic opera: questions, but few answers. *Lancet*. 1996; 347(9007):984.

Kennedy AM, Carroll S, Traynor O, Gallagher AG. Assessing surgical skill using bench station models. *Plast Reconstr Surg*. 2008;121(5):1869-1870.

Khan M, Bann S, Darzi A, Butler P. Assessing surgical skill using bench station models. *Plast Reconstr Surg*. 2007;120(3):793-800.

Larsen CR, Grantcharov T, Aggarwal R, et al. Objective assessment of gynecologic laparoscopic skills using the LapSimGyn virtual reality simulator. *Surg Endosc*. 2006;20(9):1460-1466.

Larsen CR, Grantcharov T, Schouenborg L, Ottosen C, Sørensen JL, Ottesen B. Objective assessment of surgical competence in gynaecological laparoscopy: development and validation of a procedure specific rating scale. *BJOG*. 2008;115(7):908-916.

Larsen CR, Soerensen JL, Grantcharov TP, et al. Effect of virtual reality training on laparoscopic surgery: randomised controlled trial. *Br Med J*. 2009;338:b1802.

Martin P, Martin PR, Bateson P. *Measuring Behaviour: An Introductory Guide*. Cambridge: Cambridge University Press; 1993.

Martin JA, Regehr G, Reznick R, et al. Objective structured assessment of technical skill (OSATS) for surgical residents. *Br J Surg*. 1997;84(2):273-278.

Melvin W, Johnson J, Ellison E. Laparoscopic skills enhancement. *Am J Surg*. 1996;172(4): 377-379.

Moore MJ, Bennett CL. The learning curve for laparoscopic cholecystectomy. The southern surgeons club. *Am J Surg*. 1995;170(1):55.

Ojimba TA, Cameron AEP. Drawbacks of endoscopic thoracic sympathectomy. *Br J Surg*. 2004;91(3):264-269.

Reber AS, Reber ES. *The Penguin Dictionary of Psychology*. London: Penguin Books; 1985.

Ritter EM, McClusky DA 3rd, Gallagher AG, Enochsson L, Smith CD. Perceptual, visuospatial, and psychomotor abilities correlate with duration of training required on a virtual-reality flexible endoscopy simulator. *Am J Surg*. 2006;192(3):379-384.

Rosser JC Jr, Rosser LE, Savalgi RS. Objective evaluation of a laparoscopic surgical skill program for residents and senior surgeons. *Arch Surg*. 1998;133(6):657.

Seymour NE, Gallagher AG, Roman SA, et al. Virtual reality training improves operating room performance: results of a randomized, double-blinded study. *Ann Surg*. 2002;236(4):458-463. discussion 463-454.

Smith WS, Sung G, Saver J, et al. Mechanical thrombectomy for acute ischemic stroke: final results of the Multi MERCI trial. *Stroke*. 2008;39(4):1205.

Sutherland LM, Middleton PF, Anthony A, et al. Surgical simulation: a systematic review. *Ann Surg*. 2006;243(3):291.

Sutton C, McCloy R, Middlebrook A, Chater P, Wilson M, Stone R. MIST VR. A laparoscopic surgery procedures trainer and evaluator. *Stud Health Technol Inform*. 1997;39:598.

Taffinder N, Sutton C, Fishwick R, McManus I, Darzi A. Validation of virtual reality to teach and assess psychomotor skills in laparoscopic surgery: results from randomised controlled studies using the MIST VR laparoscopic simulator. *Stud Health Technol Inform.* 1998;50:124-130.

Van Sickle K, Iii D, Gallagher AG, Smith CD. Construct validation of the ProMIS simulator using a novel laparoscopic suturing task. *Surg Endosc.* 2005;19(9):1227-1231.

Van Sickle K, Baghai M, Huang IP, Goldenberg A, Smith CD, Ritter EM. Construct validity of an objective assessment method for laparoscopic intracorporeal suturing and knot tying. *Am J Surg.* 2008;196(1):74-80.

Wherry DC, Rob CG, Marohn MR, Rich NM. An external audit of laparoscopic cholecystectomy performed in medical treatment facilities of the department of defense. *Ann Surg.* 1994; 220(5):626.

Winder J, Zheng H, Hughes S, Kelly B, Wilson C, Gallagher A. Increasing face validity of a vascular interventional training system. *Stud Health Technol Inform.* 2004;98:410-415.

Yadav JS, Wholey MH, Kuntz RE, et al. Protected carotid-artery stenting versus endarterectomy in high-risk patients. *N Engl J Med.* 2004;351(15):1493.

Chapter 8
Metric-Based Training to Proficiency: What Is It and How Is It Done?

In countries such as the UK and Ireland, high profile medical error cases had profound implications for the process under which doctors were deemed qualified to practice medicine. It also brought to the fore once again the debate about competency.

Competence Definition and Assessment

A common definition of competence is: "the condition of being capable; having *sufficient* skill and/or knowledge; *the state* of being legally competent or qualified" (Dictionary 1995). Another definition of competence is "the *minimal* level of skill, knowledge, and/or expertise derived through training and experience, required to safely and proficiently perform a task or procedure" (Marshall 1995). Pitts et al. (2006) note that there are debates about the nature or meaning of the word competence. One conceptual standpoint states that a competence is simply a demonstrable ability to do something, using directly observable performance as evidence. Another understands competence as being a: "holistic integration of understandings, and professional judgments, where 'competence' is not necessarily directly observable, rather it is inferred from performance."

One of the problems with the above definitions is that they are not really definitions but mere descriptions. In Chap. 4, we discussed the issue of operational definitions which are a pre-requisite for measurement of performance and in addition these definitions must be refutable. Falsifiability or refutability is the logical possibility that an assertion can be shown false by an observation or a physical experiment. That something is "falsifiable" does not mean it is false; rather, that if it is false, then this can be shown by observation or experiment. The term "*testability*" is related but more specific; it means that an assertion can be falsified through

A.G. Gallagher and G.C. O'Sullivan, *Fundamentals of Surgical Simulation*, Improving Medical Outcome - Zero Tolerance,
DOI 10.1007/978-0-85729-763-1_8, © Springer-Verlag London Limited 2012

experimentation alone. These descriptions of competence only give clues as to how competence might be assessed but do not specify what "capable," "sufficient," or "minimal" might mean in real terms. Falsifiability is a very important concept in *science* and the *philosophy of science*. The concept was most clearly expounded by *Karl Popper*. He concluded from his philosophical analysis of the *scientific method* that a *hypothesis*, *proposition*, or *theory* is "scientific" only if it is falsifiable (Popper 1979). This makes "competency" difficult to assess. Another problem with the understanding of the concept of competence is well demonstrated by Pitts et al. (2006). Competence is not as stated by them the capacity to demonstrate the ability to do something; rather it is the ability to demonstrate doing something to a certain standard.

Medicine has developed a wide array of techniques to assess the "competence" of doctors in training and it is from the results of these assessments that competence is inferred. The majority of these tests assess medical knowledge. However, in the 1970s, there was a move away from just assessing what the medical trainee knows, to what they could do. In 1963, Howard S. Barrows introduced the "standardized patient" into medical education and training (Barrows and Abrahamson 1964). The first standardized patients were, in fact, out-of-work Hollywood actors who were employed by the University of Southern California to play the role of patients. Playing the role of a real patient meant that each student had an opportunity to come face-to-face with the totality of the patient, his stories, physical symptoms, emotional responses to his ailments, attitudes toward the medical profession, stresses with life, work, and family. In essence, the standardized patient brought everything to the clinical situation that a real patient brings. The theory behind the practice was that the student could experience and practice clinical medicine without jeopardizing the health and welfare of a real, sick patient. The term standardized patient became adopted and widely used during the 1980s by medical education researchers who were primarily interested in clinical evaluation of performance.

In the UK, there was also considerable concern about how to assess clinical competence. Clinical competence was usually assessed by two examiners who tested the trainee's skill on a few patients. Thus, the luck of the draw played a major part in the procedure and variation in the marking standards between examiners was also a problem. Also, frequently, there was confusion about what was being tested, e.g., from being a test of skills in eliciting a history or carrying out a physical examination and a history to a test that was more about the candidates' factual knowledge than their clinical skills. In response to these problems, Harden and colleagues from the Department of Medical Education, University of Dundee developed the objective structured clinical examination or OSCE (Harden et al. 1975). In the structured clinical examination, the variables and complexity of the examination were more easily controlled. Other advantages that the OSCE had over the more traditional assessment was that it had clearly defined aims, which meant that more of the candidates' skills could be assessed with a more objective marking strategy which had been agreed with assessors in advance. The object of the OSCE is to assess basic and clinical skills in a reliable format.

It is a flexible test format based on a circuit of patient stations. At each station, trainees interact with a real patient or a standardized patient to demonstrate specific skills. These stations may be short, e.g., 5 min or long, e.g., 15–20 min and there may be as few as eight stations or more than 20. Scoring is done with a task-specific checklist, rating scales, or a combination of a checklist and rating scale. Scoring can be done by the assessors or by the standardized patients. The designing of an OSCE is usually the result of a compromise between the assessment objectives and the logistics constraints, but the content is always linked to the curriculum. If the OSCE scorers are being used for making a pass-fail decision, then it is necessary to set standards and scores. OSCEs are based on tasks that approximate performance in the clinical area of interest and the assumption is that the closer the tasks are to the clinical reality the more valid the assessment. However, there are a number of problems with this approach. The first is that each station is time limited, and so only allows trainees to perform isolated aspects of the real clinical situation. This fragmented approach provides a better opportunity to assess more performance characteristics of the trainee however; this is at the cost of degrading the doctor–patient encounter. The task-specific checklist assessment procedure for the OSCE has also been criticized. It is been proposed that checklists tend to emphasize thoroughness and may become less relevant as the experience of the candidate increases.

Assessment is like good science; once you know the questions to ask, development of the experimental design to answer the question is relatively straightforward. Medical education tends to have the same problem and once it has worked out what it should be assessing it sets about developing a sound assessment strategy. Bryant (1969) has said "examinations are about the least understood and most misused tools of education. They are used mainly to certify that the student has learned an acceptable amount of what he has been taught and to provide a grade representing that attainment. While the announced objectives of the institution may be to develop the knowledge, skills, and attitudes necessary to being a good doctor, the examination seldom measures more than the simple recall of isolated pieces of information. The student grade is usually determined by comparing their performance with the class as a whole; that is, 'grading on the curve' rather than grading according to standards carefully developed by the faculty (p. 209, 1969)." What Bryant is suggesting is that in the assessment of medical skills, the goal should be the assessment of competence rather than just assessment per se.

Competency: Accreditation Council for Graduate Medical Education

The Accreditation Council for Graduate Medical Education (ACGME) is responsible for the *Accreditation* of postgraduate medical training programs within the USA. In response to growing criticism of graduate medical education from a variety of

Table 8.1 ACGME core competencies

Competency	Definitions
1. Patient care	Provision of *timely*, effective, appropriate, and compassionate patient care
2. Medical knowledge	Uses medical knowledge for clinical problem solving and decision making Able to identify life-threatening conditions Able to formulate an appropriate differential diagnosis
3. Interpersonal and communication skills	Able to conduct an effective information exchange with patients, their families, and medical colleagues
4. Professionalism	Arrives on time, ready to work Maintains a proper appearance Inoffensive dress and appropriate cleanliness Appropriate attitudes, respect for patient autonomy, ethical behavior, probity
5. Practice-based learning and improvement	Understands patient care practices and assimilates necessary components for improvement
6. Systems based practice	Capacity to understand, access, and effectively utilize the resources of a given health care system to enable the provision of optimal emergency care

sources (including the medical community itself), the ACGME identified general competencies which all graduates should be able to meet on completion of their training (Beall 1999). The criticisms of graduate medical education center around the fact that many medical trainees were not adequately prepared to practice medicine in the rapidly changing healthcare environment. The core competencies that the ACGME developed are given in Table 8.1.

The ACGME explains in detail what performance characteristics contribute to and constitute specific competencies. It is the responsibility of a training program and the trainees to ensure that competencies are demonstrated. The ACGME reassured training program directors that the development of assessment tools would not be the sole responsibility of the training programs and that when validated assessment tools developed by ACGME or individual programs would be made available to all of them. They also assured programs that many of the assessment tools that were being used will almost certainly be appropriate. The most important factor in the continued use of these assessment systems was that they demonstrated to be valid and reliable measures of competency-based learning objectives. Initially, all training programs were encouraged to assess trainee competencies in all six domains with at least one approach in addition to global/end of rotation clinical ratings. Assessment also included direct observation and concurrent evaluation, 360° evaluation involving non-physician members of the care team, patients and families, and checklist evaluation of improvement projects and cognitive tests.

The long-term goal of the ACGME was to develop a new model of accreditation that was directly linked to the six general competencies. Furthermore, because the competencies were created in conjunction with the American Board of Medical

Specialties, it was hoped that this model of certification could be used in an ongoing basis for accreditation of physicians throughout their careers. The new competencies model was seen as a potential solution to the exponential increase in training requirements in medical education in the USA. Competency-based training offered a more innovative approach rather than the traditional prescription of what was required to be considered medically trained. However, that is not quite what has come out of the ACGME competencies program. Apart from creating general confusion among program directors as to how to achieve or implement a competency program, this new training system has probably created more bureaucracy than it replaced. For example, just some of the assessments that program directors are responsible for include 360° evaluation, chart-stimulated recall oral examination, checklist evaluation of the live or recorded performance, and global rating live or recorded performance, OSCE, Procedure, Operative, or Case logs, patient surveys, portfolios, simulations and models, standardized oral examination and written multiple choice questions (MCQ's).

Lurie et al. (2009) in a systematic review of research on the ACGME, six general competencies found that between 1999 and March 2008, 127 articles were published of which 56 met their specific review inclusion criteria (i.e., validation studies or instrument development). They found that quantitative studies of evaluation failed to develop measures reflecting the six competencies in a reliable and valid way. Overall, they concluded that the research literature provides no evidence that current measurement tools can assess the competencies identified by the ACGME independently of one another. The exception to the challenge of measuring competency was medical knowledge; measures which reliably assess medical knowledge seemed to be valid predictors of important clinical performance characteristics. This finding does not really come as a surprise as the assessment of medical knowledge has been a pillar of medical education almost since its inception. By contrast, the other five competencies reflect in varying degrees personal attributes of trainees rather than knowledge of objectively derived information. Furthermore, the relative value of these attributes is more socially and culturally determined than they are of education and training. Even concepts such as "professionalism" which predated the ACGME general competencies have "continued to defy a clearer operational definition despite several decades of attempts to derive one" (p. 306). To compound these stark conclusions is the fact that one of the specifically recommended assessment strategies proposed by the ACGME (Assessment Toolbox) is OSATS. In Chap. 7 we have explained in some detail why the published evidence on OSATS fails to meet an acceptable level of reliability for use in high stakes assessment. Overall, one of the major problems with the competencies proposed by the ACGME is that they have offered extensive detailed descriptions of what constitutes specific competencies; however, they have offered few if any operational definitions. For example, the *Practice-based Learning and improvement competency states that the trainee* "Understands patient care practices and assimilates necessary components for improvement." How is this competency falsifiable; what is it that the trainee must do, to whom and how frequently before the program director or educational supervisor decides that they do not meet this competency? Without precise operational definitions, it is not possible to reliably and validly assess performance. Simply working from the descriptions of the competencies described by the ACGME it would seem a herculean task to try and develop valid and reliable assessment tools. Lurie et al. (2009) quite sensibly conclude and recommend that the competencies identified by the ACGME should be used to guide and coordinate specific evaluation efforts rather than attempting to develop instruments to measure the competencies directly.

Competency: United Kingdom, Canada, Australasia, Ireland

Training programs in the UK, Canada, Australasia, and Ireland were under the same pressures as in the USA to examine their training and assessment practices for doctors. Rowley and colleagues (Pitts et al. 2006) stated that although the job of a surgeon cannot be neatly defined, it can at least be broken down into a series of outcomes that would lend themselves to assessment. On the matter of professionalism, the GMC detailed what it considers the constituent parts of this attribute in "Good Clinical Practice" (The principles of good clinical practice are outlined in articles 2–5 in the EU Directive 2005/28/EC (Verheugen 2005)) and Tomorrow's Doctors (General Medical Council 1993). However, Rowley (Pitts et al. 2006) from Ninewells Hospital, Dundee, Scotland suggests that the attributes of a surgeon are better captured in the work of the Canadian Medical Association outlined in their CanMED 2000 project (Frank 2005) and these are detailed in Table 8.2.

The CanMeds project suggested that competencies are "…important observable knowledge, skills and attitudes" that they chose as the central concept in planning medical education in Canada. This reflected the ultimate goal of the CanMEDs project which was to develop the abilities of physicians needed to provide the highest quality of care. The process of identifying the core abilities involved translating the available evidence on effective practice into educationally useful elements. The result was a new multifaceted framework of physician competence that comprised a number of competencies. To be useful, these were organized thematically around "meta-competencies" or physician Roles for CanMEDS (outlined in Table 8.2). Traditionally medical education has articulated competence around core medical expertise. In the CanMEDS construct, Medical Expert is the central integrative role but is not the only one. Domains of ability that have long been described or displayed by the effective physician were made more explicit and re-emphasized and articulated as a specific goal of training (Aretz 2003; Epstein and Hundert 2002; Neufeld et al. 1998).

The first step in the process of implementing these aspirations was to devise a curriculum that comprehensively detailed the qualities required and these were traceable back to categories in the CanMEDs 2000 for the nine major disciplines of surgery. One of the major parts of this curriculum was the required assessment methodologies. In the past, the knowledge and judgment of surgical trainees was

Table 8.2 CanMEDS roles and definitions

Roles	Definitions
1. Medical expert	As medical experts, physicians integrate all of the CanMEDS roles, applying medical knowledge, clinical skills, and professional attitudes in their provision of patient-centered care. Medical expert is the central physician role in the CanMEDS framework.
2. Communicator	As communicators, physicians effectively facilitate the doctor–patient relationship and the dynamic exchanges that occur before, during, and after the medical encounter.
3. Collaborator	As collaborators, physicians effectively work within a healthcare team to achieve optimal patient care.
4. Manager	As managers, physicians are integral participants in healthcare organizations, organizing sustainable practices, making decisions about allocating resources, and contributing to the effectiveness of the healthcare system.
5. Health advocate	As health advocates, physicians responsibly use their expertise and influence to advance the health and well-being of individual patients, communities, and populations.
6. Scholar	As scholars, physicians demonstrate a lifelong commitment to reflective learning, as well as the creation, dissemination, application, and translation of medical knowledge.
7. Professional	As professionals, physicians are committed to the health and well-being of individuals and society through ethical practice, profession-led regulation, and high personal standards of behavior.

assessed by summative methods, e.g., MCQs, essays, viva's or orals, and clinical examinations. In many respects, surgeons have always assessed trainees in the workplace because of the apprenticeship tradition. However, some of the problems with this approach through the years have been the lack of objectivity and some surgeons felt that undue influence may have been too important a factor in the assessment of some trainee surgeons. Nevertheless, workplace assessment offers great opportunities if the issues of reliability and validity can be resolved. Assessment tools that were developed specifically to resolve these issues were Direct Observation of Procedural Skills (DOPS) and Norcini et al. (2003) mini-CEX which could be applied in everyday situations in real-time. In the workplace, assessment tools need to be practicable as well as valid and reliable. This means that assessments should be brief and focused on small areas of activity which should limit the effect on a busy working hospital whilst capitalizing on the relevant environment. For example, during a surgical attachment, a young trainee may agree with his trainer that by the end of the attachment, he should be proficient at hernia repair. After a number of months of gradually doing more and more (and after a series of formative assessment sessions), the trainee is ready to be assessed. All the learning objectives are found to have been met, and after a 10 min debrief at the end of an operation, the trainee and the trainer agree that the trainee has demonstrated the key competence. This would be repeated in different attachments with other trainers and gradually a body of evidence from different assessors is accumulated into a growing competence portfolio.

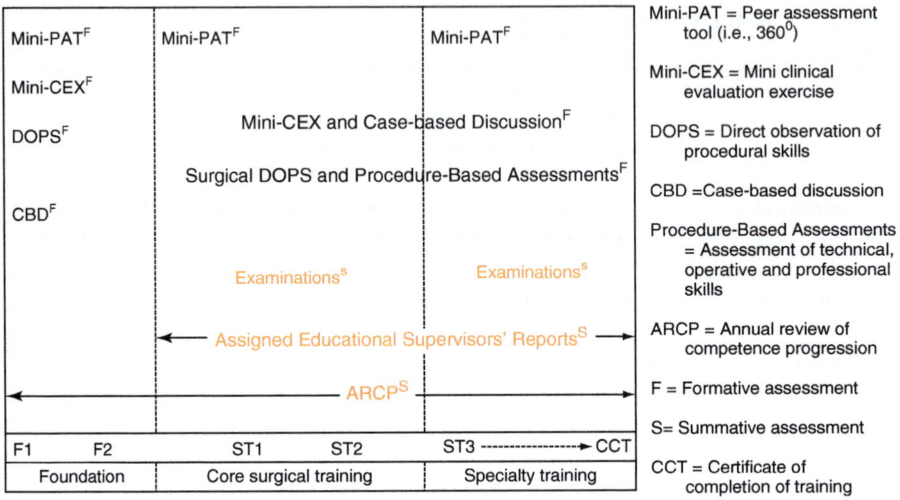

Fig. 8.1 Intercollegiate Surgical Curriculum Programme (ISCP) for training and assessment

The type of assessment depends on the stage of training of the individual. These are shown in Fig. 8.1 when the trainee enters into training at Foundation One (or F1) through Core surgical training (ST1 up to STn (can be ST7 or ST8)) and ends on receiving the Intercollegiate Surgical Curriculum Programme (ISCP) Certificate of Completion of Training (CCT). Most of the assessment process is formative, but the annual review of competence progression (ARCP) and assigned educational supervisors reports and exams are summative.

ISCP Assessments Contributing to Competency Assessment

Mini-PAT

The mini-PAT assessment is sometimes described as the 360° assessment or multi-source feedback. It is a method of assessing professional competence within a team working environment and providing development feedback to the trainee. It is first undertaken at entry-level (F1) and then every 3 years in specialty training and more frequently if there are concerns. Trainees are expected to understand the range of rules and expertise of team members in order to communicate effectively to achieve high-quality service for patients. Mini-PAT comprises a self-assessment and trainee performance assessment from a range of co-workers (range 8–12) who are chosen by the trainee and will always include the assigned educational supervisor. The assessment will not include administrators or patients. The competencies assessed map across to the Standards of Good Medical Practice and to the core objectives of the intercollegiate surgical curriculum. The assigned educational supervisor signs off on the trainee's mini-PAT assessment and makes comments for the annual review.

Mini-CEX

The mini clinical evaluation exercise (or mini-CEX) is a method of assessing skills essential to the provision of good clinical care and to facilitate feedback. It assesses the trainee's clinical and professional skills on the ward, on ward rounds, in Accident and Emergency and in outpatient clinics. Trainees are assessed on different clinical problems that they encounter in a range of clinical settings. Trainees should choose different assessors for each assessment, but one assessor must be their assigned educational supervisor. Assessors must be registered with ISCP and have expertise in the clinical problem on which the trainee is being assessed. The assessment involves observing the trainee interact with the patient in a clinical encounter. The areas of competence covered include: history taking, physical examination, professionalism, clinical judgment, communication skills, organization, efficiency, and overall clinical care. They normally take between 15 and 20 min with the patient and 5 min afterwards with the assessor. Mini-CEX should be undertaken at least six times per year in specialty training years ST1 and ST2. Their use in specialty training will depend on the specialty and level of training.

DOPS

Direct observation of procedural skills (or DOPS) is used to assess trainee's technical, operative, and professional skills in a range of basic diagnostic and interventional procedures, or part procedures during routine surgical practice. Surgical DOPS are used in some environments and procedures and can take place in wards, outpatient clinics, and the operating theater to facilitate developmental feedback. The original DOPS was developed by the UK Royal College of Physicians. The surgical DOPS can be used routinely every time the trainer supervises a trainee trying out one of the specified procedures, with the aim of making the assessment part of routine surgical practice. The assessment involves an assessor observing the trainee perform a practical procedure and then evaluating performance on a structured checklist that enables developmental feedback to the trainee immediately afterwards. An overall rating on any one assessment can *only* be completed if the entire procedure is observed and judgment will be made at the completion of the rotation as to the overall performance level achieved in each of the assessed surgical procedures. Surgical DOPS should be undertaken at least six times per year in ST1 and ST2.

CBD

Case-Based Discussions (CBD) were designed to assess clinical judgment, decision making, and the application of medical knowledge in relation to patient care in cases for which the trainee has been directly responsible. As such, the method was designed to test higher order thinking and synthesis and allows the assessor to observe how the trainee elicits, prioritizes, and applies knowledge. The function of the exercise is not focused on the trainee's ability to make a diagnosis; rather, it is more like a structured in-depth discussion between the trainee and their assigned educational supervisor about how the managed a clinical case. Challenging cases are preferred as this allows a trainee to explain the complexity involved and the reasoning behind the choices they made in the care of that patient. It also facilitates discussions on the ethical and legal parameters of clinical practice. Real patient records form the basis for dialogue, systematic assessment and structured feedback. This also allows the assessor to evaluate the quality of the trainee's recordkeeping and presentation. Assessments usually take about 15–20 min, followed by 5 min of feedback from the assessor.

Procedure-Based Assessments

Procedure-Based Assessments (PBAs) are used to assess a trainee's technical, operative, and professional skills in a range of specialty procedures or part of procedures during routine surgical practice. These provide a framework to assess practice and facilitate feedback in order to direct learning. The assessment method uses two principal components. The first is PBA form for the assessment of a series of competencies within six domains. These are content, preoperative planning, preoperative preparation, exposure and closure, intraoperative technique and postoperative management. Each one of the competencies is assessed with a number of performance characteristics, e.g., for exposure and closure these include:

E1. Demonstrate knowledge of optimum skin incision
E2. Achieved an adequate exposure through purposeful dissection in the correct tissue planes and identifies all structures correctly
E3. Completes a sound wound repair
E4. Protects the wound dressings, splints, and drains
E5. See specific PBAs

Each one of these performance characteristics is scored as, N=Not Observed or Not Appropriate; U=Unsatisfactory; and S=Satisfactory. The procedure chosen to be assessed should be representative of those that the trainee would normally be expected to be able to carry out at their level and will be one of a list of index procedures relevant to the specialty. Usually the assessor will be the trainee's assigned educational supervisor but other surgical consultants should also complete the assessments. Trainees should complete assessments on as many procedures as possible with a range of different assessors. During the assessment, the assessor can provide verbal prompts and if required intervene if patient safety is at risk.

PBAs have been adopted as the principal method of assessing surgical skills, the combined competencies specific to the procedures with generic competencies such as safe handling of instruments. They cover the entire procedure, including preoperative and postoperative planning. PBA forms have been developed for all the links procedures in all surgical specialties. The forms were designed to be quick and easy to use as assessments should be as frequent as possible when performing index procedures as a primary aid to learning. PBAs focus on index procedures in each specialty and should be used every time the index procedure is performed.

ARCP

The Annual Review of Competence Progression (ARCP) is a formal review of how well a trainee is progressing in relation to their learning agreement for their training program including their ability to go to the next level. The ARCP is underpinned by appraisal, assessment, and annual planning. The panel bases their decision on the evidence submitted by the trainee and record or the competencies attained and their progression through the training program. The ARCP panel of assessors may include the Training Program Director, other members of the relevant Specialty Training Committee, a College representative, a Deanery representative, an academic representative, an "external" representative, or a lay representative. The ARCP panel reviews a trainee's progress based on the evidence submitted and provides the trainee with an outcome. The panel is explicit about what trainees are required to submit for their review but this will include:

- Structured reports from their Educational Supervisor
- College Assessment Forms (via the ISCP)
- Clinical Logbook (via the ISCP)
- Portfolio
- (Updated Registration Form (Form R))

The outcome of the ARCP will determine the rate at which trainees progress through the training program. Possible outcomes include, incomplete evidence presented (more training time required), released from training without specified competences, inadequate progress, development of specific competencies required, and satisfactory progress, and if trainees consistently underperform or fail to supply sufficient evidence to ARCP, they may be asked to relinquish their National Training Number. The ARCP also provides a mechanism for determining certificate of completion of training (CCT) dates for trainees.

IRCP Assessments Assessed

Overall the Intercollegiate Surgical Curriculum Programme (ISCP) has done an excellent job in constructing a systematic, evidence-based, and targeted training program. Like the ACGME competencies program, they have set out the training for the performance characteristics that a well-trained doctor should possess. They have highlighted "softer" but important aspects of being a good doctor and made it clear that they are as much part of what is being assessed as medical skill. The ISCP has been much more rigorous in what they will accept as assessment of competencies in comparison to the ACGME. It is very impressive that the ISCP has PBSs already developed for every index surgical procedure. ACGME appears to be less advanced in its assessment efforts.

However, the ISCP competency assessment is not without problems. Although performance had been designed to be user-friendly, the entire process seems exceptionally bureaucratic. Perhaps this is the price that has to be paid for objectivity, transparency, and fairness in medical training at the start of the twenty-first century! The emphasis throughout training on formative feedback is good educational practice and optimizes learning opportunities for the trainee; however, there is still considerable room for subjectivity to creep into the system. This is particularly the case for the DOPS because of the Likert-scale, which we have discussed in Chap. 7. It is very difficult to achieve a high inter-rater reliability when using a Likert-scale and good inter-rater reliability levels (i.e., >0.8) are a fundamental component of a valid assessment. The PBAs are certainly one of the most impressive aspects of the ISCP assessment process, particularly as it is procedure-specific for index operations. However, the assessment metrics could certainly be made much more explicit and operational definitions of performance characteristics could be made much tighter. Definitions of performance characteristics such as optimum (without definition), adequate, sound, and purposeful leave too much room for individual interpretation and almost certainly will impact on their inter-rater reliability. However, the Intercollegiate Surgical Curriculum Programme (ICSP) has wisely not gone down the road of Likert-scale type assessments for PBAs and has instead opted for the more robust assessment process where the assessors are simply asked to assess whether performance was unsatisfactory or satisfactory. These problems are not insurmountable and will be addressed in Chap. 12.

Somewhat more worrying about the ISCP assessment systems are their definitions of the meaning of valid and reliable;

- *Valid* – To ensure face validity, the workplace-based assessments comprise direct observations of workplace tasks. The complexity of the tasks increases in line with progression through the training program. To ensure content validity, all the assessment instruments have been blueprinted against all the Good Medical Practice/CanMEDS domains.
- *Reliable* – In order to increase reliability, there will be multiple measures of outcomes. ISCP assessments make use of several observers' judgments, multiple assessment methods (triangulation), and take place frequently.

These could be put forward as one set of definitions but as discussed in Chap. 7 these are not the conventional definitions of "valid" and "reliable" in the context of assessments, particularly when used for high stakes decisions. This issue will almost certainly come under close scrutiny if a trainee who has been failed by this system chooses to challenge it legally. Another problem with the assessment process particularly in the PBAs is what constitutes "satisfactory." We assume that some type of construct validation has been conducted on the individual index PBA assessment procedures to guide this decision making. However, these studies have not been reported in the literature. Another question which needs to be addressed by the ISCP assessment system directly relates to the issue of competency; how many times must a procedure be conducted and assessed as satisfactory for the trainee to be defined as competent? Furthermore, like the ACGME, there is extensive discussion about competence and competencies but at no point does the ISCP operationally

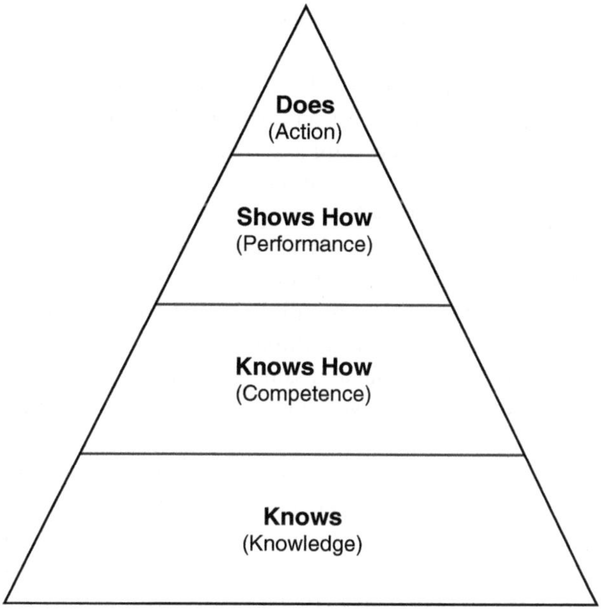

Fig. 8.2 Miller's triangle framework for clinical assessment

defined what they actually mean by competence. They give extensive descriptions of what they consider competent or what competencies are, but they do not offer a definition which is falsifiable.

Competency: Millar's Triangle Model (1990)

George E. Miller (1990) when asked to address the issue of assessment of clinical skills, competence, and performance concluded that no single assessment method could provide all the data required for a judgment of something so complex as the delivery of professional services by a successful physician. He used a triangle/pyramid model to illustrate how he construed the coalescence of performance characteristics that made a successful physician (shown in Fig. 8.2). At the base of this process is knowledge; that is, the trainee physician knows what is required in order to carry out their professional functions effectively. The trainee must also know how to use the knowledge that they have accumulated. They must develop among other things, the skill of acquiring information from a variety of human and laboratory sources. Having acquired this information, they must then be able to analyze and interpret this information so as to formulate a diagnosis and then a treatment plan. It is having sufficient knowledge, judgment, and skill that define competence (according to Webster's dictionary). Traditionally, these qualities and attributes have been assessed with medical exams. However, Miller (1990) points out that traditional academic exams failed to accurately represent how the trainee might deal with an actual patient in vivo rather than in academic examination exercise. He suggests that it is not enough for a trainee to know the way that something is done to be considered competent but they must also show how it is done. Of course one of the challenges that this question poses to the academic clinical community is how to conduct a reliable and valid assessment of that performance. Although considerable advances have been made in the assessment of clinical performance, e.g., standardized patients and OSCE's, the question remains whether what is done in the artificial examination setting is an accurate reflection and good predictor of what a successful medical graduate does when functioning independently in clinical practice. Although we have highlighted that some of the problems associated with the construction of Procedure-Based Assessments, we believe that they are a natural evolution of an optimal assessment process. They have considerably more strengths than weaknesses and we believe will prove a reliable predictor of mature clinical performance.

The problem with Miller's formulation of competency it is that is just like the other approaches we have outlined already; it simply restates the problem and reminds us how difficult it is to measure. He does not offer a definition of competence that is refutable. Furthermore, Miller (1990) appears to assume that as knowledge testing plays such a crucial role in medical education and training progression, success in overcoming that hurdle is by default, an indication of competency. Miller explicitly presents this assumption in his original paper where he aligns "KNOWS HOW" with Competence (p. S63). In reality, even in 1990, this almost certainly was not the case. Medicine to a large extent is a learned skill, and the assumption probably was that these skills were acquired at the same rate as the knowledge of how and when to practice them. High-profile medical error cases in medicine around the world have cast considerable doubt on that assumption to the point where these skills are now explicitly assessed, hence the discussion of competency. Traditionally, medical knowledge has been very well assessed, unlike medical skills. Compounding this problem is the fact that medical education practitioners now know that the same scientific and philosophical (and effort) underpinning of medical knowledge assessment and validation must also be applied to learning, assessment, and validation of procedural skills. It is no longer acceptable to assume that by the time physicians have completed their training, they will have sufficient skills to practice medicine safely. This still leaves the problem of what is sufficient?

Competency as Part of a Skill Acquisition Process

A more comprehensive account of the skill acquisition process has been proposed by Dreyfus and Dreyfus (Dreyfus et al. 1986, 2000). Both brothers were academics at Berkeley; Hubert was a professor of philosophy in the graduate School and his brother Stuart was an applied mathematician. They proposed their theory in direct opposition to much of the thinking at the time about the development and applications of computers. Dreyfus and Dreyfus analyzed the difference between

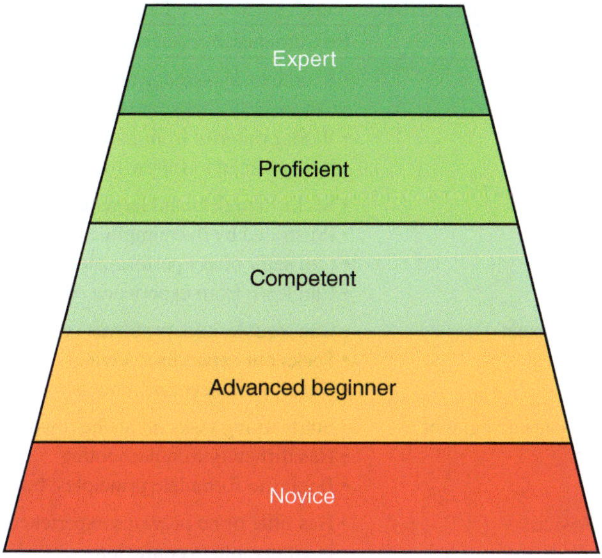

Fig. 8.3 The Dreyfus and Dreyfus (1986) model of skill development which surgery has "embraced"

human expertise and the computer programs that claimed to capture it. They proposed that much of the novelty and intuition that human beings brought to the problem-solving process could not be duplicated or replicated by computers and in particular, they argued against the concept of "computers that can think," or expert machines. In the 1980s, digital computers were basically highly complicated structures of simple switches which were either on or off. The theory on which such machines were based preceded their actual development. Philosophers like Descartes, Pascal, and Leibniz and mathematicians like Boole and Babbage sensed the potential power of combining many simple elements in rule-like ways. By the 1950s, when digital computers were just beginning to be built, logicians such as Alan Turing were already accustomed to thinking of computers as devices for manipulating symbols according to exact rules. The symbols themselves did not mean anything. Computers are general symbol manipulators and so they can simulate any process which can be described exactly.

During the 1950s when digital computers were first constructed, they were first used for scientific calculation. However, by the end of 1950s, researchers like Alan Newell and Herbert Simon began to take seriously the idea that computers were general symbol manipulators. They saw that one could use symbols to represent elementary facts about the world, then use rules to represent relationships between them and then use such rules or programs to deduce how those facts affect each other and what happens when the facts change. In this way, computers seemed to be able to simulate logical thinking. To help inform the discussion about the differences between how machines solve problems and how human beings solve problems, Dreyfus and Dreyfus (Dreyfus et al. 1986) proposed a five-stage model of skill acquisition (which is shown in Fig. 8.3). They were particularly interested in how experts solve problems, the final stage of their model.

Table 8.3 Characteristics of each stage of the Dreyfus skill development model

Stage	Performance characteristics
Expert	• Source of knowledge and information for others • Continually looks for better methods • Work primarily from intuition • Being forced to follow rules degrades performance
Proficient	• Seeks to understand larger context • Frustrated by oversimplification • Can self-correct performance • Can learn from experience of others
Competent	• Can troubleshoot problems on his/her own • Seeks out expert user advice • Develops conceptual models
Advanced beginner	• Starts trying tasks on his/her own • Has difficulty troubleshooting • Begins to formulate principles, but without holistic understanding
Novice	• Has little or no previous experience • Is vulnerable to confusion • Does not know how to respond to mistakes • Needs rules to function

In the model proposed by Dreyfus and Dreyfus (1986), the development of expertise goes through a number of developmental processes from novice through advanced beginner to competence and on to proficiency and then expert. The performance characteristics of each stage of development are outlined in Table 8.3.

There are a number of interesting aspects of the Dreyfus and Dreyfus model. It differs from Miller's model in that they concentrate on what the individual can and cannot do at each stage of skill development. There is also a clear performance hierarchy: from the novice with little or no experience who does not know the rules or how to respond to mistakes, through to the individual who is competent, who has some conceptual models of performance and can troubleshoot some problems on their own but has the insight to seek out expert advice through to the expert who is the source of knowledge and information for others and who continually looks for new and better ways to perform. Another interesting aspect of the Dreyfus and Dreyfus skill acquisition model is that they have subdivided the early parts of skill acquisition into novice and advanced beginner. During the novice stage and the acquisition of new skills, the novice learns to recognize various objective facts and features relevant to the skill and acquires rules for determining actions based upon those facts and features.

At the advanced beginner stage, performance improves to a marginally acceptable level only after the novice has considerable experience in coping with real situations. While that encourages the learner to consider more context-free facts and to use more sophisticated rules, it also teaches them more important lessons involving an enlarged conception of the world, their skill, and the boundaries of their skill capabilities. They start to recognize similar patterns in the presentation of problems and find that the skills (and experience) they have already acquired might help them solve these problems or indeed to at least recognize that they are not equipped to solve the problems. They begin to notice the subtle aspects of their own performance that lead to different outcomes. For example, when driving a needle through tissue, they notice that the angle of entry and the angle path of curvature of the hand that drives the needle through the tissue determine whether they scrape or tear tissues when suturing.

With more experience, the number of recognizable context-free and situational elements present in a real world circumstance eventually becomes overwhelming. A sense of what is important is missing. In general, a competent performer with a goal in mind sees a situation as a set of facts. The importance of the facts depends on the presence of other facts, i.e., context. They have learned that if a situation has a particular constellation of those elements, certain conclusions should be drawn, a decision made, or expectation investigated. They are no longer simply following a set of rules, but begin to perform with a goal in mind. For example, if they are performing a surgical procedure that they have been taught to carry out in a specific sequence or series of steps, they may alter the order of these steps because they believe the new way of performing is more efficient or makes a later part of the procedure easier to perform.

The proficient performer starts to move beyond the position of simply following rules and making conscious choices about goals. A degree of automation becomes apparent in their performance. Automation is the performance of a skill without conscious control (discussed in more detail in Chap. 9) and is usually indicative of a high level of skill acquisition. Although the proficient performer intuitively organizes and understands the task at hand, they still find themselves thinking about what to do. They perform the task in a sequence that they find comfortable, but they readily integrate new and more efficient ways of task performance based on salient aspects of recent performance, i.e., performance feedback (see Chap. 4). They are nearing the top of their learning curve, and in general, performance is tweaked rather than significantly altered.

The expert generally knows what to do based on a mature and practised understanding. Their matured performance which has been honed by experience has by now been largely automated. In Chap. 4 we described how the expert performer needs less attentional resources to perform routine aspects of routine tasks. They appear to perceive and understand the gross and subtle aspects of a case beyond the ability of their less experienced colleagues. Their ability to generate the correct diagnosis with evidence-based reasoning seems almost effortless as does their formulation of alternative treatment plans. These are important aspects of what it is to be an expert. As a general rule, the expanded faculties of being an expert may be considered rather routine during procedures that go routinely. However, when things go wrong during a procedure, the expert has the extra cognitive resources (i.e., attentional), the experience and the skills repertoire to deal with these situations. Dreyfus and Dreyfus (1986) point out that someone at a particular stage of skill acquisition can always imitate the performance characteristics of someone at a higher stage of development when things are going well; however, their true performance level becomes evident when things do not go well. The model of skill and development that Dreyfus and Dreyfus present is a learning model in that skill acquisition passes through distinct stages but the boundaries between these stages are not explicit. Furthermore, learning to perform any task stems from the novice stage of rule governed behavior that then advances to become more automated with experience. The rate of progression will be determined by the talent of a learner, how similar the new tasks are to the performance characteristics and the skills required for previous tasks and also the skill of the teacher.

The Dreyfus and Dreyfus model of skill development has a number of attractive features. The model is intuitively attractive because it is simple and skill acquisition as proposed by them is in a logical uncomplicated sequence. Unfortunately, learning is not that simple as more than a century of quantitative research in psychology and cognitive science has shown. It should also be remembered that Dreyfus and Dreyfus proposed their model of skill acquisition in direct opposition to the proposals of many of their colleagues during the 1970s and 1980s who were suggesting that computers would become intelligent performers of sophisticated human activities. Hubert Dreyfus (1979) argued (and was derided for many years) that human intelligence and expertise depended primarily on unconscious instincts rather than conscious symbolic manipulation and argued that these unconscious skills would never be captured in formal rules. Cognitive science knows considerably more about cognition and cognitive processes at the start of the twenty-first century than they did during the 1980s when the brothers were writing. Instinctive human performance as understood by Dreyfus and Dreyfus is probably more readily recognized as automated performance by cognitive scientists, which is somewhat less mystical than Dreyfus and Dreyfus might have conceived. The other problem with the Dreyfus and Dreyfus model is that it was not developed on the basis of experimental studies (as understood by most experimental psychologists) and so it is non-empirical. In fact, most of their formulation seems to have been based on their experience with nurses at different levels of expertise and chess players.

Proficiency: Beyond Competency

Dreyfus and Dreyfus (Dreyfus et al. 1986) propose something that is quite different from what we have discussed already. Previously we have considered competence as being either present or absent (as proposed by the different medical training bodies around the world). We have also construed it as or different levels of competence (Miller 1990). What Dreyfus and Dreyfus have proposed is that competence represents performance characteristics that are an interim level of skills development between the novice and the expert. Furthermore, the performance characteristics that are attributed to the competent performer on this scale are really not that skilled. They present the performance characteristics of an individual who is really just starting to develop just "enough" skills. While this definition conforms to the dictionary definition it us uncertain that this is the perception of medical competence held by the general public i.e., just enough. A more promising set of performance characteristics is associated with what Dreyfus and Dreyfus call proficient. At this level, the person is starting to act autonomously but at the same time being cognizant of ways to improve their performance. The dictionary definitions of proficiency are:

(a) The quality of having great facility and competence; skillfulness in the command of fundamentals deriving from practice and familiarity
(b) The ability to apply knowledge to situations likely to be encountered and to deal with them without extensive recourse to technical research and assistance

The other attractive feature about the concept of proficiency is that it is not lumbered with the same historical baggage as the concept of competency. The extensive discussion of the concept of competency has resulted in nothing more than numerous elaborate descriptions that have not resulted in closer moves to operational disprovable definitions. Another attractive feature of proficiency is that if one is proficient, one is by default competent as the model proposed by Dreyfus and Dreyfus (1986) holds that skills are developed in a progressive sequence. Although the definitions offered for proficient performance are no better operationalized than those for competence, it is easier to reach agreement on who is demonstrating proficient skills than it is to reach agreement on who is demonstrating competent skills. Even critics of the competence model of skills would agree that the vast majority of senior doctors practicing medicine are at least competent, probably proficient, and some are expert at what they do. This provides a very robust foundation on which to establish a benchmark against which performance can be judged. It means that someone who is considered to be proficient in the practice of their skills is at least competent and at best expert. A good starting point for an operational definition of proficient is "that it is what proficient individuals do." This definition may not be as elegant as might have been hoped for, but it is very difficult to argue against it. The next task is to measure what it is that individuals who are proficient do. As it turns out, this task is much easier than it might seem.

Proficiency Measured

In Chap. 7 we discussed the different types of validation efforts that were required for the validation of a simulation and the simulation metrics. We also said that one of the most important types of validation that could be undertaken was construct validation. In Chap. 5 we described how metrics were developed from the initial task analysis of the procedure to be learned through to the operational definition of performance characteristics that are associated with performing the task well or badly. If these are indeed valid performance parameters that indicate where on the learning curve someone (novice, trainee or consultant/attending) is performing, we should be able to detect qualitative and quantitative differences between these groups. These performance characteristics or metrics determine how we measure performance, whether it is in the operating room or on a simulator. It may be a single metric unit that distinguishes performance or it may be a conglomeration of metric parameters. For example, Gallagher et al. (2001) found that all of the MIST VR metric measures (time, error, economy of instrument movement (left and right instrument) and economy of diathermy) distinguished between experts and novice performance. This was confirmed by Gallagher and Satava (2002) who assessed the learning curves of experts and trainees. However, Gallagher and Satava also found that the test retest reliability of economy of instrument movement metrics did not reach a satisfactory level of reliability to be used with confidence. Despite this, they still had three robust parameters that reliably measured and significantly differentiated between the performance of experts and novices.

The next step in the scientific validation of these metrics was to establish whether these metrics predicted intraoperative performance. It should be remembered that MIST VR had been widely dismissed by many in the surgical community in the late 1990s as an interesting video game using laparoscopic surgical instruments that looked nothing like performing surgery on a patient. However, the psychomotor performance characteristics and metric measurements of performance had been derived from a task analysis on laparoscopic cholecystectomy by a surgeon, a behavioral scientist, and software engineer. To the untrained eye they may have looked nothing like surgical performance, but on closer scrutiny, the MIST VR tasks were well suited to the job. The starting position for the Yale University team that completed the first VR to OR clinical trial (Seymour et al. 2002) was a virtual reality simulator with well-validated performance metrics. MIST VR performance metrics that were used in this trial were errors and economy of diathermy. Time was excluded as a training metric because the researchers were more interested in training safe performance rather than fast performance. Economy of instrument movement (e.g., how efficiently the instrument was moved from point A to B in real terms) was excluded because of their measurement reliability issues.

There was an extensive and extended discussion within this group about how long or how many trials a trainee should be trained on MIST VR. The researchers came to the same conclusion at the end of each discussion, i.e., all that these training strategies have achieved historically was considerable variability in levels of skills. It was eventually agreed the trainees would train until they reached a benchmark; however, a similar discussion ensued about how the benchmark should be established. The parsimonious solution that was eventually achieved was that the benchmark would be established on the basis of the performance of members of the surgical team who were discussing the problem. After all, the surgeon members of the team were very experienced laparoscopic surgeons, all worked in the same department, all worked with the same surgical trainees, and that all of them recognized that they had a reasonably homogeneous skill set. From previous research, it had been shown that for experienced laparoscopic surgeons, their learning curve on the MIST VR simulator flattened out at about three trials. All of the attending surgeons participating in the study completed five trials on the manipulate-diathermy task on MIST VR on a modified difficult setting. The performance criteria or benchmarks that trainees were to be trained to was established on the basis of the mean score of the attending surgeons on trials four and five for errors and economy of diathermy (for both hands).

Proficiency Benchmarked

It was assumed by the Yale University team that the MIST VR or performance metrics of "errors" and "economy of diathermy" captured important topographical features of the performance characteristics of experienced laparoscopic surgeons. It was the team hypothesis that training a group of trainee surgeons to the benchmark represented by these metrics would impact on skills levels to the extent that there would be transference to intraoperative performance. Although this type of study had not been conducted before in medicine, there was ample evidence from other high skills industries that training in a simulated environment improved performance on a real world task. There was nothing magical or unusual about the metrics that were used to benchmark the experienced surgeon's performance. These were the metrics that had been demonstrated to be the most reliable and made the most sense, i.e., the goal of the trial was training surgeons to perform the dissection portion of a laparoscopic cholecystectomy using the electrocautery instrument. It should also be noted that the metrics used are like "time" measures, i.e., surrogate measures of skill. However, the difference between the error and economy of diathermy metrics and time is that they more accurately reflected what the trainee was doing on a second-by-second basis and therefore was a good candidate for performance feedback. The goal of training was to help trainees reach a performance criterion level which meant minimizing performance errors and maximizing efficient use of electrocautery. Information on performance errors and inefficient or erroneous use of electrocautery was given to trainees immediately after being enacted. This was achieved by the simulator with an auditory stimulus for electrocautery errors and the virtual tasks turned red to indicate an error had been enacted. As discussed in Chap. 4, augmented feedback of results such as those described here facilitates learning. In simple terms, it tells the trainee that they have just done something wrong as soon as they have done it, which allows them the opportunity to modify their behavior and not make the same mistake in the future. In contrast, a time metric would simply inform them at the end of the task that they had taken too long. This type of information is too ambiguous for the optimal facilitation of learning. If the time metric could be granularized to inform the trainee as to which parts of their performance were taking too long, this would be much better feedback. However, it would still only tell them that they were taking too long and would not give them feedback on the quality of their performance, whereas, feedback on errors and economy of diathermy does.

The mean performance level on MIST VR of the attending surgeons involved in the trial was used as the performance criterion and benchmark because it seemed the most reasonable measure. This was the first time that a performance criterion level was used as a guide for training success in a surgery clinical trial. Possible alternatives might have been using the performance of one surgeon to benchmark performance, using confidence intervals or the more traditional amount of time training or number of trials in training. The traditional approach to training was rejected fairly quickly because of the variability in skills levels. Ironically, the second clinical trial to demonstrate that virtual reality training improves intraoperative performance used precisely this approach, i.e., they trained the virtual reality subjects for ten trials rather than to proficiency (Grantcharov et al. 2004). The results show that the virtual reality–training group performed significantly better than the standard training group; however, this was more by accident than design as this approach to training is inefficient. Training to a benchmark confidence interval was also rejected as the researchers were not sure what the intervals might be based on, i.e., one standard deviation, 1.96 standard deviations, one inter-quartile range, etc. The mean level of the participating attending surgeons' performance was used because it meant that all of them had contributed to the performance criterion definition. It also meant that extreme performances (had they existed) would have been mitigated by better performances. The team were also keen to use the mean performance because they were aware of research that was ongoing in Sweden in the early 2000s which was generating results that the Swedish researchers found difficult to explain. Ahlberg et al. (2007) were investigating the learning curve of trainee surgeons performing Nissen fundoplication. They were particularly interested in whether the trainee surgeons' initial objectively assessed skill levels would be good predictors of the steepness of their learning curves and intraoperative performances. However, what they did find was that the objectively assessed measures of the senior surgeon's skills were the best predictor of their trainee's intraoperative surgical performance. Indeed, it was better than objective assessment of surgical skills on the simulator. The implication of these findings was that the trainees' skills level regress to that of their supervising surgeon (in both directions!).

Choosing the mean performance level in setting the benchmark performance criterion avoids asking difficult questions about surgeons who were not performing as well as some of their colleagues while at the same time establishing a robust skills level that is representative of a given group of surgeons as a whole. If trainees were performing to a benchmark performance criterion level, that meant that their performance was equal to or better than 50% of the performances on which the benchmark was established. Even the most ardent critic of this approach to training would have to admit that this is a much more rigorous approach to training than currently exists. However, there are a number of implications for setting a performance criterion level and how it is established (Chap. 12). The Yale team was also aware that choosing the mean performance of the attending surgeons was probably a conservative approach, but at that time, proficiency-based progression training was an unproven methodology.

Trainees on a proficiency-based progression training schedule continue training on the simulator until they reach the performance criterion level on both metrics, with both hands on two consecutive trials (for the Yale VR to OR trial (Seymour et al. 2002)). The reasons for these specifications were that laparoscopic cholecystectomy is a bimanual task and so it made sense that trainees should be adept at using instruments in both hands. VR allowed training and assessment of bimanual psychomotor performance for the laparoscopic cholecystectomy. Trainees were also required to reach the performance criterion level on both metrics because these were the metrics that best characterized the performance of the attending surgeons. They were required to reach these performance levels on two consecutive trials, because it was argued that they might reach these benchmarks on one trial by accident/coincidence, but it was unlikely that this would be the case for reaching the performance criterion levels on both metrics on both hands on two consecutive trials. Like the issue of mean performance as a benchmark proficiency level, we will return to the issue of proficiency definition in Chap. 12.

One of the advantages of using a virtual reality simulation is that machine-scored performance metrics has been demonstrated to be reliable and valid and takes a lot of the work out of establishing a proficiency level. There is a considerable effort required to develop and then validate the performance metrics but once these have been published, the surgical community can be reasonably confident in their use. However, the problem for surgery is that most of the virtual reality simulators that currently exist are for minimally invasive or image-guided procedures. This approach to surgery continues to represent a minority of surgical practice. The absence of a virtual reality simulator should not impede a proficiency-based progression training program, as demonstrated by the work of Van Sickle et al. (2008). In this clinical trial for training senior residents to perform Nissen fundoplication, no specific virtual reality simulator existed. Instead, the researchers developed novel simulations that captured essential components of the suturing and knot tying required for successful operating. They established performance criterion levels based on experienced operators' performances on these tasks, and then trained surgical residents until they reached these performance levels. The results showed that surgical residents trained to the performance criterion levels performed Nissen fundoplication more efficiently and with significantly fewer objectively assessed intraoperative errors. An important point to note about this study is contained in the discussion section of the paper. They pointed out how time consuming it was to train subjects on a non-virtual reality–based simulation program. It required one of the researchers to observe and in some cases physically score the performance of the trainee while they were training or immediately afterward. However, these are simply implementation obstacles which can be overcome with a determined approach and with innovative solutions. Another important point to note about the Van Sickle et al. (2008) clinical trial is that the researchers went through the same iterative process of metric development, operational definition, construct validation and proficiency definition, proficiency-based progression training, and blinded objective assessment of intraoperative performance to a high level of inter-rater reliability for the outcome assessment. The main point is that proficiency-based progression training quality assures the skills level at the end of the training process, i.e., the graduating trainee is performing as well as or better than 50% of the individuals on whose performance the proficiency levels are established.

Why Proficiency-Based Progression?

Some educationalists may argue that the process that we have just outlined could just as easily be called competency-based progression. However, we disagree. Competency is mired in descriptive detail that is going to make operational definitions difficult to extricate from the baggage. The main problem about competency definition is deciding where the performance criterion line should be drawn. Proficiency does not carry the same baggage. Furthermore, the vast majority of operating surgeons currently in practice operate daily in simple and complex surgical procedures. On the whole, their patients are well looked after, they get good surgical care and safe operative performance. It would be difficult to argue that this is an unreasonable target to set for trainees. The advantage of a proficiency-based approach to training is that we can quantify performance, and in so doing, we set trainees a target that they can reach in their own time-scale. Furthermore, this benchmark is based on something meaningful from the real world, i.e., experienced operating surgeons. For the talented and gifted trainee surgeons, they will reach this target quickly; for the less talented or gifted surgeon, they will take longer to reach the same target but when they do, their skills will be at the same level (at least) as their more talented colleagues. The important point is that they reach this performance criterion level within a reasonable time frame. Will the surgeon who reaches the performance criterion faster become a better surgeon? This is certainly a good research question but current subjective evidence would tend to suggest not. We know from the Yale VR to OR clinical trial team that the resident in their study, who took the longest to reach the performance criterion level performed the best intraoperatively. Furthermore, it takes more than good technical skills to make a complete surgeon.

The Meaning of Proficiency-Based Progression

The apprenticeship model of surgical training has always been credited to the program that Halsted developed at Johns Hopkins in Baltimore, USA. In Halsted's training program (which is not dissimilar to the training program that currently exists in surgery), the trainee was given increasing responsibility for the treatment and care of the patient as their training progressed. Training and progressing were at the behest of the supervising surgeon which of course could be subject to their individual whims. Proficiency-based progression as a training paradigm alters that relationship. Training progression is now determined on a trainee's objectively assessed performance benchmarked against the performance of experienced operators. This means that progression in training is based on objective, verifiable criteria, thus making the process more transparent and fair. Proficiency-based progression training also has implications for the patient. Under the Halstedian training paradigm, the operating room was used as a basic skills training environment where the trainee honed their skills during their training years. In a proficiency-based progression training program, the trainee is not allowed to operate on a patient until they have quantitatively demonstrated that they are performing at the benchmark surgical skills established by their training program. This means that the operating room is no longer a basic skills training environment but more like a finishing school where surgical technique is mastered under the apprenticeship of a senior surgeon.

Proficiency and competency are often used interchangeably; however, they are not the same. In this chapter, we have discussed the differences between proficiency and competency. Proficiency has been operationally and quantitatively defined while competency has only been described, and consequently, there is little agreement among the global medical establishment about the operational definition of competency. Furthermore, precedent has already been established with regard to the quantification and definition of proficiency (Ahlberg et al. 2007; Seymour et al. 2002; Van Sickle et al. 2008). Thus it is prudent to proceed by using a proficiency benchmark as an indicator of skills rather than competency.

Proficiency-based training as a new approach to the acquisition of procedural-based medical skills took a major step forward in April 2004. As part of the roll-out of a new device for carotid artery stenting (CAS), the Food and Drug Administration (FDA) mandated, as part of the device approval package, metric-based training to proficiency on a VR simulator as the required training approach for physicians who will be using the new device (Gallagher and Cates 2004a, b; Reinhardt-Rutland and Gallagher 1995). The company manufacturing the CAS system informed the FDA that they would educate and train physicians in catheter and wire handling skills with a high fidelity VR simulator using a curriculum based on achieving a level of proficiency. This approach allows for training of physicians to enter with variable knowledge, skill, or experience and to leave with objectively assessed proficient knowledge and skills. This is particularly important for a procedure like CAS as it crosses multiple clinical specialties with each bringing a different skill set to the training table. For example, a vascular surgeon has a thorough cognitive understanding of vascular anatomy and management of carotid disease, but may lack some of the psychomotor technical skills of wire and catheter manipulation. Conversely, an interventional cardiologist may have all of the technical skills, but may not be as familiar with the anatomical and clinical management issues. A sound training strategy must ensure that all of these specialists are able to meet an objectively assessable minimum level of proficiency in all facets of the procedure. This development helps to consolidate the paradigm shift in procedural-based medicine training and will result in a reduction in "turf wars" concerning future credentialing for new procedures. Indeed this was the approach advocated by a number of the professional medical organizations (i.e., vascular surgery, interventional cardiology, and vascular medicine and biology) intimately involved in training physicians for CAS (Rosenfield et al. 2005). As long as a physician is able to demonstrate that he or she possesses the requisite knowledge and skills to perform a procedure, specialty affiliation will become less important. Proficiency-based progression training has leveled the playing field in terms of territorial claims about specific procedures. Decisions about who carries out such procedures will be based firmly on who can perform the procedure to a safe level of skills rather than who has traditionally looked after a particular group of patients. This approach will have profound implications for the practice of medicine. Although we have shown that proficiency-based progression is a better way to train for the *in vivo* practice of procedural medicine, surgical training is about more than just procedural skills. We shall examine this issue further in Chap. 9 when we discuss how we can use the experience and knowledge gained from the development of proficiency-based progression training and augment this approach with e-learning.

Summary

Although medicine in general and surgery in particular profess to be using a competency-based training program, there seems to be no clear operationalized definition of what competency is and what it is not. There has been a considerable amount of effort made by training organizations around the world on competency; however, these efforts have mostly been directed at describing what factors are characteristic of competent performance. Efforts to measure competency appear to have been more comprehensive and systematic in the UK than in the USA. The strongest of the competency assessment procedures in the UK is the procedure-based assessment instruments which have been developed for all index surgical procedures. However, even this instrument could be considerably strengthened with more detailed assessment of the intraoperative performance of the trainee surgeon based on a task analysis as described in Chap. 5.

We have proposed that instead of using competency as the benchmark, it makes more sense to use proficiency as it is not lumbered with the same historical baggage as the concept of "competency" and is easier to establish a widely agreed upon operational definition, i.e., "proficiency is what experienced surgeons (or physicians) do." A proficiency-based training program can be developed using the following steps;

1. Perform the *task analysis* on the procedure to be learned.
2. *Metric definition*: Operationally define the key aspects of optimal procedure performance identified from the task analysis.
3. *Metric validation*: Ensure that metric-based assessment of novice trainee performance differs from experienced operator performance (i.e., construct validity).
4. *Proficiency definition*: Quantitatively assess the performance of a representative number of experienced operators (e.g., consultant/attending surgeons) on the training device/strategy to be used for trainees.
5. *Proficiency-based progression training*: Trainees train on the training device/strategy until they demonstrate the benchmark performance, consistently.
6. *Validate proficiency-based progression training*: Establish whether trainees on the training program perform better than surgeons who were traditionally trained.

The results from preliminary clinical trials using proficiency-based progression training have shown that trainees perform significantly better than traditionally trained surgeons. This approach to training has given further impetus by the FDA in the USA who in 2004 mandated training on a virtual reality simulator for carotid artery stenting. They took this decision in the interest of patient safety to ensure skills of sufficient standard are acquired by surgeons, cardiologists, and radiologists before performing the procedure on patients. Their decision set a precedent which we believe will further drive the changes in training procedural skills in medicine.

References

Ahlberg G, Enochsson L, Gallagher AG, et al. Proficiency-based virtual reality training significantly reduces the error rate for residents during their first 10 laparoscopic cholecystectomies. *Am J Surg*. 2007;193(6):797-804.

Aretz HT. How good is the newly graduated doctor and can we measure it? *Med J Aust*. 2003;178(4):147-147.

Barrows HS, Abrahamson S. The programmed patient: a technique for appraising student performance in clinical neurology. *Acad Med*. 1964;39(8):802.

Beall DP. The ACGME institutional requirements: what residents need to know. *J Am Med Assoc*. 1999;281(24):2352.

Bryant J. *Health and the Developing World*. Ithaca: Cornell University Press; 1969.

Dictionary CC. *Thesaurus*. New York: Harper Collins; 1995.

Dreyfus HL. *What Computers Can't Do: the Limits of Artificial Intelligence*. New York: HarperCollins Publishers; 1979.

Dreyfus HL, Dreyfus SE, Athanasiou T. *Mind over Machine*. New York: Free Press; 1986.

Dreyfus HL, Dreyfus SE, Athanasiou T. *Mind over Machine: The Power of Human Intuition and Expertise in the Era of the Computer*. USA: Simon and Schuster; 2000.

Epstein RM, Hundert EM. Defining and assessing professional competence. *J Am Med Assoc*. 2002;287(2):226.

Frank JR. *The CanMEDS 2005 Physician Competency Framework. Better Standards. Better Physicians. Better Care*. Ottawa: The Royal College of Physicians and Surgeons of Canada; 2005.

Gallagher AG, Cates CU. Approval of virtual reality training for carotid stenting: what this means for procedural-based medicine. *J Am Med Assoc*. 2004a;292(24):3024-3026.

Gallagher AG, Cates CU. Virtual reality training for the operating room and cardiac catheterisation laboratory. *Lancet*. 2004b;364(9444):1538-1540.

Gallagher AG, Satava RM. Virtual reality as a metric for the assessment of laparoscopic psychomotor skills. Learning curves and reliability measures. *Surg Endosc*. 2002;16(12):1746-1752.

Gallagher AG, Richie K, McClure N, McGuigan J. Objective psychomotor skills assessment of experienced, junior, and novice laparoscopists with virtual reality. *World J Surg*. 2001;25(11):1478-1483.

General Medical Council. *Tomorrow's Doctors: Recommendations on Undergraduate Medical Education*. London: GMC; 1993.

Grantcharov TP, Kristiansen VB, Bendix J, Bardram L, Rosenberg J, Funch-Jensen P. Randomized clinical trial of virtual reality simulation for laparoscopic skills training. *Br J Surg*. 2004;91(2):146-150.

Harden RM, Stevenson M, Downie WW, Wilson GM. Assessment of clinical competence using objective structured examination. *Br Med J*. 1975;1(5955):447.

Lurie SJ, Mooney CJ, Lyness JM. Measurement of the general competencies of the accreditation council for graduate medical education: a systematic review. *Acad Med*. 2009;84(3):301.

Marshall JB. Technical proficiency of trainees performing colonoscopy: a learning curve. *Gastrointest Endosc*. 1995;42(4):287-291.

Miller GE. The assessment of clinical skills/competence/performance. *Acad Med*. 1990;65(9):S63.

Neufeld VR, Maudsley RF, Pickering RJ, et al. Educating future physicians for Ontario. *Acad Med.* 1998;73(11):1133.

Norcini JJ, Blank LL, Duffy FD, Fortna GS. The mini-CEX: a method for assessing clinical skills. *Ann Intern Med.* 2003;138(6):476.

Pitts D, Rowley DI, Marx C, Sher L, Banks T, Murray A. *A Competency Based Curriculum for Specialist Training in Trauma and Orthopaedics*. London: British Orthopaedic Association; 2006.

Popper KR. *Objective Knowledge: An Evolutionary Approach.* Oxford: Clarendon Press; 1979.

Reinhardt-Rutland AH, Gallagher AG. Visual depth perception in minimally invasive surgery. In: Robertson SA, ed. *Contemporary Ergonomics*. London: Taylor & Francis; 1995:531-536.

Rosenfield K, Babb JD, Cates CU, et al. Clinical competence statement on carotid stenting: training and credentialing for carotid stenting–multispecialty consensus recommendations: a report of the SCAI/SVMB/SVS Writing Committee to develop a clinical competence statement on carotid interventions. *J Am Coll Cardiol*. 2005;45(1):165-174.

Seymour NE, Gallagher AG, Roman SA, et al. Virtual reality training improves operating room performance: results of a randomized, double-blinded study. *Ann Surg*. 2002;236(4):458-463; discussion 463-454.

Van Sickle K, Ritter EM, Baghai M, et al. Prospective, randomized, double-blind trial of curriculum-based training for intracorporeal suturing and knot tying. *J Am Coll Surg*. 2008;207(4): 560-568.

Verheugen G. (2005) *Good Clinical Practice.* Retrieved. from http://eur-lex.europa.eu/LexUriServ/LexUriServ.do?uri=OJ:L:2005:091:0013:0019:en:PDF. (accessed 10 July 2010).

Chapter 9
Didactic Education and Training for Improved Intraoperative Performance: e-Learning Comes of Age

E-learning

E-learning comprises all forms of electronically supported learning and teaching which are aimed at imparting or facilitating the construction of knowledge. E-learning is perceived by many as made up of the computer and network-enabled transferor of knowledge. Applications that facilitate this process include web-based learning, computer-based learning, virtual classrooms, and digital collaboration. The vast and extensive development of the Internet has facilitated what many individuals perceive as the engine of e-learning. However, e-learning has been available long before the widespread availability of the Internet. The Open University (OU) in the United Kingdom was one of the developments that came out of Harold Wilson's government which was elected in 1967. The OU was the world's first successful distance teaching university and was founded on the belief that communications technology could bring high-quality degree-level learning to people who had not had the opportunity to attend campus universities. Prof Walter Perry, who had been a professor of Pharmacology at Edinburgh and a member of the Medical Research Council staff, was appointed as the first vice chancellor of the OU (or as it was then known "University of the Air"). Perry was convinced to become involved because he believed that the standard of teaching at conventional universities was pretty deplorable. One of its initial ambitions was to use the media and other devices to deliver course materials that would allow students to learn by themselves. This, he believed would inevitably effect – for good – the standard of teaching at conventional universities. The university expanded during the 1980s and harnessed new technologies for the delivery of course material. These new methods included the use of computers and multimedia mix. Courses were delivered in written form, via radio programs and some television programs. In the mid-1980s, there was a rapid expansion in the growth and use of personal computers which enhanced the possibilities for the delivery of OU courses. Students, mostly adults, embraced learning on personal computers, CD-ROM, and web-based media with enthusiasm. By the mid-1990s, the university began a massive exploitation of the Internet which made the OU the world's leading e-university.

A.G. Gallagher and G.C. O'Sullivan, *Fundamentals of Surgical Simulation*, Improving Medical Outcome - Zero Tolerance,
DOI 10.1007/978-0-85729-763-1_9, © Springer-Verlag London Limited 2012

E-learning Benefits

Early e-learning systems and computer-based learning packages often attempted to replicate autocratic teaching styles whereby the role of the learning system was assumed to be simply the transfer of knowledge. However, pioneers such as Graziadei (1997) realized that e-learning could be much more than this. The potential benefits of an e-learning system are enormous and include:

- *Increased access*: Via whatever type of electronic technology (but usually the Internet), students can access academics from around the world, thus acquiring knowledge that is not constrained by physical distance, political ideology, or economic boundaries. In surgery, this gives trainees access to information and courses in centers of excellence. What is true for the student is also true for the academic institution. This means that they can deliver large amounts of their academic content to anywhere in the world.
- *Convenience of access*: The development of e-learning means that course content is available at any time of the day to anywhere in the world and is not bound by the size of a lecture theater. While there are many constraints on operating room access, the same rules pretty much hold true as well, i.e., only so many observes can be accommodated in an OR.
- *Convenience of use*: Users of e-learning can access the materials from a location that suits them whether this is their home, the hospital library, or indeed their own desk. The reverse is also true where users can access the same materials from a variety of locations. The usual constraint is access to the Internet.
- *Distributed training*: As we shall see later in this chapter, knowledge and skill are optimally acquired when spread out over a period of time rather than massed into an intense course. E-learning facilitates this process.
- *Facilitates the development of computer skills*: Modern medicine cannot be practiced effectively and efficiently in the absence of good computer skills. E-learning enforces varied and continued practice of the these skills.

The Traditional Lecture

A lecture is an oral presentation intended to present or convey critical information or teach an audience about a particular subject. Although the use of lectures is much criticized as a pedagogical method, (most) universities have not yet found a practical alternative teaching method to deliver the vast majority of their courses. Lectures delivered by a talented speaker can be highly stimulating. They have also survived in academia for some considerable period of time probably because they are quick, flexible, cheap, and efficient at introducing large numbers of students to a particular field of study. The practice in the medieval university was for the instructor to read from an original source to a class of students who took notes on the lecture. The reading from original sources evolved eventually into reading from lecture notes. Throughout much of history, the spread of knowledge through hand-written lecture notes was an essential element of academic life. Unfortunately, some lecturers today are accustomed to simply reading their own notes from the lectern much as 500 years ago. The use of multimedia presentation software such as Microsoft PowerPoint has changed the form of the lecture which can now include video presentations, animated graphics and web-based material. Most lectures continue to be presented verbally and augmented with PowerPoint bullet points.

Traditional e-Learning Packages

When virtual reality simulation was first thought of in surgery, it was widely perceived to be a panacea for many of the ills of surgical training. It has taken almost two decades for the surgical community to realize that virtual reality simulation and indeed simulation per se is simply a tool for the efficient and effective delivery for part of the curriculum. Unfortunately, e-learning suffers from the same misperception. For some it is perceived as a new and trendy way to deliver educational material; for others, it is simply a way of delivering a lecture to more people in more diverse locations. E-learning may be all of these things, but more importantly, it is potentially a very powerful and effective tool for the efficient and effective delivery of the curriculum. There seems to be considerable effort put into the content of e-learning packages, i.e., what it looks like, eye catchy material such as grand rounds delivered by a famous surgeon in a famous hospital half-way around the world. Content is only part of what makes a good e-learning package. Of equal importance is how the content is configured, delivered, and assessed so as to optimize learning in an efficient and effective manner. To achieve this end requires an explicit understanding of where and how it can be used to gain the greatest effect. Human beings are not passive recipient vessels for information no matter how enthusiastic or committed they are to the learning process. Likewise, human beings are not empty vessels which we fill full of skills in our skills laboratories and operating rooms. As shown in Chaps 3 and 4, human beings are active information processors. Although they process vast quantities of information from their immediate environment, this information is filtered from the outset. Initially, by a perceptual system that filters and organizes the information that is sensed and then by the working memory system that decides whether or not to attend to the information. The information that does reach short-term memory is then organized and "chunked" before storage in long-term memory. The information that is chunked and stored can be of multiple sensory modalities and this is particularly likely to be the case in learning material related to clinical surgery. For example, trainees are likely to have to learn information by listening to instructions (auditory information) about a surgical procedure that they are watching (visual information) being performed or that they themselves are actually performing (kinesthetic information).

E-learning Optimized

E-learning is naturally suited for the delivery of multisensory information such as material associated with learning to perform surgery. It can provide a flexible learning environment that can be used as an adjunct to face-to-face teaching, skills laboratory training, and clinical surgery training for both novice and very experienced operators. E-learning offers particularly exciting opportunities for augmenting the learning process in surgery and procedural medicine. For example, in a well-delivered traditional lecture, the academic has very few ways of knowing how effectively they have imparted the information that they are trying to communicate. Furthermore, it would be unrealistic to expect that all of the audience would be learning at the same pace, but the traditional lecture is delivered in the standard 40–50 min time period to the individuals sitting in the same room. The hope is that by the time of the exam, everyone is at a sufficient standard to at least pass the course. If the material is delivered on an e-platform, the progress of each individual can be tracked with a formative assessment process. This means that individuals who learn at a slower pace can have their education supplemented automatically or they can be flagged for direct academic intervention.

The education and training of a surgeon is all about one thing, i.e., preparing trainee surgeons to take care of patients, nothing more and nothing less. As seen in Chap 8 there are multiple aspects to this in terms of professional behavior, interpersonal behavior, etc. However, as identified in the CanMeds, at the core of this process is the assumption that the surgeon is a safe operator. Another core assumption is that what the surgeon is taught will prepare them for operating and taking care of patients. In other words, it is hoped that knowledge and skills acquired in the classroom and skills laboratory will generalize to the operating room specifically and to patient care generally.

Transfer of Training

In Chap 4 we discussed the different types of factors that affect the efficiency of psychomotor skill acquisition. These factors or, more accurately, these contingencies should be optimally configured for efficient learning. We proposed that virtual reality simulation affords an ideal opportunity to marshal and to configure these variables for optimal effect. By and large, the variables which are important for learning on a virtual reality or physical model simulator are also important in an e-learning package. The end goal of the process is the same, i.e., a proficient surgeon. Generalization is one of the most powerful learning processes where knowledge or skills acquired in one context have positive effects on another similar situation. It is the application of a skill learned in one situation to a different but similar context. For example, in Chap 6 we described the process of training on the MIST VR system until a predefined level of technical skills proficiency was reached. When surgical trainees had acquired this objectively defined performance criterion level, they were then allowed to perform the surgical procedure on the real patient. Although the MIST VR tasks looked nothing like the anatomy of a gall-bladder, the assumption was that skills acquired on MIST VR would generalize to the LC. The reasons were: (1) MIST VR trained the appropriate psychomotor coordination of laparoscopic instruments; trainees were required to hold a target object in (virtual) three-dimensional space with one hand while applying electrocautery with an instrument in the other hand and pressing a foot-pedal when the electrocautery instrument was touching the target object. (2) MIST VR trained the surgical trainee what to do, but more importantly what not to do; to successfully complete the task, the target object had to be held in a stable position within a predefined virtual space and then small cubes on the surface of the target object had to be burned off with the electrocautery instrument. Electrocautery could only be applied when the target object was within the predefined space; otherwise, an error was scored; if electrocautery was used when the instrument was burning non-target objects, an error was scored; an error was also scored if electrocautery was used when the instrument was not touching any object. This may seem somewhat abstracted from performing a LC; however, on closer scrutiny, it is not. This task taught appropriate use of surgical instruments, choreographed use of surgical instruments to complete the task, practice in hand-eye-foot coordination, and trainees were also taught how to perform the task with a minimum of errors and using electrocautery efficiently. They were also given feedback on their performance with formative feedback proximate to errors and summative feedback when they had completed the task. The results of this training speak for themselves; surgeons trained on MIST VR to a level of proficiency made six times fewer objectively assessed intraoperative errors when operating *in vivo* on real patients than subjects traditionally trained (Seymour et al. 2002).

The lesson to be learned from this example is that a great deal of learning can take place on appropriate training tasks that have good feedback on performance and are configured in a way that they emulate the crucial aspects of the real world task. Training on these tasks generalizes to real world tasks and there is good evidence to support this conclusion. The general rule is that the closer the simulation or the emulation is to the real world task the greater the amount of skills that will be transferred. One would expect even greater transfer of skills from a high fidelity simulator such as VIST in comparison to MIST VR. It should also be noted that the higher the risk of adverse events from the procedure to the patient, the higher the fidelity and more accurate the simulation should be. We must emphasize here that we are not simply referring here to the fact that a simulator "looks" like the real procedure. Rather, we would expect that the simulators for training high-risk procedures look, feel, and behave like operating on a real patient (or close as possible). It will never be possible to devise a VR simulation that looks, feels, and behaves EXACTLY like the real patient but a full physics simulation environment such as VIST will provide a very realistic approximation.

The function of e-learning should be the same as training on a simulation model, i.e., support for delivery of the curriculum. E-learning and simulations are not something apart from the curriculum but should be viewed as tools for the efficient and effective delivery of the curriculum. Virtual or physical model simulations afford the opportunity for hands-on interactive training, which is a particularly powerful way for the acquisition of procedural skills. However, e-learning can also be a powerful tool, if used in the correct way.

One of the goals of e-learning and simulation training is to have the trainee as well prepared as possible for their training in the operating room. Although minimally invasive surgery has been blamed for many of the problems facing surgeons in training, one of the major positive changes that it brought about is that it forced medical educators to systematically think about the entire training process. Traditionally, the operative surgical training started and ended in the operating room. With the advent of MIS, it very quickly became clear that the operating room was an inappropriate environment to acquire basic skills for this type of surgery. The surgical community realized that before trainees could commence their clinical training in the operating room, they had to at least have the basic psychomotor skills with which to operate. This meant that the early part of MIS skills training took place in the skills laboratory rather than the operating room. Compounding these training difficulties was the reduction in work hours in the United States and Europe. The surgical community looked for new training devices and strategies with little systematic understanding of why particular strategies or devices were effective, e.g., more training is better! This was despite the fact that there was more than 100 years of research data and knowledge that was directly applicable to this problem. In our review of this literature in Chap 4 we outlined the strategy that can be implemented in a curriculum via a simulation device to overcome these problems. Although surgery developed training solutions for the skill acquisition problems posed by MIS, these solutions were not developed from first principles, but rather, intuition. Furthermore, devices such as MIST VR which were developed and did adhere to sound behavioral principles for training and learning were frequently dismissed as not looking like they would do the job they were designed for.

Elements of Transfer of Training from e-Learning

Verified Pre-learning

Virtual reality simulation provides a very good interim opportunity for hands-on skill acquisition. However, technical skills for surgery are not practiced in a vacuum. They need to be learned and practiced in the context. One of the problems currently faced by skills laboratories around the world is that trainees turn up for their 1 or 2 days skills training course with considerably variable preparation. Some candidates turn up very well prepared and have done the appropriate reading on the disease process or the organ system on which they are to be taught to operate on; they know the anatomy and physiology, surgical instruments to be used, and possibly some of the operative techniques. Other candidates turn up, with little or no preparation at all, and consider it fortunate that they turned up at all!. Unfortunately, the trainers organizing this type of skills laboratory are tied to the level of the candidate who turns up with no preparation. E-learning allows for the situation to be completely avoided. At the Royal College of Surgeons in Ireland, surgical trainees pay an annual fee that runs into thousands of Euros for access to courses in the skills laboratory. The skills laboratory has courses scheduled for the entire year. This means that training time in the lab must be used effectively. The problem of the ill-prepared trainee could be dealt with by scheduling study and assessment of online material prior to attending the skills laboratory. Candidates wishing to train in the skills laboratory would not only have to study the online material, they would also have to pass a predefined level, before even applying for a training slot. This would mean that candidates turning up for training would be well prepared. This process could also help to optimize the training they do receive in the skills laboratory. For example, all candidates attending training would have passed the online didactic component for the course. However, across members of the class, a consistent aspect of the didactic material, e.g., anatomy and physiology, laboratory tests, operative procedure etc., may have been poorly understood as indicated by the number in the class who got that part of the assessment wrong. In light of this information, the course leaders could investigate why it was that the trainees found this aspect of the material difficult to understand and cover the material in more detail in the classroom. The advantage of this approach is that it guarantees a sufficient level of knowledge to ensure that skills laboratory training progresses in a timely fashion; it highlights potential weaknesses in a candidate's knowledge that can be rectified, and it ensures the course faculty that the trainees are motivated, i.e., they made the effort to undertake study and assessment of the online material as it related to the skills course. This is considerably more information than is currently available to course faculty. Furthermore, it puts the onus of knowledge acquisition clearly on the trainee. The faculty and the training body have provided sufficient and appropriate learning material to prepare for the course and the trainee is not allowed to attend until they have passed the online didactic material.

Pre-learning: Declarative Memory

To get the most out of training on a simulator, the trainee should know background information on the task/procedure they are learning, i.e., context. They should also know when, where, how to do it, and what with. The trainee can either learn this information in the skills lab just prior to participating in hands-on training on a simulation model or they can acquire this information before they attend for training. All of this information can be delivered prior to training.

When a surgeon performs an operative procedure, the skills that they apply are based on information that they have retrieved from their long-term memory, which

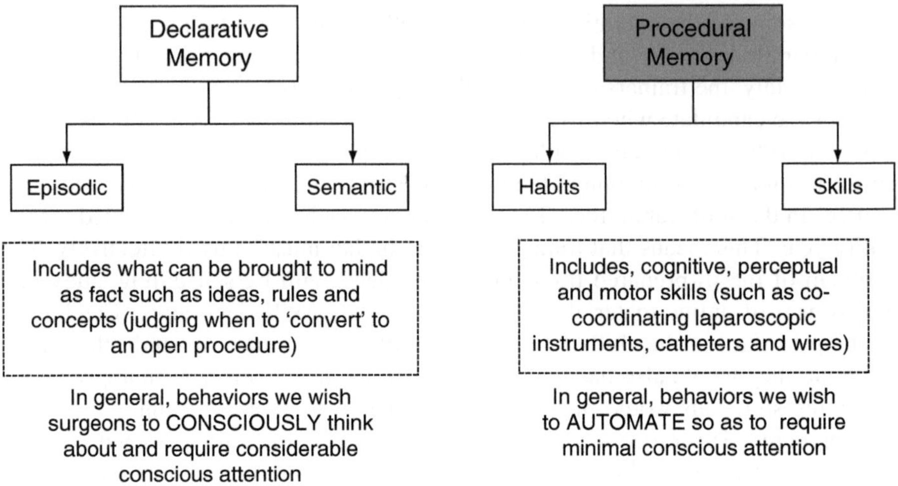

Fig. 9.1 Different types of attributes of declarative and procedural long-term memories

they have learned from didactic teaching, reading, and probably skills practice on simulation models. They may also have acquired information from observing others or from what others have told them. This information, retrieved from long-term memory, is one of two types of human long-term memory, i.e., declarative memory and non-declarative or procedural memory. These two types of memories are crucial for skilled performance. Declarative memory refers to information which can be consciously recalled, such as facts and events (Keane and Eysenck 2000). Non-declarative or procedural memory refers to unconscious memories such as those pertaining to skills and habits like riding a bicycle or driving a car. Figure 9.1 shows a diagrammatic representation of the different types of long-term memories and their attributes.

Declarative memory can be subdivided into two different types; semantic memories contain factual knowledge that is independent of the individual's personal experience. Types of semantic information in surgery would include signs and symptoms, anatomy and physiology, laboratory test norms, etc. Episodic memories are those that are idiosyncratic and personal to the individual experience. Semantic memories may consist of information remembered from a particular course attended by the individual and the information on a particular disease system. However, episodic memories relating to the same course may contain information on who they attended a course with, whether they enjoyed the course or not, what they did badly on the course, or on what they excelled. Episodic memory information concerns fairly sharply circumscribed concepts. Furthermore, episodic memory is believed to be the system that supports and underpins semantic memory (Tulving and Thomson 1973). Episodic memory appears to apply meaning to information and situations and appears to make information easier to recall. Semantic information can be learned but it seems to be less "easily" learned than episodic information. One of the tactics in optimizing memorization of information is to facilitate the learner applying episodic "tags" to the information. This means that the information is more "meaningful" and hence easier remembered.

E-learning can facilitate the application of these strategies to enhance the storage and to facilitate the retrieval of information necessary for the learning and practice of surgical skills. For example, information on gallstones and cholecystectomy could be linked to a famous British Prime minister, Anthony Eden. A medical mishap would change the course of Eden's life forever. During an operation in 1953 to remove gallstones, Eden's bile duct was damaged, making him susceptible to recurrent infections, biliary obstruction, and liver failure. He required major surgery on three occasions to alleviate the problem and his handling of the Suez crises has been directly linked to the medication he was taking to alleviate postoperative symptoms (Dutton 1997). Having set the context, the presenting symptoms of the disease that Eden first presented with could be recounted, then a lesson in the anatomy and physiology of the gallbladder and cystic structures. Trainees could then be shown how the operation is approached and performed using the traditional open surgical approach and what caused the complications in Eden's case and how alleviation would be approached. This would then lead on to the development of laparoscopic cholecystectomy and the complications that ensued with its introduction. The important anatomy, physiology, signs, and symptoms information about cholecystectomy is tagged on to the information about Anthony Eden. This otherwise bland information is made more colorful and hence more memorable by real world association and implications for a great British Prime Minister.

Pre-learning: Procedural Memory

Procedural memory is our memory for how we do things. In Chap 4 we described the process of skill acquisition outlined by Fitts and Posner (1967). They proposed that learning a new skill involves three stages. The Cognitive stage involves the learner developing an understanding of what the skill comprises. This process involves understanding the units of behavior and performance characteristics in the sequence that occur in the construction of a skilled performance. In the second stage, the Associative phase, they practice and hone performance based on what they know, and their experience in the application of what they know, until efficient patterns of performance emerge. It is during this stage that ineffective characteristics are dropped and performance starts to become automated. Larger and larger chunks of activity are put together to form smoothly executed sequences. It also becomes possible to carry out other tasks at the same time, leading to better dual task performance. This is an extremely important aspect of skill acquisition and is crucial for the intraoperative performance of safe surgery. An important aspect of the training of surgeons is to have as much of their procedural skills developed to the stage where they are automated before they enter the operating room. The reason for this is simple; the performance of clinical surgery makes multiple cognitive demands particularly on attentional resources, i.e., what the surgeon can consciously attend to by automating where possible skills such as, psychomotor coordination of instruments. It leaves more attentional resources available for higher-level tasks such as intraoperative problem solving.

The final phase outlined by Fitts and Posner (1967) was the Autonomous phase. This is when the learner perfects their skill usually with practice. It leads to what many individuals consider the essence of what is meant by skilled performance, i.e., performance that is automatic, unconscious, or instinctive. None of these descriptions stand up to close scrutiny given the difficulties in operationally defining "automaticity" but they convey the idea of performance that is carried out in a very different way from that of previous phases of skill acquisition. Not all performances evolve to this level of skill and many will remain at Phase 2. The differences between Phases 1 and 2 are that the learner "knows that" and in Phase 3 they "know how." This difference is probably a good example of what best distinguishes between declarative (Phase 1 and 2) and procedural knowledge (Phase 3). The fundamental idea is that as a skill is learned there is a change in the type of knowledge that underpins performance. The early stages (Phase 1 and 2) are typified by a reliance on declarative forms of knowledge and on explicit rules for carrying out the task. However, as the learner becomes more familiar with the task and develops efficient and effective performance sequences, they begin to refine their performance to suit themselves. They can perform the task to a high level of quality even in the presence of distracting events. Performance seems almost immune to disruption and they have the ability to accurately prioritize and sequence events during un-planned-for intraoperative events. Skill application appears to be done without conscious awareness almost as if the knowledge has been compiled (just as in computer programming) into something akin to machine code (Anderson 1993).

As mentioned, one of the advantages of developing skills to the point where they are automated means that there are more attentional resources available to allocate to other aspects of task performance. However, one of the disadvantages is that the declarative knowledge that well practiced skills were based on are lost to the practitioner. Unfortunately, this means that the skilled practitioner may not necessarily make the best trainer. It also means that they may have difficulty identifying performance characteristics that need to be operationally defined (see Chap 8). However, this is not an absolute situation and many surgeons can be trained to identify aspects of performance that they have automated. Another problem associated with skills automation is probably more serious and that is the problem of acquiring bad habits during training. This is a particular weakness of poorly designed or badly monitored simulations. For example, some virtual reality endoscopy simulations allow the trainee to pass the endoscope straight down past the vocal cords into the esophagus. Unfortunately, in real patients, navigating the endoscope past the vocal cords is rarely straightforward. If the trainee learns on the simulator that this part of the task is straightforward that is precisely what they may do on the patient on whome they perform the procedure thus risking an injury.

Memorizing Strategies

One of the goals of lecturers, handouts, and notes is to help an individual to remember the material they have learned. This material in turn will be used to inform the trainee about appropriate aspects of the surgical procedure. Cognitive psychologists have built up a considerable understanding of useful strategies for helping people to remember information they have learned. This knowledge is based on over a century of quantitative research.

Organization

Miller (1956) developed the term "chunking" in a classic paper concerning the capacity of immediate memory. In this study, he asked subjects to remember strings of the digits. In keeping with what was known at the time about the usual span of apprehension, the subjects recalled only about seven digits correctly. However, Miller also showed that people can remember a greater number of digits by organizing the digits into higher-order groups, i.e., 0911, 2004, 2506, 1959, 1690, 1966, 1603, which consecutively are the date of the World Trade Center terror attack in New York, the birth year of one of our children that was born in the USA, the date of birth of one of our children, the date of birth of one of us (the prettier one!), the date of the Battle of the Boyne, the year England won the World Cup and the year Queen Elizabeth I died. Miller argued that the chunking method worked by allowing the subjects to use their limited cognitive capacity more efficiently. This finding is important because it established that human beings were limited capacity information processors. The estimated capacity of immediate memory has been established as 7 ± 2 chunks, but this is probably best viewed as a rough approximation. This is because the capacity of immediate memory reflects the limits of a potential capacity and because the amount of capacity available can vary depending on the type of task, and the level of fatigue; therefore, the capacity of immediate memory can vary across situations (Baddeley et al. 1975). The most that we can say is that the capacity of immediate memory is limited but not fixed and that organization facilitates immediate memory. In presenting information on an e-learning platform, it is best to impose organization on the material to be learned and remembered. In operative surgery, most procedures lend themselves to ready organization in terms of anatomy and physiology, signs and symptoms, diagnosis, intervention and follow-up. The surgical procedure itself also lends itself to the process of chunking, e.g., preoperative preparation, the procedure itself, and postoperative management. Performance of the procedure is also usually already organized into manageable chunks by experienced surgeons. Surgeons have already worked out the steps in the procedure and they are likely to allow trainees to perform certain parts of the procedure depending on their level of training and experience. These naturally occurring organizational chunks should be utilized in the organization of e-learning information. If there is no agreed-upon intraoperative steps for the surgical procedure, a set of procedure steps should be imposed for the purpose of facilitating learning. However, it should be pointed out to the learner that there is no uniform agreement on the steps or the order of the steps in the procedure that they are being taught. An even better strategy would be to have agreement among surgical supervisors of a "reference procedure" approach within the surgical training program. This would ensure consistency from online learning, the skills laboratory training, and intraoperative supervision. After the trainee is comfortable in the performance of the procedure, they can hone their procedural skills based on the wisdom of their more senior supervising surgical colleagues.

Understanding

An optimal approach in trying to memorize something is to first understand it. A good way to do this is to try helping the learner make connections between what they have already learned and experienced and the new information. As we have pointed out earlier, episodic memories (that is memories idiosyncratic to the individual) are usually remembered better than semantic memories. The easiest way to do this is to help the learner relate the new information to what they already know. Educationalists constructing the e-learning package will have a very good idea of what the learner knows based on the level of training and the contents of the program curriculum which is almost certainly based on a national or international curriculum. Not only should the designers of an e-learning package consider what knowledge and experience the learner brings to the learning situation, but they should also check the understanding of the learner as they work through the e-learning package. This type of assessment (e.g., either formative or summative) is important not just for the quality assurance of trainee performance, but they can also be used to ensure that the trainee does not progress to more difficult parts of their online education package without a thorough understanding of the material they have already covered. If this is not done, the trainee will find subsequent parts of the learning increasingly more difficult and it also increases the probability gross misunderstandings of the material being learned. It is very important to avoid a chain of apparently inconsequential misunderstandings and errors which could lead to catastrophic consequences for a patient. As we have pointed out earlier, it is very easy to develop bad habits and bad behavior. Once these have become automated and integrated into the knowledge and practice system of the individual doctor, they are very difficult to extinguish. It is better to ensure that they do not occur in the first place and a way to avoid them is with formative assessment. We shall say more about assessment of e-learning performance later.

Graphic Organizers

These tools help the learner to see things as they are trying to learn and they also help organize information. There are many different types of strategies that can be used as graphic organizers. These can be as simple as a PowerPoint slide with a diagrammatic representation of the anatomical structure or the disease process that the individual is trying to learn. It could be an animated PowerPoint presentation showing cause and effect relationships or a cycle of relationships. Graphic representation of information is easier to recall for a number of reasons. It helps to organize the information into a coherent format. It can also present and summarize the information in an anatomically correct visual format, which has greater power to convey knowledge than words.

Visualization

Visualization means that the learner is helped to see a mental image of what it is they are trying to learn. Developing mental imagery can be facilitated with the use of animated films or actual video recordings of what it is we are trying to get the learner to remember. If a picture paints 1,000 words, animated films are even better. The availability of these demonstrations has become extremely common with the increased power of computer presentations and the amount of information that can be transmitted in real time over the Internet. Films have the advantage of organizing information to be learned and presenting it in an interesting way, showing the order and sequence in which events occur and also showing the context in which they occur. As such, they are very powerful aids to help the learner remember complex information. Another advantage of this approach is that it explicitly relates information to be learned with that which has been very well learned, probably years ago, e.g., anatomy and physiology. Establishing relationships between new ideas and previously existing memories dramatically increases the probability that the new information will be remembered. The more interesting the visualization strategy, the more coherent and integrated it is, the greater the facilitation of memory storage. Developing a coherent strategy is not complex or difficult; however, it does take forethought, organization and improvisation.

Repetition

The more times repeats something, the better memory will be for that information. However, each time that information is gone through, a different angle should be used so that the learners are not just repeating exactly the same activity. Varying the approach will create more connections in long-term memory. Frequency of repetition affords the opportunity for the material to become better integrated and associated with information that has already been learned. Retention of information depends on the elaborateness of its processing. The elaborate processing can occur by relating incoming items to other incoming items as well as information that has been learned previously. In studies of free recall, people spontaneously organize words into groups, and this elaborate processing was correlated with higher levels of retention (Anderson and Reber 1979). Further retention can be facilitated by inducing trainees to organize the information themselves so that it is distinctive; their understanding of it is complete and idiosyncratic.

Formative Assessment

In 1967 Michael Scriven coined the terms "formative" and "summative" evaluation (Scriven 1991). The purpose of formative assessment is to enhance learning and not to allocate grades. Formative assessments are considered part of instruction and instructional sequence and are thus non-threatening methods used to score performance rather than to grade it. Results of formative assessment given immediately enhance learning. Thus, formative assessment used in an e-learning package provides a very powerful learning tool. Assessments should occur when content is being taught and learned and should continue throughout the period of learning. Formative feedback lets the trainee know how well they are doing and this information should also be available to the trainer. For the trainee, it reinforces their progress and rewards success. For the trainer, it gives them valuable information on how well a cohort of trainees are progressing but it also highlights material that may need to be revisited, to provide better explanation or subsidiary information. Formative assessments also serve another function, and that is enforced repetition of material that is being learned or has been learned. Thus, formative assessment facilitates the "effortful" recall of learned information which encourages the elaborateness with which information is encoded in long-term memory. Furthermore, the more frequently a piece of information is retrieved from long-term memory in different contexts, the easier it is to retrieve that information on future occasions. Figure 9.2a and b gives examples of what an online component of teaching and assessment might look like. Figure 9.2a (the teaching slide) shows the anatomical landmarks of the colon that the trainee should know and be able to freely report before performing the examination on a real or virtual patient with a flexible endoscope. In Fig. 9.2b, the goal is to assess the trainee's knowledge of anatomical landmarks of the colon. The landmarks are highlighted by the arrows and the task for the trainee is to drag with the computer mouse one of the labels on the right-hand side to the appropriate arrow on the left-hand side of the figure. If a trainee drags a landmark name to the correct position on the figure, the label stays in position indicating that they are correct. In contrast, if they drag a landmark name to an incorrect position, it immediately and automatically returns to the list of landmark names, indicating that the attempted positioning was wrong.

Memorizing: Stress and Sleep

It is important that the context in which the current of information is taught to individuals is taken into consideration. This is particularly so for surgeons. It has been found that declarative information is less likely to be recalled if learning is

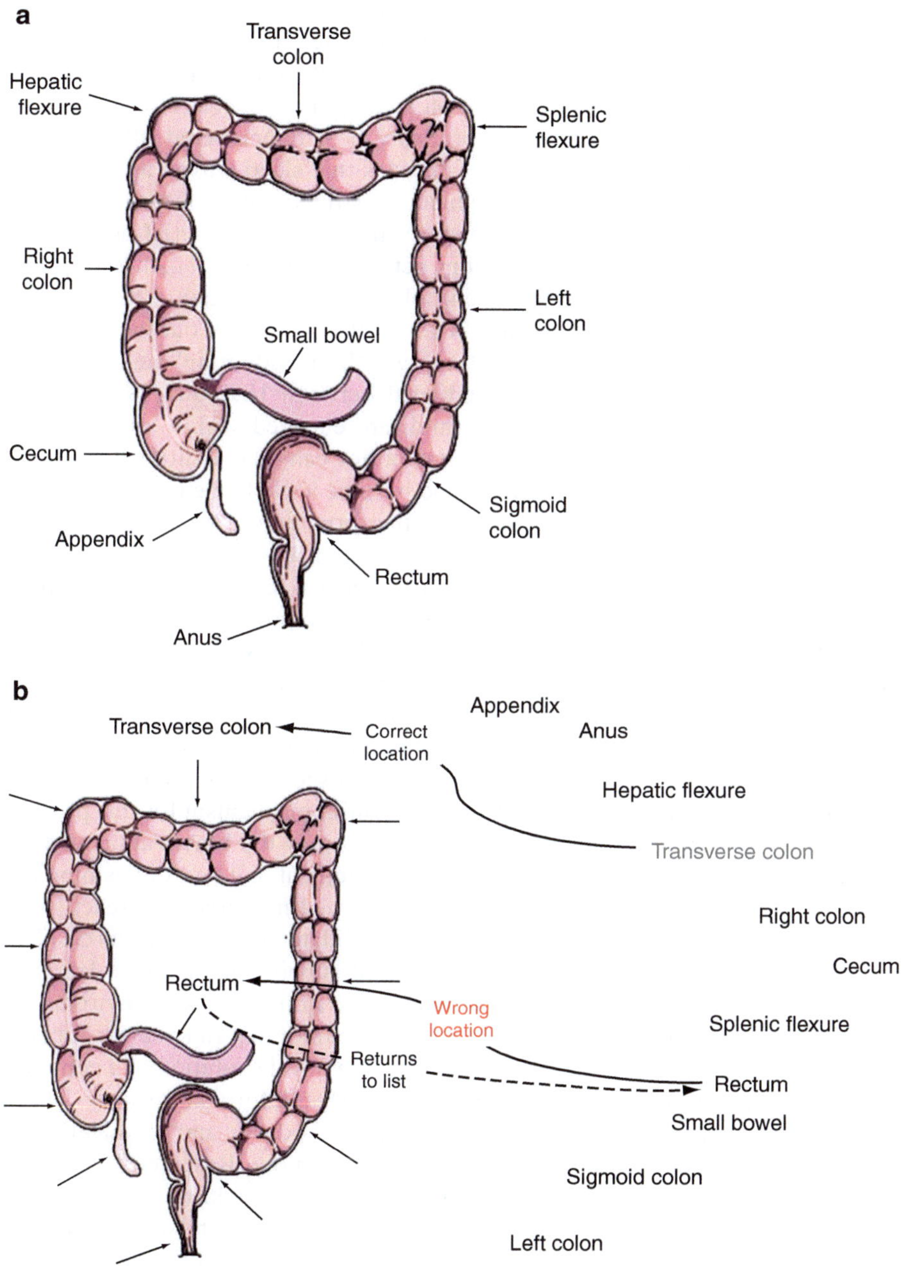

Fig. 9.2 (**a**) Anatomical landmarks of the colon for colonoscopy training. (**b**) Anatomical landmarks of the colon for colonoscopy training formative assessment component

followed by a stressful experience. Surgical trainees who attend a very interesting and informative grand rounds and then go immediately to the operating room or a busy emergency room are less likely to remember the information they learned from grand rounds, than those who are on a study day (Lupien et al. 1997). In contrast, the information learned is probably best remembered after a good night's sleep. It was believed for many decades that sleep played an important role in the consolidation of declarative memory. Memory consolidation is a category of processes that stabilize a memory trace after the initial acquisition (Dudai 2004). Although the relationship between sleep and remembering has been known for centuries, the term "consolidation" is credited to the German psychologists Georg Elias Müller and Alfons Pilzecker. They outlined the idea that memory takes time to fixate or undergo "Konsolidierung" and it is discussed in relation to their studies conducted between 1892 and 1900 (Dudai 2004). As noted in Chap 3 sensory stimuli are encoded within milliseconds; however, the long-term maintenance of memories can take additional minutes, days, or even years to fully consolidate and become a stable memory (i.e., resistant to change or interference). Therefore, the formation of a specific memory occurs rapidly, but the evolution of a memory is often an ongoing process. These findings help to account for an observation that post-sleep performance of some trainees in the skills labs seem to show significant improvement in the absence of practice. It has been suggested that the central mechanism or consolidation of declarative memory during sleep is the reactivation or reverberation of newly learned memories. The idea originates from Donald Olding Hebb's (1904–1985) theory that a cell, functioning as a whole unit, continues to respond or reverberate after the original stimulus that initiated its response has been terminated. More recently, it has been suggested that the central mechanism for this process of declarative memory consolidation during sleep is the reactivation of hippocampal memory representation. Neuropsychological and neurophysiological PET studies have now shown that the newly learned memories are reactivated during sleep and through this are helped consolidate (Ellenbogen 2005). The implications for these findings are obvious and support the use of e-learning platforms for learning didactic information remote from a stressful environment by a well-rested trainee. For surgical device companies that run courses for surgeons on how to use newly developed devices or a novel evolution of a common surgical device, these findings probably make less comfortable reading. These courses are usually run over 2 days and involve both didactic and technical skills training with a course dinner in the intervening evening. Research has shown that even moderate alcohol consumption shortly before bedtime catalyzes disruptions in sleep maintenance and sleep architecture. This can have deleterious effects on knowledge storage, maintenance, and retrieval. This means that minimum alcohol consumption and early to bed might make these courses less attractive to both senior and junior surgeons. However, these variables are much easier to control in the comfort of the trainee's own accommodation, i.e., learning at home.

Procedural Training

In a virtual reality simulator or emulator, the handles of real instruments are used as effectors for virtual instruments to interact with virtual tasks or simulated tissues. The question arises: when does an online education and training package seep into the function of a simulator. Consider the following example. In Fig. 9.3a–c, we have

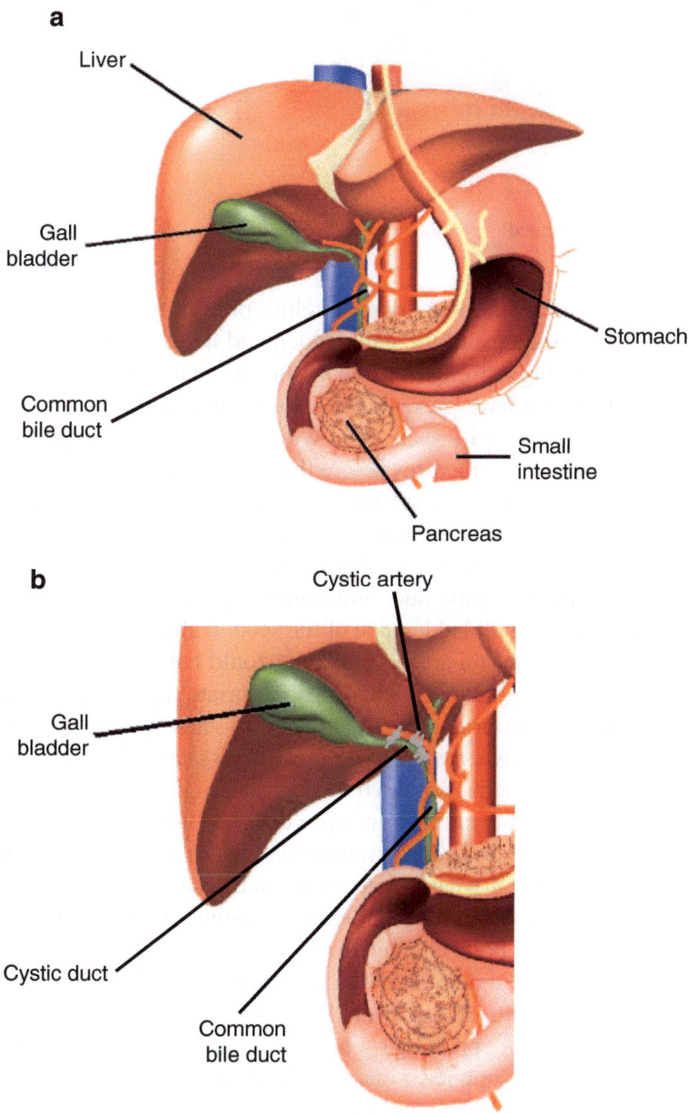

Fig. 9.3 (**a**) and (**b**) Diagrams illustrating the anatomy of the gallbladder in relation to other organs and clips application over the cystic duct and artery during cholecystectomy. (**c**) Figure illustrating the anatomy of the gallbladder and the trainee is asked to apply the surgical clips over the cystic duct and artery using the computer mouse

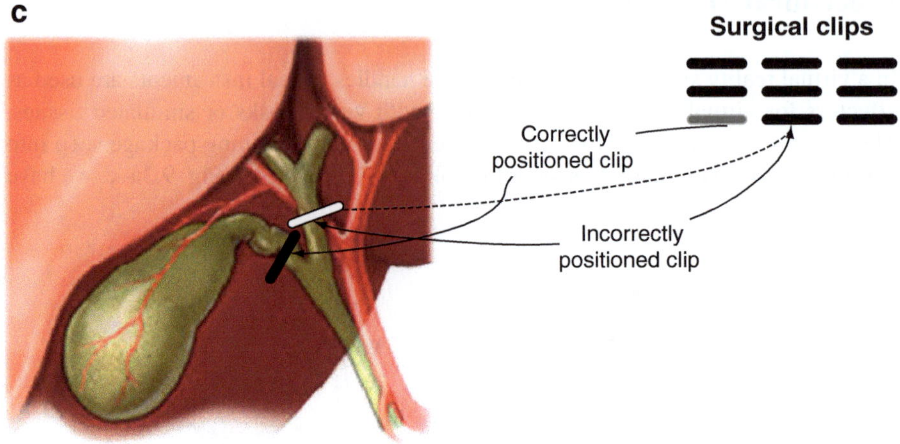

Fig. 9.3 (continued)

presented the anatomical organs in close proximity to the gallbladder. We have also shown the structures of the gallbladder, and in Fig. 9.3b, we have shown the correct location of surgical clips on the cystic duct and cystic artery for safe dissection. In Fig. 9.3c, we have presented the trainee with a novel image of a gallbladder and cystic structures and tasked them with placing the appropriate number of surgical clips on the cystic structures before they can be safely dissected. The task could have been made slightly more difficult by requiring the trainee to choose the appropriate clip applicator from a range of surgical tools. The description of the task could also have required the trainees to identify where on the cystic structures they would dissect, i.e., clip the cystic duct with three clips and then dissect between the 2nd and 3rd clip (on the gallbladder side of the second clip). They might have done the cystic duct before the cystic artery. This then could have been assessed much the same as the task described in Fig. 9.2b. The appropriate regions of on the cystic duct and the cystic artery appropriate for clipping and dissection could have been liberally defined with spacing between clips. The area of dissection between clips could also have been defined and errors enacted by the trainee could have been immediately fed back to them had. Is this online education or procedural training? We would suggest that this is the start of procedural training and that in reality there is no clear demarcation boundary between what is education and what is training. All of these aspects of education and training lie on a fidelity continuum where possibly the lowest level of fidelity might be book chapters or text and an intermediate level of fidelity might be a MIST VR type simulator all the way up to the highest fidelity training opportunity, i.e., a real patient. The goal of the surgical curriculum is the training of safe and effective skills for operating room performance. Whether something is taught online, in the classroom, in one-to-one tutorials or in the skills laboratory is somewhat academic. They should be taught and trained in the most efficient (including cost-efficient) way possible. The question should not be should we do it, rather it should be what do we want to achieve by using this education/training platform and is this the best use of the trainers and trainees time? We emphasize trainer's time because e-learning modules will require preparation and even with dedicated technical support, they will still require considerable academic effort to prepare or storyboard the didactic material, validate it, and then monitor its implementation and the trainees progress. Validation of these systems is essential and these studies should be conducted to the same level of rigor as VR simulations (Chap 7).

Trainees need to be presented with multiple examples of the same task, which ideally should increase in complexity commensurate with their passing formative assessments. Subsequent tasks might include good quality images of the cystic structures preoperatively. The task of trainees would be to identify the cystic structures for exposure, clipping, and dissection. The reason for this is simple: it has been proposed that one of the major reasons for complications associated with laparoscopic cholecystectomy is failure to accurately identify the cystic structures (Way et al. 2003). Training could continue online until the trainee was able to accurately identify cystic structures consistently. This would considerably improve their operative safety.

The facility of being able to link laparoscopic instruments in a MIST VR type frame to the Internet to perform virtual reality tasks is not widely available. However, it is possible to perform certain basic tasks using a simple computer mouse that almost certainly will have beneficial effects that transfer to skills laboratory training sessions. For example, in a study by Jordan et al. (2001), they trained subjects to trace a groove in a "U" or a "Z" shape with a stylus. The end of the stylus was monitored by the subject via an endoscopic camera. This meant that the stylus had a "fulcrum" on it as seen in laparoscopic surgery instruments. If they touched the edge of the groove, an alarm sounded and this was classified as an error. The reason these two shapes were chosen was that the "U-shape" had one fulcrum along the *x*-axis and the "Z-shape" had two. They found that subjects who trained on the "Z-shape" performed significantly better on a novel laparoscopic task. They concluded that this was because the "Z-shape" training group had more exposure or training to the *x*-axis fulcrum which transferred to improved performance in the novel laparoscopic task. In an online training component, instead of using a stylus, a computer mouse could be used instead. The goal of this task would be to help the trainee to automate the apparent movement inversion on laparoscopic instruments caused by the fulcrum effect. Trainees could trace a variety of shapes where the action of the computer mouse has been inverted, i.e., the trainee moves the computer mouse to the right and the arrow on the screen moves to left and vice versa. The same would also apply to *y*-axis movements. In another study using the same task, researchers found that trainees benefited most from the feedback they had on the accuracy of their stylus tracking performance and transfer of training to a novel laparoscopic task was greatest for the group who had the most performance feedback during training (Van Sickle et al. 2007). The data from these studies tell us that considerable benefits can be accrued from skills training in fairly basic tasks. These data would suggest that a simple training task could make skills training on their simulation in the skills laboratory much more efficient as subjects would automate to the fulcrum effect much quicker after pre-training. As suggested earlier, educationists should continuously question how, when, and where is the most effective and efficient platform to deliver education and skills training. It is our belief that e-learning is currently underutilized and could be used much more effectively and probably less expensively to supplement skills laboratory training and make it more efficient. It is highly probable that e-learning could be effectively used as part-task trainer. Which parts of a particular task are suitable for part-task training could almost certainly be worked out during the task analysis process of a given procedure for the identification of performance metrics. It has been our experience that while addressing these questions, the task analysis team usually considers training platforms as well.

Observational Learning

"Live" Cases: Basic

A very powerful learning strategy touched on briefly in Chap 4 is observational, vicarious or modeling (Bandura 1982). Observational learning occurs when an individual observes another person (referred to as the model) engage in a particular activity. The observer sees the model perform that activity but does not engage in that activity, for example, watching another surgeon perform a specific procedure. The observer learns the behavior merely by watching the model. The modeled behavior is assumed to be acquired by the observer through cognitive or covert coding of the observed events. Unlike traditional learning situations, there are no active contingencies impinging on the learner/observer. Observational learning is assumed to have taken place when the observer exhibits performance characteristics which have not been explicitly trained. This very powerful education and training method is widely used in medicine from ward rounds in the morning, to observing in outpatient clinics and in the operating room. However, as highlighted in Chap 4, not all behaviors modeled by more experienced surgeons are necessarily behavior that we would wish the trainee to develop, i.e., some senior surgeons may have developed poor procedural habits! E-learning affords an ideal opportunity to use this powerful learning methodology minus the bad habits.

Given the availability of video recording facilities in operating rooms and other centers where procedural care is delivered, recording index cases for use on e-learning packages should be relatively straightforward. The training program would not require a large volume of these procedure recordings; however, they should be chosen strategically. Furthermore, it is probably inefficient to show the entire procedure and it would probably be more beneficial to edit the recording so that it correlates well with the organizational structure that has been detailed in the didactic procedure outline. This means that the recorded procedure should follow in the same sequence order or procedural steps as the didactic module states. This reinforces the cognitive model that the learner has for the procedure and helps to consolidate the information that they have acquired with the new information they get from the video recording. Although it is common for very experienced or expert surgeons to talk through the surgical procedure as they are performing it, this is probably not ideal for general-purpose teaching and training. A better alternative would be to get the operating surgeon to do a voice-over of the recording. This voice-over should be clearly scripted and correlate closely with the organizational and procedural structure outlined in the didactic component. This would be relatively straightforward if the operating surgeon has been involved in the preparation of the didactic component from the outset. It is important that education and training materials concord as closely as possible so as to facilitate learning.

Live Cases: Advanced

The edited and live cases, just outlined, are probably best utilized for basic surgical training. Recorded cases of more advanced procedures for more senior surgeons would also be a useful adjunct for training and continuing professional development. The case mix that surgeons in training or indeed surgeons in practice are going to encounter in the future will continue to reduce (Crofts et al. 1997). This is a consequence of reduced work hours, more skills training taking place online, in the classroom or the skills laboratory and increased hospital and unit specialization. On the one hand, this will have beneficial effects for the patient as the surgeon has more experience and a greater volume of similar cases which can only improve the quality of care. However, we believe that the constriction on the variety and mix of cases that consultants and probably trainees are exposed to may have negative consequences on the development of wisdom. Many of our surgical and medical colleagues argue that the most important attribute that trainee surgeon can develop is decision making. Decision making is a constituent part of a spectrum of performance characteristics that constitute a "good" surgeon or a "good" doctor. Wisdom is a deep understanding and realizing of people, things, events, or situations, resulting in the ability to choose or act to consistently produce the optimum results with a minimum of time and energy. Wisdom is the ability to optimally (effectively and efficiently) apply perceptions and knowledge to produce the desired results. Wisdom is comprehension of what is true or right coupled with optimum judgment as to action. In Chap 8 we outlined the efforts made by the major medical and surgical training organizations around the world to defining competence and competency. However, we believe that wisdom is the overarching goal which these organizations aspired to train. While they have done a relatively good job of describing the constituent parts of a good doctor, there is concern that the sum of the parts may not add up to what is hoped, i.e., a wise doctor. We will return to the issues of wisdom acquisition in Chaps 11 and 12.

Learning Management System

A learning management system (LMS) is software for delivering, tracking, and managing training/education. LMSs range from systems for managing training/educational records to software for distributing courses over the Internet and offering features for online collaboration. Probably the single most important decision in this process and also one of the most difficult decisions will be about the LMS. There are many commercially available LMSs and it is difficult to choose between them. The decision about which learning management system to choose should not be taken by educationalists in isolation from other members of the team. Just like decisions about metric development, the decision about which LMS to choose should be informed by a computer scientist who is very familiar with the different systems that are commercially available. This individual should also be very well acquainted with the needs of the surgical training program. The surgeons on the decision team should have a good idea about the types of material that they wish to deliver on an e-learning platform. A behavioral scientist or psychologist should also be included in the decision-making team as they would have a fairly good knowledge about the types of metrics that they wish to implement in the formative and summative assessments and the sort of data that they want reported back to the course administrator. The LMS chosen to deliver and manage the e-learning content should make considerable time savings for the academics providing the course content. This may not be the case in the short term but it certainly should be a medium-term goal. A learning management system should not simply "look pretty." It should be an efficient and effective tool for the delivery and assessment of online learning content. Most of the commercially available LMSs are more than capable of delivering content. However, close scrutiny should be paid to the ability of the system to deliver and to manage formative and summative assessment. If this aspect of the LMS is not chosen well, the academic program could end up with a system that is not much more functional than a DVD. The same rules for choosing a simulator apply to choosing an LMS. Purchasers must look beyond the sales pitch and ask to see working examples of systems that would be ideal for their purposes or aspects which might be suitable for online education and training of surgeons. Unfortunately the commercially available LMSs that do exist have not been designed or developed with the functionality that we have outlined in this chapter. This does not mean that it cannot be developed relatively quickly.

The surgical training program would need to know or at least be confident that the person completing the online education and assessment units was the person that it was supposed to be. This is not a difficult feature request; it may have to be implemented in a novel way, such as intermittent requests for identity confirmation. The LMS should also provide a straightforward course authoring methodology that is relatively easy to learn for the multiple academics that will be using the system and contributing to content development and content libraries. The LMS should also provide a relatively straightforward content management system which is easily configurable for multiple specialties. It should also provide straightforward administrative reporting and tracking of individual trainees and groups of trainees as they progress through the content. Very importantly, the LMS should administer and manage the formative and summative assessment process. This means that the system also needs to be able to manage the content library and exam engine. Another feature, which we suggest is crucial, is ensuring that trainees demonstrate the performance criterion or proficiency level before being allowed to progress. This process should not be managed on a day-to-day basis by an academic supervisor. It should be overseen by an academic supervisor whose function is to identify individuals who are struggling with module content and to investigate and intervene when appropriate. Likewise, the LMS would manage trainee course compliance and more importantly failure to comply. Over the longer term, the system should track individual and group performance through the different years and modules of the course. This type of LMS use is relatively novel, particularly in high stakes education and training programs such as surgery. That means that results on almost everything that is done with the LMS system need to be reported in the peer-reviewed literature, particularly on the reliability and validity of the system and the amount of transfer of training. Currently, we can only guess what the transfer of training rate might be. In an ideal world, the most valuable data that could be reported on are gross system errors. However, we are not confident that this information will be reported completely and publicly.

Summary

E-learning platforms hold enormous potential for the delivery and management of curriculum material in surgical training programs. They should not be used as a novel way of delivering a traditional lecture. The power and flexibility of e-learning should be harnessed to augment and facilitate the learning process based on sound principles. These dictate that material to be learned is organized in a format that relates to previously learned material and requires the learner to interact with the material and to problem solve. Learners' performance on these problem solving or assessment exercises should be assessed formatively on an ongoing basis with feedback given to the learner in a proximate fashion, i.e., close to performance. There should also be a summative assessment component to the learning process and individuals should not be allowed to progress until they have demonstrated the requisite performance criterion level. This will have implications for satisfactory trainee progress which should be implemented and managed with a Learning Management System (LMS). These LMSs need to be validated to the same level of rigor as VR simulations.

References

Anderson JR. *Rules of the Mind*. Hillsdale: Lawrence Erlbaum; 1993.

Anderson JR, Reder LM. An elaborative processing explanation of depth of processing. In L. Cermak, F. Craik (Eds.), *Levels of processing and human memory*. New York: Lawrence Erlbaum Associates; 1979:385-404.

Baddeley AD, Thomson N, Buchanan M. Word length and the structure of short-term memory. *J Verbal Learn Verbal Behav*. 1975;14(6):575-589.

Bandura A. Self-efficacy mechanism in human agency. *Am Psychol*. 1982;37(2):122-147.

Crofts TJ, Griffiths JMT, Sharma S, Wygrala J, Aitken RJ. Surgical training: an objective assessment of recent changes for a single health board. *Br Med J*. 1997;314(7084):891.

Dudai Y. The neurobiology of consolidations, or, how stable is the engram? *Ann Rev Psychol.* 2004;55:51-86.

Dutton D. *Anthony Eden: A Life and Reputation*. London: A Hodder Arnold Publication; 1997.

Ellenbogen JM. Cognitive benefits of sleep and their loss due to sleep deprivation. *Neurology.* 2005;64(7):E25.

Fitts PM, Posner MI. *Human Performance*. Belmont: Brooks/Cole Publishing Co; 1967.

Graziadei, WD. 1997. Building Asynchronous & Synchronous Teaching-Learning Environments: Exploring a Course/Classroom Management System Solution. Retrieved 9th July, 2011, from http://eric.ed.gov/ERICWebPortal/search/detailmini.jsp?_nfpb=true&_&ERICExtSearch_SearchValue_0=ED405842&ERICExtSearch_SearchType_0=no&accno=ED405842

Jordan JA, Gallagher AG, McGuigan J, McClure N. Virtual reality training leads to faster adaptation to the novel psychomotor restrictions encountered by laparoscopic surgeons. *Surg Endosc.* 2001;15(10):1080-1084.

Keane MT, Eysenck MW. *Cognitive Psychology: A Student's Handbook.* London: Psychology Press; 2000.

Lupien SJ, Gaudreau S, Tchiteya BM, et al. Stress-induced declarative memory impairment in healthy elderly subjects: relationship to cortisol reactivity. *J Clin Endocrinol Metab.* 1997;82(7):2070.

Miller GA. The magical number seven, plus or minus two: some limits on our capacity for processing information. *Psychol Rev.* 1956;63(2):81-97.

Scriven M. Beyond formative and summative evaluation. In: McLaughlin MW, Phillips DC, eds. *Evaluation and Education: A Quarter Century*, vol. 90. Chicago: National Society for the Study of Education; 1991:19-64.

Seymour NE, Gallagher AG, Roman SA, et al. Virtual reality training improves operating room performance: results of a randomized, double-blinded study. *Ann Surg.* 2002;236(4):458-463; discussion 463-454.

Tulving E, Thomson DM. Encoding specificity and retrieval processes in episodic memory. *Psychol Rev.* 1973;80(5):352-373.

Van Sickle K, Gallagher AG, Smith CD. The effect of escalating feedback on the acquisition of psychomotor skills for laparoscopy. *Surg Endosc.* 2007;21(2):220-224.

Way LW, Stewart L, Gantert W, et al. Causes and prevention of laparoscopic bile duct injuries: analysis of 252 cases from a human factors and cognitive psychology perspective. *Ann Surg.* 2003;237(4):460.

Chapter 10
Simulation Training for Improved Procedural Performance

A Simulation Strategy: Preliminary Steps

The use of simulators to train surgical skills was ushered in as a consequence of the difficulties in acquiring the skills to practice minimally invasive surgery (Satava 1993). This revolution in surgical training forced the surgical community to think about training in general. Haluck et al. (2007) has suggested that when the field of medical simulation first started, it seemed quite straightforward. It has evolved into a highly complex field impacting on almost every discipline in medicine. While one of the major drivers of these changes has been concerns about patient safety the greatest impetus has come from medicine itself, and in particular surgery. In the spring (March) of 2002, a closed-door meeting between educational leaders in surgery was held at Boston College. The purpose of the meeting was to discuss what position the American College of Surgeons (ACS) should take regarding the emergence of surgical simulation as it related to surgical training in the USA. The meeting was chaired by Prof Gerry Healy (later President of the ACS but at that time one of the most senior Regents of the ACS (Healy 2002)). Healy opened the conference by giving a very clear account of where the ACS stood regarding surgical simulation. They, as an organization, were observing the developments in surgical simulation with great interest; however, they were not sure what position they should take in relation to it. Dr Steve Dawson (from CIMIT, MGH/Harvard), one of the leading thinkers and lead developer of simulation, gave the opening address to the conference. He gave a very lucid account of the development that had taken place in simulation in the last decade (many of them elegant developments emanating from or originating in his laboratory). However, he concluded that an ingredient for helping to make simulation training a success in surgery was lacking, i.e., clinical trial data.

One of the conference delegates interjected and pointed out that the first prospective, randomized, double-blind clinical trial on virtual reality training for the operating room would be presented at the American Surgical Association (ASA) annual meeting in April 2002. He summarized the main findings of the clinical trial,

A.G. Gallagher and G.C. O'Sullivan, *Fundamentals of Surgical Simulation*,
Improving Medical Outcome - Zero Tolerance,
DOI 10.1007/978-0-85729-763-1_10, © Springer-Verlag London Limited 2012

i.e., case-matched, virtual reality trained surgeons made six times fewer objectively assessed intraoperative errors than the standard trained group. After some denial that this type of a clinical trial was even possible, Prof Jo Meekins (then Chairman of Surgery at Montréal, Quebec, Canada) questioned the individual who had summarized the results of the clinical trial. After a brief period, Meakins explained to Healy that in his opinion, the results sounded very promising and reliable. He understood the clinical trial design, the assessment procedure and the outcome measures. He was also aware that the clinical trial was the "Education Paper" of the ASA annual meeting in 2002. The ASA is the oldest and probably the most distinguished surgical organization in the USA, and to have a paper accepted at their meeting is very difficult. It was even more difficult to have an education paper accepted as it would have been subjected to rigorous scrutiny. On hearing this, Healy very bravely took the leadership initiative to change the direction of the meeting at Boston College from "What position should the ACS take in relation to simulation?" to "How does the ACS implement a simulation strategy in surgery?" (Healy 2002).

Creation of a Simulation Center

During the first decade of the twenty-first century, there was rapid growth of interest in the use of simulation for education and training in surgery. Although there were still skeptics about the value of surgical simulation, the leadership in surgery had taken the strategic decision to support the implementation of a simulation strategy. This included the launch of a program backed by the ACS to accredit education institutes which included the use of surgical simulation. After pilot testing in July 2005 to validate the ACS accreditation system, the program was launched during the ACS Clinical Congress in October 2005. The accreditation program was voluntary, with two levels of accreditation offered: I comprehensive and II basic (Pellegrini et al. 2006). Creation of an ACS-accredited skills training center was perceived to be a substantial endeavor. Even without financial and logistical considerations, education, skills training, and simulation technology are independent, fully developed disciplines (Haluck et al. 2007). One of the goals of the ACS program was to facilitate the establishment of a training center network with a coherent set of standards across the USA. However, a more informal goal was to facilitate the sharing of experiences, successes, and failures regarding the implementation of simulation in medical education and training. In the initial tranche of members that sought accreditation, the majority were from the USA. However, there were a number of international applicants, which included Imperial College, (London, UK), Lund, (Sweden), Karolinska, (Stockholm, Sweden), University of Western Ontario (Canada), Athens (Greece), Tel Aviv (Israel), and Montréal (Canada) (American College of Surgeons, 2011).

The creation of dedicated training space for surgical or medical simulation is a fundamental pre-requisite for any medical training program, anywhere in the world.

Minimally invasive surgery forced the surgical community to examine in detail how they were training the surgeons of the future. As a result of this self-examination, surgery very quickly realized that there were fundamental problems with how they were conducting training per se. Other interventional disciplines such as gastroenterology, gynecology, cardiology, radiology, emergency medicine and anesthetics have come to the same conclusions as surgery as evidenced by the radical changes in training programs in these disciplines around the world. The way that these groups practice medicine is changing radically and the skills that were acquired by them to successfully navigate their apprenticeship and early years as a consultant/attending will not suffice for their career. They will have to learn to use new medical devices and to perform procedures in new ways. Furthermore, these changes will occur under greater and greater scrutiny and accountability. Lastly, these changes must be managed within a shorter working week, immaterial if that is in the USA, Europe, or Australia.

Sharing Resources (Issues)

All of the separate disciplines in medicine would prefer to have bespoke training and a simulation laboratory for their own discipline; this possibility is simply a non-starter. Individual disciplines can construct as many arguments as they like against shared facilities and equipment, but the facts of the matter are very clear, as we have tried to emphasize in this book. How doctors learn the practice of medicine whether it be surgery, cardiology, or anesthetics is not some mystery yet to be discovered. Human beings are not some unfathomable quantity; they process information that they acquire from their environment through their sensory organs, which is then organized by their perceptual system and filtered by a cognitive system which stores the information in long-term memory for use later. Psychologists have developed considerable knowledge based on more than a century of quantitative research about how these human attributes function and break down. They also know how to get the multi-factorial systems functioning optimally. The problems that the different disciplines in medicine have with the process of training safe doctors have more in common than they have differences. This means that they should develop a core of expertise within training centers that can be utilized by the different medical disciplines. We have commented on this issue specifically in Chap. 5 with reference to the development of metrics. This team should almost certainly be the foundation stone of most of the educational activities within the Center be that training goals or scientific and validation goals. The reason for this is that this team should have a very detailed understanding of the training problem, the procedures or skills that are to be trained and how these should be assessed and then validated. The same principles lie at the heart of development of a proficiency-based progression training paradigm within all of the procedural disciplines in medicine. Likewise, precisely how the different types of validation are done with discipline-specific procedures may vary, but the science of the cause-and-effect relationships will remain the same. Also, the underlying methodology for the establishment of a proficiency level will flow from these developments. In this book, we refer specifically to surgery because it is the discipline we work in. However, we are aware that the methodology and strategies that we are describing are applicable to any area of procedural medicine as well as subjects allied to medicine.

As we will show later in this chapter, the technology used for training different procedural skills can be used by multiple disciplines in medicine. The training and assessment of suturing and knot tying will be discussed here in the context of training surgeons to tie intracorporeal sutures during a Nissen fundoplication. The methodology could also be used for training and assessing most types of intracorporeal knots and sutures. We will also discuss the acquisition of endovascular skills for carotid artery stenting. The catheter and wire skills necessary for the safe performance of carotid artery stenting are also necessary in interventional cardiology, interventional radiology, vascular surgery, interventional neuroradiology and neurosurgery, and lately anesthetics for intraoperative peripheral nerve block. That means that in all probability the same simulator should be capable of training some level of endovascular skills in all of these disciplines. The same is true for simulators that train basic laparoscopic surgical skills. Why would a training authority or a hospital pay for the duplication of these resources (and the space that they are housed in along with technical support staff)? Just as we have emphasized that the training of a surgeon should be efficient, effective and to a transparent, fair standard of performance, we also think that the equipment purchased for this training should be used optimally. This almost certainly will mean that multiple disciplines will use the same platform to train. While we understand that some of the "suspicions" that many of the disciplines within medicine have toward each other, the prospect of sharing the same space and training devices is not really that awful! It has been our experience that when different disciplines are forced to work together (for whatever reasons) and they make the decision to make it work, they invariably learn a lot from each other which helps them develop their clinical skills and ultimately helps the patient. We will not discuss this issue in detail here, but readers should be mindful that simulation education and training resources are almost certainly going to be shared resources.

Choosing a Simulator (Issues)

Dr. Matt Ritter provides a useful overview of most simulators currently available for training surgical skills (Haluck et al. 2007). He gives information on a range of simulators in relation to who can be trained on them, what they cost to buy, and maintain. One of the useful insights he provides is that shopping for simulators is like shopping for most electronic goods; there is usually a difference between what is desired, what is needed and what we can afford. In deciding which simulators to purchase, a number of basic questions should be asked. These include: Who is to be taught? What is to be taught? How will instructions be delivered? When will the training occur? Where will training occur? An additional consideration should be the number of people who will be trained on the simulator. If the trainees are large classes of junior surgeons learning to perform basic laparoscopic maneuvers, a high-end procedural simulator is probably inappropriate. However, if the class is a large number of consultant/attending surgeons learning to perform an advanced endovascular procedure, a full procedural simulator is entirely appropriate. Both of these scenarios have considerable potential cost implications. If the training program sponsor is enormously wealthy and willing to spend millions of GB pounds, EUR euros, or US dollars in purchasing dedicated training space and equipment, there will not be a problem. In our experience, this has never been the case. In fact, it has been our experience that even training programs that can easily afford the cost of simulation and training facilities rarely want to pay for them. This is no small matter and we will discuss this issue in greater detail in Chap. 12. At this point, it is sufficient to say that the establishment of simulation and training laboratories is going to happen and someone certainly is going to pay for it. What needs to stop are the endless delays and obstacles put in front of well thought-out and costed proposals for simulation and training facilities completed by surgeons.

A good approach to choosing which simulators to purchase is to be mindful of the training that the device is to be used for and the amount of feedback on performance which the trainee needs for optimal improvement of performance. This information is presented in Fig. 6.7, Chap. 6. The more information that is required for performance feedback, the higher the fidelity of the simulator has to be (and the more expensive it will be as well). For example, if information is simply required on task completion, very simple simulation or emulation models will suffice. Doctors have been using these types of training devices for decades for acquiring skills such as suturing and knot tying. Most trainees normally carry suture material and tying instruments in their pocket and practice suturing and knot tying wherever and whenever possible, e.g., on a chair railing for knot tying or on a rubber glove for suturing. This is a very simple but effective approach to training. In contrast, preparing trainees to perform a full surgical procedure requires considerably more preparation to ensure that skills learned in the training environment transfer to operating room performance in vivo.

Transfer of Training (Issues)

The goal of any training program is to ensure that skills acquired in the training environment are transferred to the working environment in vivo. This is a relatively straightforward and important concept that was derived from Thorndike and Woodworth's (1901) transfer of practice. We have discussed this concept in Chap. 4 but the basic idea is very simple; Thorndike and Woodworth explored how individuals would transfer learning in one context to another context that shared similar characteristics. However, the concept has become somewhat clouded with the

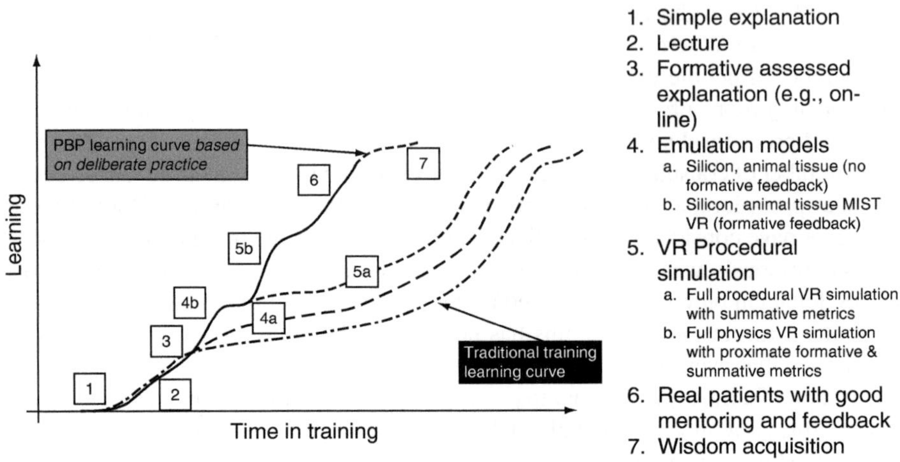

Fig. 10.1 Diagrammatic representation of the "estimated" speed of learning with proficiency-based progression (PBP) training and traditional training as a function of time in training

involvement of Human Resources Departments, "Learning Organizations" and "Corporate Universities" investigating the amount of employee training that transfers directly to work practice. This is an important concept within all large and small organizations as their future success depends on the speed with which people within their organization can learn and transfer good ideas into practice. While we completely understand corporate interest in this phenomenon, we have some doubts about the utility of some of the methods that they have used to assess transfer of training. In particular, we were surprised to discover that one of the methods used by organizations that have attempted to assess transfer of training effect has been surveys of employees to ascertain their "opinion" or their "feelings" on the amount of transfer of training that occurred in their experience. In industry, the most commonly cited estimate of transfer of training to job performance is 10% (Broad 2001)! These estimates (or probably more accurately "guestimates") of the transfer of training might just possibly be due to the way that the researchers operationally defined transfer of training and how they assessed it. What we are more confident about is the amount of transfer of training occurring in surgical simulation training programs that have been conducted under somewhat more rigorous training and testing conditions (Seymour et al. 2002). Furthermore, the transfer of training effect that we are focusing on in this book is task or procedure specific (Chap. 6) and the assessment methodology is much more robust (Chap. 5) than that used by large corporations.

Figure 10.1 shows a graphic representation of the estimated proportion of transfer of training that occurs from different targeted educational and training activities as a function of the emulation/simulation fidelity. There is relatively little transfer of training from a simple explanation (1) of how to do something such as tying a surgical knot. A well-organized formal lecture (2) elicits a greater but still modest amount of transfer of training. Although the information provided by a lecturer is probably the same as an online didactic explanation on how to tie a surgical knot, it elicits a greater transfer of training because of the formative and summative assessment that are elements of the didactic material (3). As explained in Chap. 4, one of the most powerful learning aids in the acquisition of skill is feedback on performance to the learner. This is difficult to provide in a formal lecture situation, but relatively straightforward to provide in an online didactic education package. Performance feedback is somewhat easier to give during actual training using physical or virtual training models (4a) because it is easy to see what the trainee has done right and what they have done wrong and to check that this is the case. However, this assumes that the trainer has a well-developed set of performance metrics that are actually valid performance indicators (Gallagher et al. 2008). Even with these performance metrics, feedback on some emulation/simulation models is only provided after the task has been completed. While this information is valuable and facilitates learning, it would be more effective if it had been delivered proximate to the performance error being enacted by the learner (e.g., a MIST VR type emulator). That is why we have speculated that greater transfer of training occurs with emulation/simulation models that have formative assessment as well as summative assessment (4b). Both of these types of simulations provide more information to the trainee and the trainer than previous levels of education and training materials. The same problem occurs with higher fidelity, full procedural simulations. Although fidelity of these simulators (5a) is greater and the individual can be required to perform an entire procedure, the same rules apply about performance feedback as with the lower fidelity emulation/simulations. These simulations will allow the trainee to complete a full procedure in the appropriate and fairly realistic anatomical context, in the correct sequence with the correct instruments in the correct order. Whilst this information provides a valuable procedural organizational structure for the learner which they can peg previously learned information (e.g., online, see Chap. 9) and newly acquired information, it is not as powerful a learning tool as a virtual reality simulation that provides all of these facilities and on top of that gives detailed (proximate) formative feedback on device handling performance (5b). Two of the simulators that we will discuss later in this chapter fall under categories 5a and 5b. For example, a high fidelity full procedural simulator for left side hemi-colectomy allows the surgeon to complete the entire procedure. It ensures that the procedure is conducted in the correct order using the correct surgical instruments, but the trainee only gets feedback on their performance when they have finished the procedure (Neary et al. 2008). In contrast, some of the virtual reality simulations for endovascular procedure, such as carotid artery stenting, will give formative feedback on catheter and wire manipulation skills throughout the procedure (Gallagher and Cates 2004b).

Of course one of the most powerful approaches to training that has been used for decades is on-the-job training on patients (6). The apprenticeship model that has served surgery well for more than a century has been based on graded responsibility in the operating room while performing procedures on actual patients. We are not suggesting that the patient is a simulator; what we are explicitly stating is that no amount of training on a simulator will replace some proportion of training in the operating room while actually operating on a patient. However, the operating room should no longer be used as a training environment for the acquisition of basic surgical skills. Rather, it should be considered more akin to a finishing school where the skills that the trainee surgeon has already acquired are put into practice on real patients while being supervised by a master surgeon. This allows the trainee to hone their skills further, while being bombarded with naturally occurring operating room distractions such as the wrong instrument pack being left out, learning to work with a new scrub nurse, or intraoperative complications, minor and major. Better education and training online and in the skills laboratory can supplant much of the early part of the learning curve that would normally be experienced in the operating room. However, it will never completely replace it. The transfer of training that occurs on real patients is at the top end of the learning curve (7). For example, it allows the trainee to generalize or transfer skills acquired on a patient requiring elective laparoscopic cholecystectomy to a patient requiring emergency laparoscopic cholecystectomy. This process of learning continues throughout the entire career of the practicing surgeon and we refer to it as the acquisition of wisdom. We shall discuss this concept in greater detail in Chaps. 11 and 12, but it is fair to say at this point that we are concerned that this important attribute of mature procedural performance is ill-defined and poorly understood at this crucial time, just as the training paradigm in procedural medicine is changing radically.

Transfer of Training: Good and Bad

In Fig. 10.1, a general rule of thumb regarding transfer of training is that the greater the fidelity of the simulator and the better the formative and summative assessment, the greater the proportion of skills that will be transferred. However, as the fidelity of the simulation increases so also does the cost. The assumption that we make in general is that transfer of training is a good thing and we have speculated that greater transfer goes with higher fidelity. However, transfer of training can be bad as well. If the simulator trains or reinforces bad or poor operative performance characteristics and these go unchecked, the probability is that this is what the trainee surgeon will do on a real patient. The "cracker" obvious simulation blunders are easy to spot, i.e., being able to pass an endoscope straight down through the vocal cords or being able to pass a catheter and wire up through the carotid artery into the brain unhindered, are probably less problematic than the more subtle simulation blunders. These are simply poor-quality simulations. Equally, simulators can analyze and score these unsafe behaviors as having occurred and then score them unambiguously in formative assessment. This is precisely what happens in a full physics virtual reality simulation training environment. The trainee can make almost any type of error, but they will be scored and given feedback immediately that they have enacted an error. Furthermore, if a trainee is unsure precisely what operative error they have enacted, the simulator can give them this information as well. The more problematic simulators are ones that have high face validity (with a matching price tag) that look and feel like the real procedure and use the same instruments. However, in training and assessment mode, the trainee is allowed to enact procedural errors that are either not scored at all or are scored in a summative manner. This means that the trainee only gets feedback after that particular training trial has been completed. Unfortunately this means that there is no guarantee that the trainee will have learned that this aspect of their performance is unsafe. Even worse, the trainee may develop an unwarranted self-belief in their ability to perform the procedure due to the lack of proximate formative feedback. At this level of simulation fidelity, these types of situations are probably unacceptable. If the simulator is not capable of providing intraoperative formative assessment of the trainees' performance, this deficit must be made up with close supervision by a proctor or surgeon. This type of scenario makes for very expensive training.

Full physics virtual reality simulators currently exist but mostly for training endovascular procedures, e.g., VIST. Furthermore, it has been shown that patient-specific data can be formatted and downloaded into the simulator so as to allow the rehearsal of an advanced skills procedure, e.g., carotid artery stenting (Cates et al. 2007). The authors formatted the angiographic data from a 64-year-old man with severe chronic obstructive pulmonary disease, prior right carotid endarterectomy, and recent transient ischemic attacks. The right internal carotid artery had an ulcerated lesion with 80% stenosis. They practiced the case on the simulator (VIST) and when they performed on the real patient, they found that virtual reality–simulated and live-patient cases showed a high degree of similarity to the angiographic anatomy. They also found that catheter movement and handling dynamics, catheter-catheter interaction, wire movement and dynamics, and embolic protective device deployment and retrieval demonstrated a one-to-one correlation of device movement in virtual reality compared with the live-patient case. Decisions about catheter selection (correct sizing of balloon, embolic protective device, and stent) and catheter technique (catheter- and wire-handling dynamics) transferred directly and correlated with the live-patient procedure. This means that full physics virtual reality simulation environments could potentially be used as decision support devices (Fig. 10.1). For example, after receiving the CT or MR images of a patient, the surgeon may be unsure whether to operate or not. They could have the patient-specific data formatted and downloaded into a simulator and then attempt the step or part of the procedure that they perceived as posing the most difficult. This would help them ascertain whether they could successfully complete that part of the procedure, and decide on the approach and surgical devices. They may then decide that attempting the procedure poses too great a risk to the patient. By identifying optimal patient-specific techniques prior to the actual procedures, virtual reality simulation has the enormous potential for improved patient safety. Unfortunately, to download and format patient-specific data currently takes a minimum of 2–3 days. We believe that this functionality will be reduced to a period of hours rather than days in the very near future and will facilitate the performance of high-risk procedures such as thrombectomy in acute stroke cases.

Transfer of Training Examples

MIST VR: Lessons Learned

The first study to use a proficiency-based progression training paradigm on a virtual reality simulator was completed by Seymour et al. (2002). This study adhered to the vast majority of principles and practices that we have outlined in this book. Trainees were randomized to train on the simulator and trained until they met a pre-defined performance criterion level. This performance criterion level was based on the quantitatively assessed performance of five very experienced attending laparoscopic surgeons in the Department of surgery at Yale University USA. Trainees' intraoperative performance was assessed using the methods detailed in Chap. 5. In many ways, this study was relatively straightforward. The researchers concentrated training and assessment on one part of the laparoscopic cholecystectomy surgical procedure, i.e., dissection of the gallbladder from the liverbed. This part of the surgical procedure was well emulated in task six of the MIST VR simulator and the performance metrics of the simulator had already been developed by the company that had conceived of MIST VR (Virtual Presence Ltd., London, UK). Despite the fact that MIST VR had been dismissed by many in the surgical community as "not a proper surgical simulator," the MIST VR tasks and metrics were parsimonious and provided formative and summative feedback. An added advantage was that the metrics had been very well validated and so the researchers knew how to establish proficiency (i.e., error scores and economy of diathermy and *not* economy of instrument movement). They were also aware of research findings on the distribution of training; so none of the subjects trained on the simulator for longer than 1 h periods until they reached the quantitatively defined level of proficiency on two consecutive trials. Furthermore, all subjects trained on the simulator performed their index surgical procedure within days of completion of training. If trainees had not completed their index surgical procedure, they would have been required to re-demonstrate proficiency. Skills that are not utilized will very quickly extinguish and the rate of extinction is even faster for newly acquired skills. Thus, it is important to get trainees to use their skills as soon as possible after the proficiency level has been demonstrated. This probably accounts for a large proportion of the failure of transfer of training in industrial settings. Seymour et al. (2002) were also aware of the role of knowledge in skilled performance. An individual who knows how to perform a particular procedure is considerably more likely to be able to perform that procedure well than an individual who does not know how to perform the procedure. However, knowing how to perform the procedure does not guarantee that the individual is capable of performing the procedure in practice. To exclude knowledge of procedure performance as a performance-predicting variable, all of the trainee surgeons in this clinical trial were taught what to do during this portion of the laparoscopic cholecystectomy, what not to do, and their knowledge of this was assessed; both groups scored 100% in the post-didactic assessment. Furthermore, as there was no difference between the groups in their objectively assessed, perceptual, visuo-spatial and psychomotor performance at the start of the trial, intraoperative performance differences between the groups could only be accounted for by the training they had received.

The study by Seymour et al. (2002) has been criticized for only completing and assessing part of a laparoscopic cholecystectomy rather than the entire procedure and that only senior surgical trainees were used. In a separate study, McClusky et al. (2004) developed the metrics for the entire laparoscopic cholecystectomy using the same methodology which was used in the Yale study and as described here in Chaps. 5 and 6. In contrast to the Seymour et al., study, all surgical trainees in this study were in postgraduate years 1 and 2 (i.e., relatively junior surgical trainees). They found that VR-trained subjects completed the full LC 20% faster than controls (31 min vs. 39 min), made half as many errors while exposing cystic structures (5.3 vs. 10), and one-third fewer errors in dissecting the gallbladder (5.5 vs. 8.2). Overall, the VR-trained group made 60% fewer, objectively assessed intraoperative errors (11.7 vs. 19.7) than the standard trained surgeons. Both of these studies used the MIST VR as their training platform. In another study conducted at the Karolinska Institute in Sweden, the researchers completed another VR to OR study for the entire laparoscopic cholecystectomy (Ahlberg et al. 2007). They used the entire procedural metrics developed by McClusky et al. (2004) for the assessment of intraoperative performance. The Karolinska team had been trained at Emory University in Atlanta, Georgia, USA in the application of the objective assessment metrics. They had also been trained to identify the intraoperative assessment metrics to an inter-rater reliability >0.8. There were two important differences in the Ahlberg et al. (2007) study in comparison to the Seymour et al. (2002) and McCluskey et al. (2004) studies. The first major difference was that the virtual reality–trained surgeons trained on the LapSim VR simulator (Gothenburg, Sweden) rather than MIST VR. The second major difference was that all of the subjects included in the study completed ten full laparoscopic procedures. Not surprisingly, they found that proficiency-based progression trained surgeons made significantly fewer objectively assessed intraoperative errors in comparison to the standard trained group of surgeons. By this stage and with accumulating scientific evidence, there is good reason to believe that proficiency-based progression training on a virtual reality simulator provides a superior method of training surgical skills (for junior surgeons performing a straightforward laparoscopic surgical procedure such as cholecystectomy).

Nissen Fundoplication Simulation: Complex Skills

The skills training that we have described thus far has been on commercially available virtual reality simulators and training was for a relatively common elective laparoscopic surgical procedure, i.e., cholecystectomy. The question remains whether the same training and assessment paradigm would be as effective in training advanced laparoscopic skills for procedures such as Nissen fundoplication. Laparoscopic technical skills such as intracorporeal suturing and knot tying are of

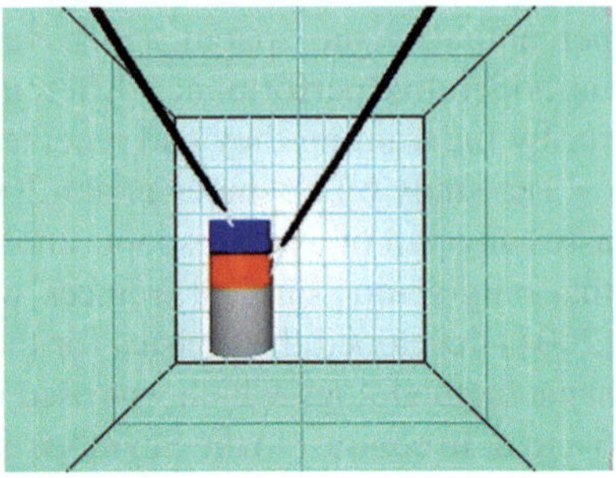

Fig. 10.2 Preliminary bimanual MIST VR psychomotor training used in the Van Sickle et al. (2007) proficiency-based progression clinical trial on intracorporeal suturing for Nissen fundoplication

fundamental importance to perform advanced laparoscopic skills. Unfortunately, no commercially available virtual reality simulator has been developed which trains the necessary skills for intracorporeal suturing and knot tying. Training programs for teaching intracorporeal suturing and knot tying exist (Rosser et al. 1998); however, their metric-based assessments are crude and rely mainly on completion time. At Emory University in Atlanta, Van Sickle and colleagues (Van Sickle et al. 2005, 2008a, b) developed a complete training and assessment program for intracorporeal suturing and knot tying based on the principles and practices that we have described in Chaps. 5–8.

Before specialized laparoscopic skills training for intracorporeal suturing commenced, simulation-trained subjects were schooled on a simple bimanual virtual reality task (shown in Fig. 10.2). This task was on the MIST VR simulator and required subjects to traverse the virtual cylinder with two virtual laparoscopic instruments grasping alternative segments of the task until completed.

Subjects were trained on this task until they demonstrated the quantitatively established level of proficiency. Subjects then received a didactic module which explained the details of laparoscopic suturing. They were also taught to tie a three-throw, slip-square intracorporeal knot because this is what is used to complete the fundal suturing portion of a laparoscopic Nissen fundoplication.

During this phase, subjects in the simulation-trained group received supervised training on both intracorporeal knot tying and suturing in a staged fashion, beginning with suturing. Foam models with rubber tubing on a standard suturing board were used to simulate the esophagus and fundus of the stomach for suturing practice (Figs. 10.3 and 10.4). A 6-inch 2–0 silk suture was passed through the rubber and foam model in a manner identical to that used in full-or partial thickness bites of the fundus and esophagus in a Nissen fundoplication. In Fig. 10.3 subjects were first taught to drive the needle through one piece foam tubing before progressing to the three bite model (Fig. 10.4) which more closely resembled the surgical task. Once proficiency on suturing was established, subjects progressed to the knot tying phase of training.

The knot tying sequence from performing the initial knot and sliding it down to approximate the tissues and then re-squaring it and adding the final throw is shown in Fig. 10.5. A novel model for training this technique was developed and is shown

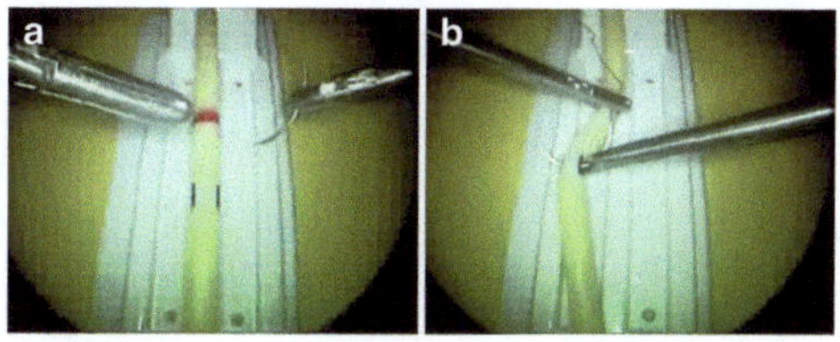

Fig. 10.3 (**a, b**) Simple suturing training model used in the Van Sickle et al. (2007) proficiency-based progression clinical trial on intracorporeal suturing for Nissen fundoplication. Trainees are taught the optimal way to hold the needle (**a**), and then drive it atraumatically through the target (**b**)

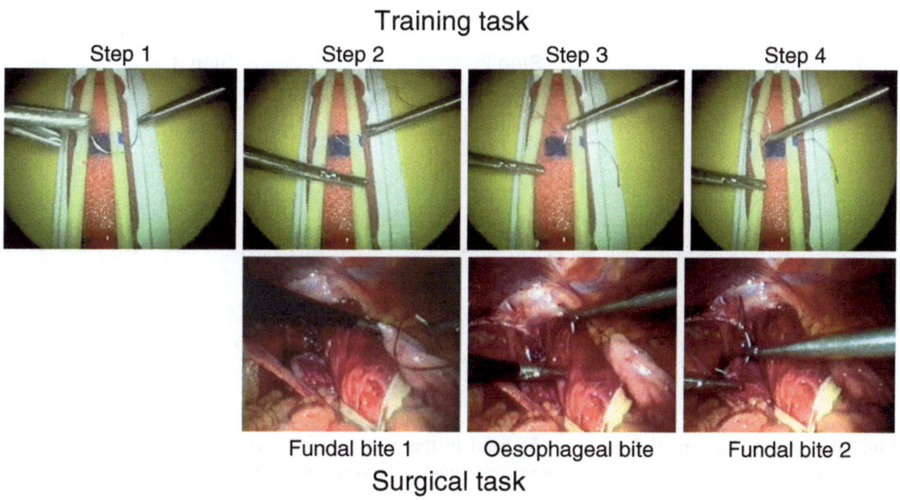

Fig. 10.4 Simple suturing training model used in the Van Sickle et al. (2007) proficiency-based progression clinical trial on intracorporeal suturing for Nissen fundoplication

in Fig. 10.6. This simple model involved a plastic tube covered in foam which was placed inside a sponge. The sponge was then fixed on the floor of a box trainer and trainees practiced intracorporeal suturing until they reached the proficiency level. If the subjects pulled the foam-covered tube out of the sponge, they automatically failed the task and started over. The goal of this part of the training program was for a trainee to learn to tie intracorporeal knots that would not slip but without putting tension on the foam-covered tube. Subjects practiced knot tying using 2.0 silk suturing, a laparoscopic needle driver, and an atraumatic grasper under laparoscopic visualization in a standard box trainer.

Formation of the knot was timed, beginning with the first grasp of a suture and ending with cutting of the suture tails. The tied ligature was then removed from the foam model by dividing it at its midpoint opposite the knot and analyzed using a tensiometer and software. The force-extension curves for each knot were determined, and a knot

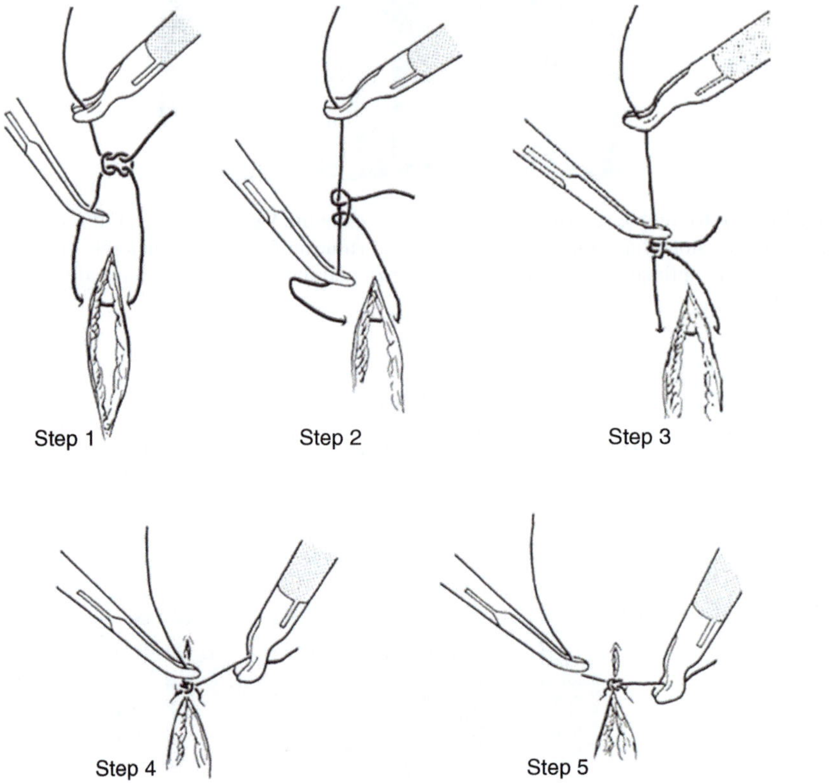

Fig. 10.5 Knot tying model steps (1–5) used in the Van Sickle et al. (2007) proficiency-based progression clinical trial on intracorporeal suturing for Nissen fundoplication

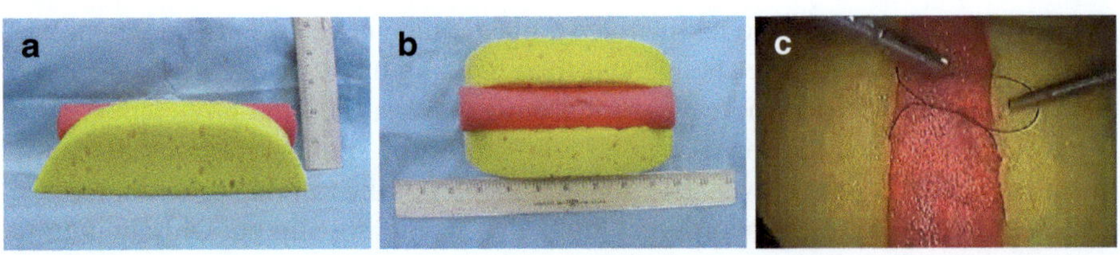

Fig. 10.6 (**a–c**) Knot tying model used in the Van Sickle et al. (2007) proficiency-based progression clinical trial on intracorporeal suturing for Nissen fundoplication: (**a**) side view; (**b**) plane view, and (**c**) being used for knot tying training

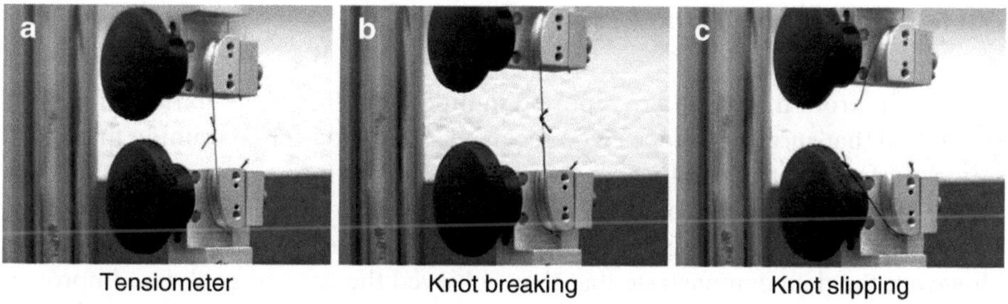

Fig. 10.7 Surgical knot tensiometer (**a**), assessment technique used in the Van Sickle et al. (2007) proficiency-based progression clinical trial on intracorporeal suturing for Nissen fundoplication showing the stretched suture breaking (**b**), and slipping (**c**)

quality score (KQS) was calculated by expressing the strength of the knotted suture as a percentage of the strength of the intact suture based on the following equation:

$$\text{KQS} = \frac{\text{Knot breaking/slipping force} \times \text{integrated force for the knot}}{\text{Suture breaking force} \times \text{integrated force for the suture}}$$

The knot quality was then expressed as a function of execution time, generating a performance quality score (PQS) for the knot:

$$\text{PQS} = \frac{\text{KQS} \times 100}{\text{Execution time (s)}}$$

The simulation group of subjects trained on this task until they were able to make the knots in the correct sequence and achieve PQS performance criteria on two consecutive knots (Fig 10.7).

Subjects in both the simulation and standard trained groups performed the fundal suturing portion of a laparoscopic Nissen fundoplication with an attending/consultant surgeon blinded to training status. Attending/consultant surgeons were instructed to behave no differently toward the trainee than they would during a normal case. A standardized three-suture fundoplication was performed with the first and most cephalad suture being placed by the attending/consultant surgeon. The remaining two sutures were placed by the trainee surgeons. The first subject-placed suture consisted of fundal-esophageal-fundal bites followed by the tying of the previously described slipknot. On the second subject-placed suture, the esophageal bite was omitted. The entire subject performed portion of the procedure was video recorded for future analysis by blinded reviewers as has been described in Chaps. 5, 6 and 8.

Nissen Fundoplication: Lessons Learned

The results from this study are reported in more detail in Chap. 6. In summary, it was found that surgical trainees who received simulation-based training made significantly fewer intraoperative errors during the performance of a highly complex surgical skill, in comparison to the standard trained group. This study is interesting because it involves the development of bespoke, homemade simulations. However, the data demonstrate that they achieved the desired goal, i.e., improved intraoperative performance during intracorporeal suturing. This goal was achieved at a fairly high price. The methodology applied in this study was rigorous as it was always intended to publish the results and to extend the data on proficiency-based progression training for an advanced laparoscopic surgical procedure. In addition to the development of new simulation models, the researchers also had to develop new intraoperative metrics for assessment during the training phase and during the live surgical skills application in a real patient. This meant that the study took almost 3 years to complete. One of the major problems in completing this study was getting access to surgical trainees. The subjects were recruited as part of their normal rotation through surgical service and many of them reported difficulty extracting themselves from their normal ward and operating room duties to go and train in the skills laboratory. If this type of training is to become standard practice in surgical training programs, training program directors must prioritize the facilitation of this type of training. Van Sickle et al. (2008a) have demonstrated that this approach to training produces superior technical skills than the traditional approach but to harness the benefits this approach to training has to be championed.

Another issue with this type of training is the proficiency level that trainees had to reach before they could complete the part of the surgical procedure they had been trained for on a patient. Two subjects failed to reach proficiency on one of the three measures. Not surprisingly, they performed considerably worse than their colleagues who did demonstrate proficiency. Under ideal circumstances, these two subjects should have been excluded from the study. However, even with their inclusion, the simulation-trained group performed significantly better than the standard trained group. At the time of conducting the study, there was some concern that the proficiency level might have been set at too high a level. However, the proficiency level had been established on the quantitatively assessed performance of surgeons who were experienced in the performance of Nissen fundoplication. It is very difficult to construct arguments against that benchmark.

The metrics applied in this study were developed from first principles as detailed in Chap. 5. They were developed by the research group from a task analysis of multiple video-recorded Nissen fundoplication procedures by experts and novices. This meant that the researchers had a very good idea about what types of performance characteristics they should concentrate on during training and what types of simulation models might be appropriate. It also meant that they were very experienced in the application of those metrics during training and during the assessment of intraoperative performance. However, that assessment process, particularly during training, was an enormous drain on human resources. As we have indicated previously, formative assessment is one of the most powerful attributes that should be included in an efficient and effective training program. The vast majority of the training that took place in this trial was conducted on novel simulation and assessment devices. This meant that apart from the MIST VR training component, one of the researchers had to always be available to provide proximate formative feedback to trainees. This is a very expensive way to conduct training and provides very strong support for the development of training programs that have a more automated assessment process. Initially, this would appear to indicate the necessity for an assessment device such as ICSAD (Smith et al. 2002) or OSATS (Martin et al. 1997), Chap. 5, coupled to the novel simulations that were developed for this study. However, on closer scrutiny, neither of these assessment devices will suffice as they both provide summative assessment. Furthermore, ICSAD only provides abstract data which only makes sense when contextualized, i.e., some type of procedure assessment of the surgical task being performed, and there are considerable questions about the reliability of OSATS assessments. The only viable alternative which can fulfill all performance-assessment criteria is a virtual reality simulation device and the MIST VR simulator, it should be able to provide the formative as well as summative assessment of performance. This would eliminate the necessity for a continuous (rather than intermittent) supervision and assessment of trainees during training a much more efficient solution to training highly complex surgical skills.

Left-Sided Laparoscopic Colectomy: Complex Procedural Skills

In an ideal world, virtual reality simulation would be the preferred option for technical and procedural skills training. In the long run, it is a less expensive and more efficient solution to the problem of training surgical skills. It reduces the amount of intensive supervision required for trainees and avoids much of the subjective assessment problems. It also eliminates the problem of task re-use. However, as the previous example on Nissen fundoplication has shown, in the absence of an alternative solution, homemade simulation and assessment programs can be effective at training advanced laparoscopic surgical skills. The simulation training solution that we have discussed may not have been efficient, but it has certainly demonstrated very clearly proof of concept for training and assessing advanced laparoscopic skills. It is precisely these skills that are required for the performance of advanced laparoscopic surgical procedures such as colorectal surgery. Although laparoscopic surgery was introduced in the early 1990s, the surgical community is still in the process of establishing which procedures are viable from a minimally invasive approach. In 2004, the COST trial assessed the safety of laparoscopically assisted and open colectomy for colon cancer (Nelson et al. 2004) and found that the outcomes from both approaches to surgery were equivalent. The laparoscopic group returned to normal activities quicker and used less analgesia. The 5-year follow-up data on these patients showed that laparoscopic colectomy for curable cancer was not inferior to open surgery based on long-term oncological endpoints. The overall survival rate for the open surgery group was 74.6% and 76.4% for the laparoscopic group. The overall recurrence rates were 21.8% of the open group and 19.4% for the laparoscopic group (Fleshman et al. 2007). However, the problem with expanding the application of the laparoscopic approach to colorectal cancer is training the surgeons to perform the procedure proficiently.

Virtual reality simulation of abdominal organs is not yet at a sufficiently advanced stage to simulate (in a clinically realistic and acceptable way) the properties of organs and surgical instrument interaction that would be of value for the training and assessment of procedural skills for colorectal surgery. However, a hybrid solution might be possible. Haptica Ltd. (Dublin, Ireland) developed a hybrid simulator which tracked the movement of laparoscopic surgical instruments in a three-dimensional space inside a box trainer. This meant that a surgical task could be placed in the simulator (i.e., the boxtrainer) and instrument movement (e.g., path length and smoothness) could be assessed relative to task performance. Assessment was very similar to the data produced by ICSAD (Smith et al. 2002) (Chap. 5). The assessment system suffered from the same shortcomings as the ICSAD system in that surgical performance on the actual task needed independent assessment. However, it did offer a good interim solution in the absence of full virtual simulation. Figure 10.8 shows the colorectal simulator (or CRS) developed by Haptica for training hand-assisted, left-sided colectomy. Also shown are the different steps in the performance of the surgical procedure and the images for the didactic component of training for the procedure. The surgeons would receive the didactic training either online or on a CD. The actual surgical task consisted of an anatomically correct tray (Fig. 10.9) constructed from silicone type material. They would be mentored through a case with an experienced proctor and at the end of the case, that tray was removed and assessed against predefined intraoperative errors with the trainee present during the assessment process (i.e., they were shown scoring criteria and it was explained to them why they were marked correct or incorrect). The errors are shown in Table 10.1. Tray errors were much more explicitly defined than reported in Table 10.1. For example, Error 1, *Incomplete division of the inferior mesenteric artery* was defined as follows. An error will be recorded if the mesenteric artery is *not*:

- divided between its origin at the aorta and its first branch (the left colic artery);
- transected and the ends sealed with either a complete staple line or two laparoscopic clips;
- divided completely and both free ends separated without any residual tissue remnant connecting the free ends

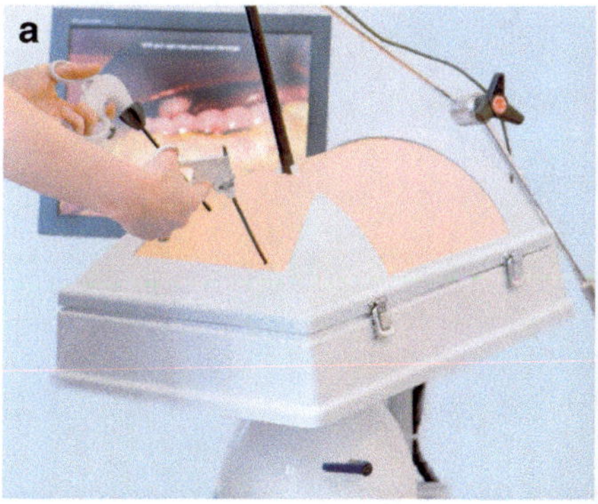

b

- Step 1: Tilting Bodyform
- Step 2: Identification of the IMA
- Step 3: Identification of the left ureter
- Step 4: Transection of the IMA
- Step 5: Mobilization of Sigmoid
- Step 6: Mobilization of descending colon
- Step 7: Take down of splenic flexure
- Step 8: Creation of intracorporeal anastomosis
- Step 9: Testing anastomosis

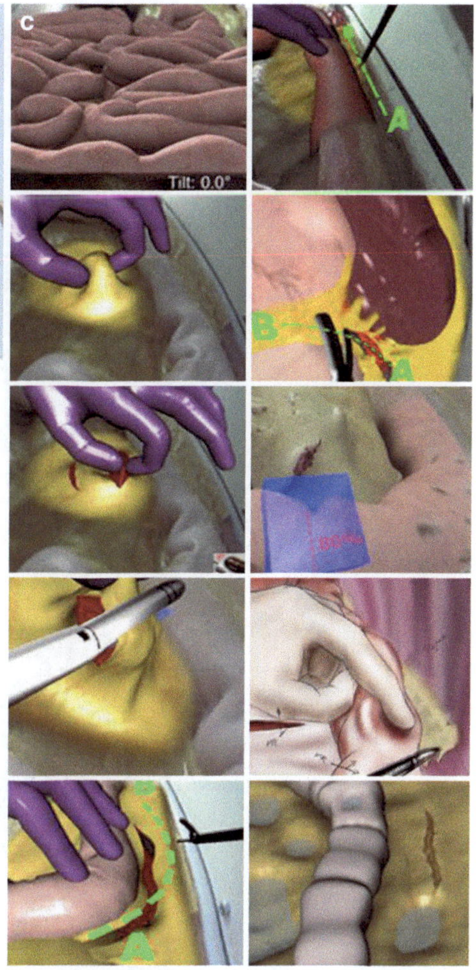

Fig. 10.8 CRS simulation (**a**), which was modified for hand-assisted left-sided colectomy. The procedural steps for hand-assisted left-sided colectomy (**b**), and the didactic module included with the simulation showing these steps (**c**)

Preliminary assessment of the simulator for construct validity (for the procedure performed entirely laparoscopically) showed that the metrics distinguished between novice and expert colorectal surgeons (Neary et al. 2008). It should also be noted that the novice surgeons in this study were in fact very experienced consultant surgeons but novice to laparoscopic colectomy. Experts performed the simulated procedure significantly faster and were more efficient in the use of surgical instruments. They also made fewer objectively assessed intraoperative errors on the tray.

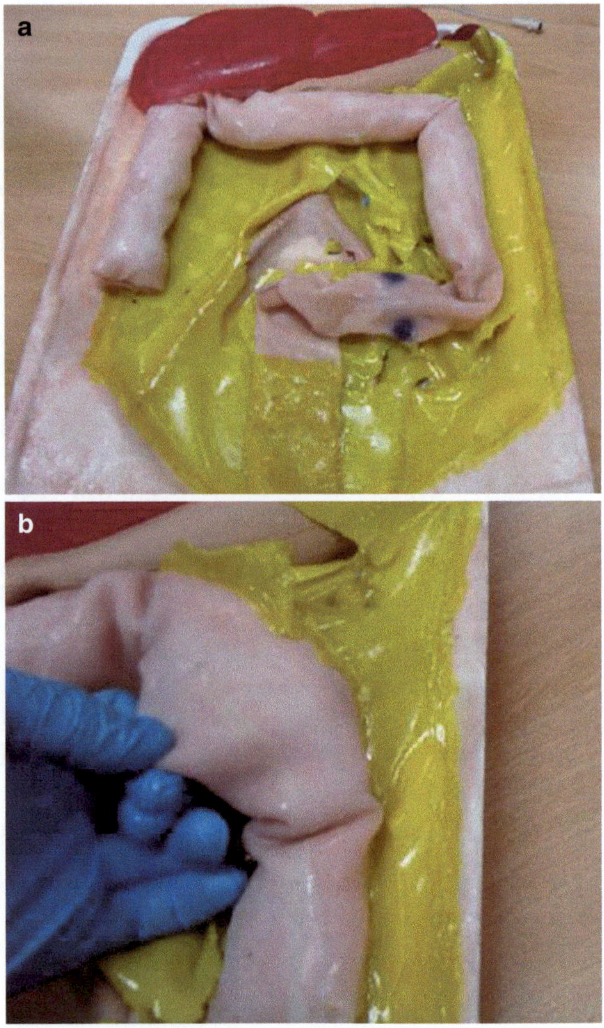

Fig. 10.9 CRS simulation for hand-assisted anatomically correct (**a**, **b**) surgical task for left-sided colectomy

Left-Sided Laparoscopic Colectomy: Lessons Learned

The CRS simulator was a good interim solution for a difficult training problem. Traditionally, training would have been conducted on an animal model or a cadaver. These are very resource intensive training solutions. In contrast, the CRS could be used in a wide variety of spaces with very few specialized requirements other than electrical power connections and possibly an Internet connection. The trays were "supposed" to be relatively clean; however, in reality, they were quite messy and the person conducting the assessment of the tray had to wear rubber gloves and a

Table 10.1 CRS simulation hand-assisted, left-sided colectomy tray errors

Error number	Anatomy tray metric errors
1	Inadequate division of inferior mesenteric artery *Critical error*
2	Inadequate division of inferior mesenteric vein
3	Mesenteric injury
4	Inadequate exposure of left ureter *Critical error*
5	Inadequate division of sigmoid mesentery
6	Inadequate mobilization of left colon
7	Inadequate mobilization of splenic flexure
8	Inadequate division of mesorectum
9	Inadequate rectal transection *Critical error*
10	Inadequate anastomotic alignment *Critical error*
11	Anastomotic tension
12	Anastomosis not centered
13	Organ injury *Critical error*
14	Specimen left in place *Critical error*

disposable gown. These were not major problems in comparison to traditional training solutions but they do indicate that matters are never as clear-cut as they first appear. A more important point about the trays was their cost; they were quite expensive and could only be used once. As should be clear from discussions in Chaps. 6 and 8, the whole point of training on the simulator is that the trainee continues training until they quantitatively demonstrate the level of proficiency established prior to training. This means that each trainee is going to use a minimum of two trays (i.e., proficiency must be demonstrated twice in two consecutive trials for training to considered complete). In reality, the vast majority of surgeons take considerably more than two trials to reach proficiency. As the number of trainees required for training to proficiency increases, so also does the cost of training. The simulator and the box trainer are reusable, but not the trays. Of course, there is also the problem of disposing of the trays that have been used. The researchers considered keeping the trays that had been used for archiving purposes, but they very quickly discovered that each tray took up considerably more space than a simple DVD recording of the procedure. The problem with a DVD recording of the procedure is that it gave incomplete information on surgical performance during the procedure, i.e., performance could only be scored reliably and accurately by physically examining the tray.

There was also the problem of the formative feedback. The instrument tracking metrics scored by the simulator reliably distinguished between experts and novices; however, these scores were only available after the procedure had been completed. Furthermore, error scores on the tray were also only available when the procedure was complete. Formative feedback and guidance could be given to the trainee intra-operatively; however, this meant that the person doing the proctoring had to be very experienced on the simulator (so as to guide trainees performance) and they also had to be very familiar with the surgical procedure so that they could reliably map the steps of the simulation training to the actual operative procedure. This in turn means that the proctors have to be very well trained in surgery and in implementing a standardized curriculum. The ideal solution would be to have very experienced laparoscopic colorectal surgeons acting as proctors, but in reality, this is not feasible, probably not even in centers of excellence. The alternative is to have skills laboratories with technicians conducting the proctoring. The problem with this approach is that trainees, who are in real life fairly senior surgeons, may not always be receptive to the guidance and suggestions of a well-trained lab technician!

Another potential problem with this approach to training, i.e., using a hybrid simulator, is the potential for subjectivity to creep in to scoring. However, if the metric errors are unambiguously and fully operationally defined and proctors are trained to be able to identify errors to a high-level of inter-rater reliability, this should not be a problem. Indeed, this problem has never occurred on any course that we have taught on. One of the more interesting aspects of the implementation of metrics that evolved from this study was the introduction of critical errors. In Chap. 5 we explained that it was very difficult to train individuals to reliably score intraoperative performance using a Likert scale. It is not impossible, but it is very difficult because it takes a long time. During the development of metrics for this procedure, it became clear relatively quickly that not all the intraoperative metric errors could be treated the same. The possibility of using a Likert scale assessment was excluded from the outset. Weighting of metric errors was discussed but was also excluded as a possibility because of the level of complexity that this would add to validation studies. It would also make the calculation of performance scores much more difficult. What the researchers decided on was to define particular intraoperative errors as critical errors. A critical error was defined as an error enacted in the simulation that if enacted during an *in vivo* surgical procedure would expose the patient to significant risk of harm. This meant that no matter how well the trainee did in their performance of the rest of the procedure, they automatically failed to demonstrate proficiency if they enacted a critical error during that training trial. This very parsimonious scoring solution has clinical validity and unambiguously makes the point to trainees. We have since integrated this concept into much of the rest of our work.

Full Physics, Full Procedural Virtual Reality Simulation

Endovascular procedures confer similar benefits to MIS, such as minimum invasion of the body cavity, reduced pain, less recovery time, etc., but also share similar problems (Cotin et al. 2000). Endovascular procedures use catheters or other devices inserted through blood vessels to diagnose and treat vascular disease, but present similar proprioceptive-visual conflict issues as MIS and is further complicated by x-ray imaging involving only two-dimensional visualization with only gradations of gray scale in the images. Angioplasty is a common endovascular procedure, where a balloon catheter is inserted into an artery then inflated causing the plaque blockage to be compressed against the artery wall, thus clearing the obstruction (with catheter/devices from outside the body exiting through the groin). Other endovascular techniques to maintain open the artery include the placement of a stent (i.e., tiny metal lattices that are compressed tightly over a deflated catheter balloon). When the balloon is inflated, the stent widens the vessel. However, clinicians must operate using an x-ray image on a monitor, i.e., a fluoroscope. They must also guide the catheter(s) along a vessel in three-dimensional space using two-dimensional gray-scale visual cues from the fluoroscopic image. Other complicating factors in endovascular procedures are the size of the devices (wires can be as thin as 0.014″) and the long distance from manipulation site location to the operating site. A further problem is that there is a time/x-ray exposure factor (Kelly and McArdle 2001). Radiologically guided procedures generate some of the highest radiation exposure doses in medical imaging. One of the most recognized complications is skin injury, caused by prolonged fluoroscopy (Koenig et al. 2001a, b). A major determinant of fluoroscopic imaging time is the experience of the operator. Clearly, the ability to decrease this imaging time would confer significant benefits for this patient group. Conventional endovascular training methods include training on animals, cadavers, or mechanical models using real medical devices and x-rays. In the United Kingdom, inherent problems with these strategies include the ethical and legal problems of training on animals, risks posed with repeated exposure to x-rays, and the expense of using real interventional medical devices. Most endovascular training still occurs on patients with one-on-one training with experienced trainers during a clinical procedure. Virtual reality simulation offers a very powerful training alternative.

One of the VR simulators that physicians can train on is the Vascular Interventional Training System (or VIST, see Chap. 2), which simulates the physics and physiology of the human cardiac and vascular system. It also provides visual and haptic feedback, similar to what a physician would see on the fluoroscope and feel if they were operating on a patient. Also included in the package is a graphical–user interface coupled to an instructional system that provides a framework for learning from the simulation. The complete package represents one of the most advanced VR packages for medical simulation currently available in the world today. Not only does it allow physicians to train with no risk to patients, but it also facilitates objective assessment of performance. It provides both formative and summative assessment which can be used to help the surgeon reach an objectively defined level of performance before using this technique on patients. The implication of having these objective metrics readily available in a full VR, full physics simulator is that only surgeons/physicians who clearly demonstrate proficiency on the simulator should/could be approved to carry out the procedure on patients.

Figure 10.10 (top panel) shows fluoroscopic images from a carotid artery stenting procedure from the VIST simulator. These are the images that the operating surgeon/physician would see when they are operating on the patient. The images in the bottom panel show different stages in the carotid artery stenting with embolic protection procedure. One of the early problems with the VIST simulator was that it could potentially measure ANY aspect of tool anatomy interaction; however, it had few if any clinically relevant procedure-specific metrics.

A group of researchers at Emory University in Atlanta developed clinically relevant metrics for carotid artery stenting. Carotid artery disease is the buildup of atherosclerotic plaque in the major neck vessels delivering blood to the brain, a major cause of stroke. Carotid artery stenting (CAS) is a minimally invasive, nonsurgical

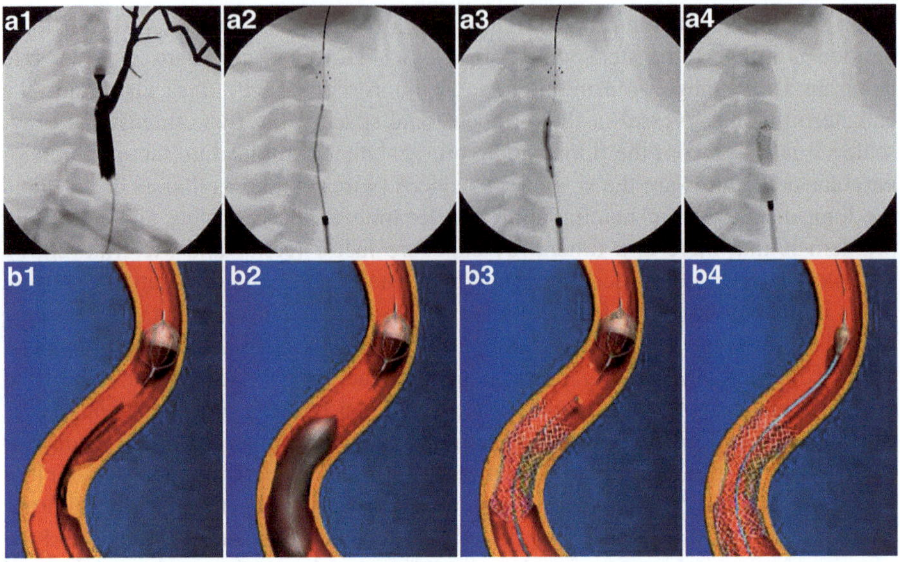

Fig. 10.10 (**a1–a4**†, **b1–b4**‡) Simulated fluoroscopic images (**a**1–4) showing the carotid lesion (**a1**), the fluoroscopic image of the deployment of the embolic protection device (**a2**), the angioplasty (**a3**) and the successful deployment of the carotid stent with the embolic protection device extracted (**a4**), and cartoons (**b**1–4), depicting the carotid lesion with the embolic protection device deployed (**b1**), the angioplasty (**b2**), in vivo deployment of the carotid stent with the embolic protection device capturing plaque (**b3**) and the embolic protection device being extracted post-deployment of the carotid stent (**b4**)

procedure intended to improve blood flow to the brain while helping prevent debris from entering cerebral circulation, and an important alternative for patients who are ineligible for the traditional surgical approach to treatment of carotid endarterectomy (CEA). Risk factors for carotid artery disease include advanced age, family history of stroke, plaque buildup in other areas of the body, high blood pressure, and diabetes. The American Heart Association has estimated that 20–30% of strokes are associated with carotid artery disease, caused by particles of atherosclerotic plaque travelling into the vessels that supply the brain with oxygen and vital nutrients. The traditional non-medical treatment for this problem was for a vascular surgeon to open up the diseased carotid artery and extract the occluding plaque manually. However, this is a clinically risky procedure for the patient as the operation itself may in fact precipitate a stroke. In 2004, a multicenter clinical trial showed that at 1 year, 12.2% of patients who had CAS had adverse outcomes (i.e., stroke, myocardial infarction, ipsilateral stroke, or death) in comparison to 20.1% in the CEA group. Also, at 1 year, carotid revascularization was repeated in fewer patients who had received stents than in those who had undergone endarterectomy; cumulative incidence, 0.6% vs. 4.3% (Yadav et al. 2004).

† Vascular Intervention Simulation Trainer (VIST), Courtesy of Mentice AB, Gothenburg, Sweden
‡ Courtesy of © Cordis Corporation 2011

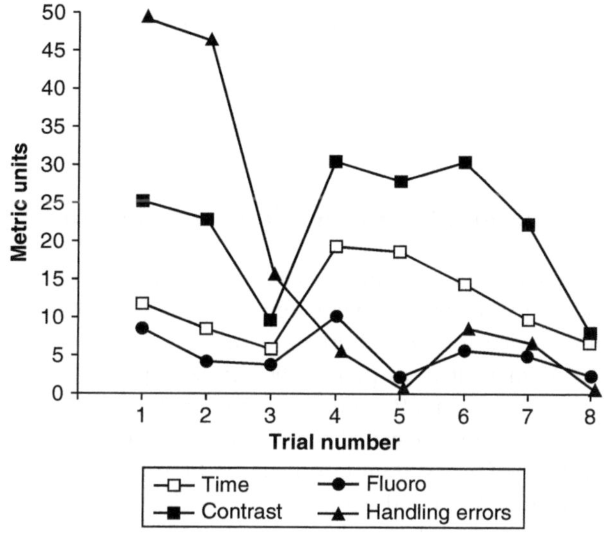

Fig. 10.11 Traditional clinical measures (operating time, amount of contrast agent used, fluoroscopy time) during carotid angiography that gives only a crude indication of learning and skill acquisition across training trials. In comparison to metrics measuring intraoperative instrument handling errors

The reason that the Emory University researchers were interested in developing metrics for CAS simulation was that the procedure could potentially have been performed by vascular surgeons, interventional cardiologists, and radiologists. There needed to be a training strategy that would ensure that all of these groups of physicians could hone their skills outside the operating room and catheterization laboratory. After developing the clinical metrics and ensuring that (some of) them were built into the simulator, they then proceeded to validate these metrics. They found that the simulated sequence of using guidewires and catheters was rated to be nearly identical to actual carotid artery stenting by 100 very experienced physicians (vascular surgeons and interventional cardiologists). They also reported that VIST looked, felt, and behaved similar to working on an actual patient (Nicholson et al. 2006). In a separate study, they assessed the reliability and validity of metrics that they had developed as well as the traditional metrics of time to perform the procedure, fluoroscopy time, and the amount of contrast agent used (Patel et al. 2006). They demonstrated that the metrics had high internal consistency, good test re-test reliability, and were sensitive to trainee performance improvements, i.e., demonstrated their learning curves. In particular, they found that catheter and wire handling metrics were the most sensitive to performance improvements. Figure 10.11 shows the VR performance data from one trainee across eight different training sessions. The traditional performance metrics of time, contrast, and fluoroscopy appear to show minimal learning by the trainee when clearly the trainer saw improvement in the trainee's performance. In contrast, the handling errors category shows a fairly typical learning curve. On trial one the trainee was making lots of technical errors, but by trial three, they had been reduced dramatically and were eliminated by trial eight. This category of metric included the tip of the catheter scraping against the vessel wall, advancing the catheter without a guide-wire in front of it, and allowing the catheter too close to the carotid lesion. In contrast to the more traditional metrics, these measures do show a very clear learning curve pattern. Furthermore, these are formative as well as summative metrics and were in fact used by the team to establish a level of proficiency for carotid artery angiography.

Developments, Implications, and Lessons Learned

Proficiency-based training as a new approach to the acquisition of procedural-based medical skills took a major step forward in April 2004. As part of the roll-out of a new device for carotid artery stenting (CAS), the Food and Drug Administration (FDA) mandated, as part of the device approval package, metric-based training to proficiency on a VR simulator as the required training approach for physicians who would be using the new device (Gallagher and Cates 2004a). The company manufacturing the CAS system informed the FDA that they would educate and train physicians in catheter and wire handling skills with a high fidelity VR simulator using a curriculum based on achieving a level of proficiency. This approach allowed for training of physicians who entered with variable knowledge, skill, and experience to leave with objectively assessed proficient knowledge and skills. This is particularly important for a procedure like CAS as it crosses multiple clinical specialties with each bringing a different skill-set to the training table. For example, a vascular surgeon has a thorough cognitive understanding of vascular anatomy and management of carotid disease, but may lack some of the psychomotor technical skills of wire and catheter manipulation. Conversely, an interventional cardiologist may have all of the technical skill, but may not be as familiar with the anatomical and clinical management issues. A sound training strategy must ensure that all of these specialists are able to meet an objectively assessable minimum level of proficiency in all facets of the procedure. This development helped to consolidate the paradigm shift in procedural-based medicine training and in the long run will result in a reduction in “turf wars” concerning future credentialing for new procedures. As long as a physician is able to demonstrate that he or she possesses the requisite knowledge and skills to perform a procedure, specialty affiliation will become less important. Indeed this was the approach advocated by a number of the professional medical organizations intimately involved in training physicians for CAS (Rosenfield et al. 2005).

The implications of the FDA decision for simulation and medicine are far-reaching. One of the main functions of the FDA is to protect the public and to ensure that the new medical devices/products are sagely introduced into the marketplace. In the case of carotid artery stenting with embolic protection, the FDA was very aware that different medical disciplines were competing to perform the procedure. The FDA was also aware that the different disciplines brought different skill-sets to performance of the procedure. To ensure that this did not compromise patient safety in the performance of this high-risk procedure, they agreed that doctors who wished to perform the procedure should objectively demonstrate that they had adequate clinical experience (i.e., sufficient patient numbers on whom they had completed CAS already) or they could train on a simulator until they reached a predefined level of proficiency. This was the first time that a skills benchmark had ever been imposed (by a very powerful government agency) on medicine. We believe that the long-term implications of this decision on procedural-based medicine will be far-reaching. The FDA have now realized that they do not have to take the word of an individual doctor or a company manufacturing a new medical device about the skills of the practitioners using the device; they can check the skills level of the operator, probably on a simulator. This decision also offers great opportunities for simulation device manufacturers. It means that manufacturers have the opportunity to facilitate medical device manufacturing by getting approval from the FDA for their device without first testing it on patients and before the operators have been trained. Also, training to use the device on real patients is minimized and instead surgeons can prepare to perform the procedure on a device that measures their performance and is objective, transparent, and fair. Furthermore, the manufacturers of medical devices can now offer additional quantitative support on the safety and efficacy of their device before ever testing it on a single patient, which will certainly make the decision of the FDA to go to full clinical trial much easier. This also means that large manufacturers of new medical devices should now, in all probability, plan for the development of a simulation as part of the role of their new technology. We believe that this technology is now beginning to change the training paradigm in all of procedural-based medicine. Simulation training to an objectively determined level of proficiency offers a superior skill acquisition process that is objective, based on real world skill-sets, and removes professional politics from the credentialing equation. It also means that the physicians performing the procedure on patients for the first time will have a more homogenous skill-set which in well-controlled studies of MIS procedures has led to safer objectively assessed intraoperative performance (Ahlberg et al. 2007; Seymour et al. 2002; Van Sickle et al. 2008a).

The most sophisticated virtual reality simulators currently available in medicine are for endovascular procedures such as carotid artery stenting, coronary stenting, renal stenting, and other vascular procedures. We have experience of the vast majority of these and we have a number of observations to make. The first is that the simulators are very expensive. The price ranges from about \$100,000 to about \$1.3 million. There is also the cost of maintenance cost and technical support. These simulators run on the most sophisticated widely available computer platforms available and the engineering technology which is used to detect device performance is at the very edge of what is possible. This means that these devices are usually fairly fragile. In our experience, they need substantial technical support to keep them running reliably. The manufacturers assure us that things have improved in terms of reliability, but in our experience, it is preferable to hope for the best, but plan for the worst. The simulator that we tend to opt for in this group is the VIST system. It is a full physics–based virtual reality simulation of the cardiac and vascular system. This means that when the system was being developed, the simulated anatomy was based on the actual measured physical properties of the real anatomy and the anatomy-device interaction is about as realistic as is currently possible. There are "prettier" simulators available that have the look and feel of the cath lab environment; however, the anatomy–device interaction is not particularly realistic. Furthermore, the formative feedback on device–anatomy interaction is not based on real-time data derived from the performance of the trainee. Some of the simulation manufacturers may argue that they do provide formative feedback metrics in their simulation. The types of metrics that we believe are most valuable in the learning process for the trainee are proximate performance metrics on how they are performing with the surgical instrument on a second-by-second basis, e.g., handling error data shown in Fig. 10.11. Performance feedback on the percentage of a lesion covered by the stent, whether the right catheter and wire, was chosen and whether they were chosen in the correct order, etc. are important pieces of procedural information that can be used for formative feedback. Their impact on device handling learning will be minimal. Also, some manufacturers claim that their simulators are full physics and we do not doubt them. However, neither of us are computer scientists and so we usually have this fact checked independently to avoid confusion in ensuing discussions. We have not always corroborated the claims of the manufacturers.

Despite being advocates of full physics virtual reality simulation, it has been our experience that they are not without their problems. For example, in theory, it should be possible to measure any aspect of technical performance as all other data are included as part of the simulation. The reality is somewhat different. As part of the development of metrics for CAS, the team at Emory University in Atlanta, USA, developed an extensive list of intraoperative performance characteristics that they wished to measure. Although they had developed explicit performance characteristic definitions that characterized the operative procedure particularly well, the simulation manufacturers were not able to capture the essence of these metrics. Furthermore, some other metrics that the simulator was able to capture and characterize did not appear to be reliable indicators of performance characteristics even based on simple laboratory verifications studies. This did come as a surprise to the Emory team but they were reassured (from their own trainee performance data) by the fact that they did not need to measure all of the performance characteristics that they wanted in order to facilitate the learning process in an efficient and effective manner. Metrics, such as scraping the catheter against the vessel wall, advancing the catheter without a guide-wire in front it, having a catheter too close to the lesion (as well as multiple other performance metrics) etc., clearly discriminated between experts and novices and clearly showed the effects of learning which they saw transfer to intraoperative performance. They could also be used to give performance feedback on a second-by-second basis during training. The amount of time taken to perform the procedure, the amount of contrast agent used, fluoroscopy time, as well as information on devices used, the order they were used in and proportion of lesion covered by the stent etc., could also all be given as summative assessment.

Another problem with high-end simulation stems from the physician and not the simulator. Some physicians attend training courses and expect the simulator to behave and respond just like real patients. Simulators are not real patients, and although the simulation experience will continue to improve, they will never entirely mimic the human patient exactly. Also, we find some of the attitudes toward simulation training by physicians somewhat perplexing. They have the opportunity to train on the full procedure using the exact same devices that they would on a real patient and they are not satisfied with this. Not infrequently, they complain that simulators are not the same as the patient; at this stage, we usually point out to them that porcine or animal models are even more dissimilar and do not even have the advantage of anatomical correctness, nor formative feedback.

Another problem that we have on training courses is feedback from (usually fairly senior) physicians or surgeons that their assessment metrics do not accurately reflect what they believe to be their performance on the simulator. Ten years ago, these comments may have caused more concern. However, in light of data that is emerging from clinical studies and simulation studies on the objective assessment of technical skills, we are more inclined to accept the data as measured by the simulator. This almost certainly is the case if the simulator we are using has had their metric assessments well validated. One of us has been known on these occasions to point out to the trainee (no matter how senior they are) that they (the surgeon or trainee) are the individuals at the end of the operating instruments and that the other trainees are not experiencing the same performance-assessment disparities!

Another not so insignificant problem which also stems from the trainee is feedback on what the simulation feels like. These problems stem from fundamental human factors of sensation and perception, which we discussed in Chaps. 3 and 4 as they relate to human performance and skill acquisition. In a sense, what the trainee is reporting is correct. However, the explanation is somewhat complex. If we could exactly know the physical forces, moments, pressures, and shear applied to the hands/fingers during exact activities, we could replicate them precisely and people feeling it should have the exact same experience that they have in real life. The problem is that it is very difficult to build sufficiently instrumented tools and/or sensorize hands to measure all the subtle aspects of what we feel. And then it is just as difficult to build sufficiently capable devices to put this out as haptic information interfaced with a computer simulation. The whole intermediate processing layer of the brain probably comes in here. We suspect that human beings get multiple aspects of haptic and tactile sensory inputs which at low levels fuse and interpret. Our high-level functions then interpret that to mean something driven by our conscious perception of the fused information. The problem is that people (surgeons and physicians) do not realize that they are fusing multiple inputs, some obvious, some subtle. So we get generalized statements like "it's too soft," "it's too hard," "it should be slicker," "it should be rougher," and so on. Full physics procedural simulation is based on what we can measure about what the human sensory system actually detects. Unfortunately, sensation and perception in human beings are correlated but they are not the same and do not correspond on a one-to-one basis. This problem is likely to persist for some considerable time and will take advances in cognitive/behavioral science coupled with engineering solutions to solve the problem. At the time of writing, these solutions are not apparent. It is our belief that this will not significantly impede the deployment of simulation to learning how to operate as it is an order of magnitude better solution than acquiring early learning curve skills on patients.

Summary

Proficiency-based progression simulation training significantly improves objectively assessed intraoperative performance. Cumulating clinical trial data demonstrates this for straightforward as well as for complex surgical skills, mostly in the minimally invasive surgery environment. There is a lack of virtual reality simulators for complex surgical procedures such as Nissen fundoplication and laparoscopic colectomy. In one of the studies that we considered here, a group of researchers from Emory University in Atlanta developed their own metric-based simulations for training intracorporeal suturing knot tying for Nissen fundoplication. The data showed that their simulation models were effective at training the skills targeted. However, the absence of computer-scored performance meant that training had to be closely supervised in order to provide informative feedback to trainees. A hybrid virtual reality simulator for minimally invasive colectomy had similar problems; but both were good interim solutions in the absence of a virtual reality simulator. Full physics–based virtual reality simulators are available for endovascular procedures, but they tend to be expensive and fragile. Despite this, endovascular simulators represent the leading edge of virtual reality simulation. In 2004, the FDA in the USA mandated training on a simulator to an objective level of proficiency for surgeons and physicians who wanted to perform carotid artery stenting with embolic protection. This decision set precedent in procedural-based medicine. We believe that it will have far-reaching implications for medicine and for simulation.

References

Ahlberg G, Enochsson L, Gallagher AG, et al. Proficiency-based virtual reality training significantly reduces the error rate for residents during their first 10 laparoscopic cholecystectomies. *Am J Surg*. 2007;193(6):797-804.

American College of Surgeons. (2011, Revised July 6, 2011). ACS Accredited Education Institutes. Retrieved 9th July 2011, from http://www.facs.org/education/accreditationprogram/news.html

Broad M. *Transfer of Training: Action-Packed Strategies to Ensure High Payoff from Training Investments*. Cambridge: Perseus Books; 2001.

Cates CU, Patel AD, Nicholson WJ. Use of virtual reality simulation for mission rehearsal for carotid stenting. *J Am Med Assoc*. 2007;297(3):265.

Cotin S, Dawson S, Meglan D, et al. ICTS, an interventional cardiology training system. *Stud Health Technol Inform*. 2000;70:59-65.

Fleshman J, Sargent DJ, Green E, et al. Laparoscopic colectomy for cancer is not inferior to open surgery based on 5-year data from the COST Study Group trial. *Ann Surg*. 2007;246(4):655.

Gallagher AG, Cates CU. Approval of virtual reality training for carotid stenting: what this means for procedural-based medicine. *J Am Med Assoc*. 2004a;292(24):3024-3026.

Gallagher AG, Cates CU. Virtual reality training for the operating room and cardiac catheterisation laboratory. *Lancet*. 2004b;364(9444):1538-1540.

Gallagher AG, Neary P, Gillen P, et al. Novel method for assessment and selection of trainees for higher surgical training in general surgery. *ANZ J Surg*. 2008;78(4):282-290.

Haluck RS, Satava RM, Fried G, et al. Establishing a simulation center for surgical skills: what to do and how to do it. *Surg Endosc*. 2007;21(7):1223-1232.

Healy GB. The college should be instrumental in adapting simulators to education. *Bull Am Coll Surg*. 2002;87(11):10.

Kelly B, McArdle C. *Imaging the Acutely Ill Patient: A Clinician's Guide*. London: WB Saunders Company Limited; 2001.

Koenig TR, Wolff D, Mettler FA, Wagner LK. Skin injuries from fluoroscopically guided procedures: part 1, characteristics of radiation injury. *AJR Am J Roentgenol*. 2001a;177(1):3.

Koenig TR, Mettler FA, Wagner LK. Skin injuries from fluoroscopically guided procedures: part 2, review of 73 cases and recommendations for minimizing dose delivered to patient. *AJR Am J Roentgenol*. 2001b;177(1):13.

Martin JA, Regehr G, Reznick R, et al. Objective structured assessment of technical skill (OSATS) for surgical residents. *Br J Surg*. 1997;84(2):273-278.

McClusky DA, Gallagher AG, Ritter EM, Lederman A, Van Sickle KR, Smith C. Virtual reality training improves junior residents' operating room performance: results of a prospective, randomized, double-blinded study of the complete laparoscopic cholecystectomy. *JAMA*. 2004;199(3):73.

Neary PC, Boyle E, Delaney CP, Senagore AJ, Keane FB, Gallagher AG. Construct validation of a novel hybrid virtual-reality simulator for training and assessing laparoscopic colectomy; results from the first course for experienced senior laparoscopic surgeons. *Surg Endosc*. 2008;22(10):2301-2309.

Nelson H, Sargent DJ, Wieand HS, et al. A comparison of laparoscopically assisted and open colectomy for colon cancer. *N Engl J Med*. 2004;350(20):2050-2059.

Nicholson WJ, Cates CU, Patel AD, et al. Face and content validation of virtual reality simulation for carotid angiography: results from the first 100 physicians attending the Emory NeuroAnatomy Carotid Training (ENACT) program. *Simul Healthc*. 2006;1(3):147-150.

Patel AD, Gallagher AG, Nicholson WJ, Cates CU. Learning curves and reliability measures for virtual reality simulation in the performance assessment of carotid angiography. *J Am Coll Cardiol*. 2006;47(9):1796-1802.

Pellegrini CA, Sachdeva AK, Johnson KA. Accreditation of education institutes by the American College of Surgeons: a new program following an old tradition. *Bull Am Coll Surg*. 2006;91(3):8-12.

Rosenfield K, Babb JD, Cates CU, et al. Clinical competence statement on carotid stenting: training and credentialing for carotid stenting–multispecialty consensus recommendations: a report of the SCAI/SVMB/SVS Writing Committee to develop a clinical competence statement on carotid interventions. *J Am Coll Cardiol*. 2005;45(1):165-174.

Rosser JC Jr, Rosser LE, Savalgi RS. Objective evaluation of a laparoscopic surgical skill program for residents and senior surgeons. *Arch Surg*. 1998;133(6):657.

Satava RM. Virtual reality surgical simulator. The first steps. *Surg Endosc*. 1993;7(3):203-205.

Seymour NE, Gallagher AG, Roman SA, et al. Virtual reality training improves operating room performance: results of a randomized, double-blinded study. *Ann Surg*. 2002;236(4):458-463; discussion 463-454.

Smith SG, Torkington J, Brown TJ, Taffinder NJ, Darzi A. Motion analysis: a tool for assessing laparoscopic dexterity in the performance of a laboratory-based laparoscopic cholecystectomy. *Surg Endosc*. 2002;16:640-645.

Thorndike EL, Woodworth RS. The influence of improvement in one mental function upon the efficiency of other functions. *Psychol Rev*. 1901;8(3):247-261.

Van Sickle K, Iii D, Gallagher AG, Smith CD. Construct validation of the ProMIS simulator using a novel laparoscopic suturing task. *Surg Endosc*. 2005;19(9):1227-1231.

Van Sickle K, Gallagher AG, Smith CD. The effect of escalating feedback on the acquisition of psychomotor skills for laparoscopy. *Surg Endosc*. 2007;21(2):220-224.

Van Sickle K, Ritter EM, Baghai M, et al. Prospective, randomized, double-blind trial of curriculum-based training for intracorporeal suturing and knot tying. *J Am Coll Surg*. 2008a;207(4): 560-568.

Van Sickle K, Baghai M, Huang IP, Goldenberg A, Smith CD, Ritter EM. Construct validity of an objective assessment method for laparoscopic intracorporeal suturing and knot tying. *Am J Surg*. 2008b;196(1):74-80.

Yadav JS, Wholey MH, Kuntz RE, et al. Protected carotid-artery stenting versus endarterectomy in high-risk patients. *N Engl J Med*. 2004;351(15):1493.

Chapter 11
Simulation In and For Medicine: Where Next?

In the previous chapters, we discussed the reasons why certain types of surgical skills such as those for laparoscopic surgery are difficult to learn. The processes of skill acquisition for laparoscopic surgery, are precisely the same processes involved in skill acquisition per se. Skill acquisition can occur coincidently (but not necessarily efficiently or optimally). For at least a century, surgery has had the luxury of being able to acquire the required operative skills by operating on real people over a lengthy period of time (e.g., duration of training in the UK and Ireland is about 13 years). In the USA, a surgeon is considered trained after a five year apprenticeship (6–7 years if the trainee studies for Fellowship). Questions have now been asked in the UK and Europe regarding why there is such a difference between how long it takes to train a surgeon in the USA and in the UK or Europe. However, globally not only is the number of years which are required to train a surgeon being questioned but also the number of hours that surgical trainees and indeed surgeons should work is under consideration. These questions originated from high-profile patient safety issues such as the Libby Zion case in New York (1988). As a result of this case, the training/working hours of junior doctors were reduced to 80 h/week and are due to fall still further. In the EU, the number of hours worked by junior doctors is even lower, i.e., 48 h. As well as these pressures, the practice of surgery (and by default training) has come under closer and closer scrutiny also as a function of high-profile medical error cases such as the Bristol Case (Senate of Surgery 1998) in the United Kingdom and the To Err is Human report (Kohn et al. 2000) in the USA. These reports claimed that a considerable number of deaths in hospitals were due to medical error and had the effect of focusing more and more attention on the practice of surgery.

In the light of these contentious issues, surgery was required to develop a mature understanding of why certain types of surgical skills were more difficult to learn than others. In many respects, the development and widespread application of minimally invasive surgery during the 1990s was a fortuitous event for the surgical establishment. It meant that surgery could no longer afford the luxury of coincidental learning. They had to systematically work out why a well and trusted training paradigm was failing some surgeons in the acquisition of skills for the practice

A.G. Gallagher and G.C. O'Sullivan, *Fundamentals of Surgical Simulation*, Improving Medical Outcome - Zero Tolerance,
DOI 10.1007/978-0-85729-763-1_11, © Springer-Verlag London Limited 2012

of minimally invasive surgery. We are not trying to trivialize the decades and centuries of knowledge which were transmitted from one group of surgeons to the next via the apprenticeship model. However, the apprenticeship model on its own as developed by Halsted at Johns Hopkins was by the late twentieth century inefficient, and in some cases ineffective at preparing surgeons for the practice of modern surgery. We are also not arguing that the apprenticeship model does not work because clearly it does and has done so for at least a century. The majority of surgeons (and other procedural-based practitioners), who were trained under the apprenticeship model, currently practice medicine safely. One of the goals which we set ourselves in writing this book was to put down on paper the factors implicit in the apprenticeship model which make it an effective education and training strategy. In previous chapters, we described and discussed many of these. In terms of cognition, the training program should teach trainees what they need to know to be able to perform the task safely and proficiently. This information needs to be organized in a way that facilitates storage in long-term memory for retrieval at the appropriate time. Technical skills need to be taught in the context of this clinical knowledge and trainees need to be informed proximal to their performance how well or how badly they performed. Knowledge and skills can be taught, trained and acquired by the trainee in a variety of ways, including, notes, lectures, online learning, cadavers, animal models, simulation models including virtual reality. However, all these methods of learning are simply different ways for the effective and efficient delivery of a curriculum. It is the curriculum that was delivered by Halsted and his descendants that directly links education and training in surgery today to the education and training in surgery 50 or 100 years ago. The knowledge base has evolved as have the tools for delivery of the curriculum, but the curriculum remains a constant. Halsted's greatest contribution to surgical education and training was the systematic formulation and delivery of a curriculum for training a surgeon. This also lay at the heart of his graded patient care and the operative responsibility which he gave to his trainees. What we intend to achieve in this book is to draw together the disparate scientific findings (which are a lot) and how they relate to effective and efficient learning and how best to deliver it using twenty-first century knowledge of education, learning, and technology. As stated previously, we have applied this knowledge to surgery because that is our work area. However, the science of behavior that we have outlined applies to the learning of any area of procedural-based medicine.

Deliberate Practice in the Acquisition of Skill

The view in surgery and other high skill occupations is that merely "engaging" in a sufficient amount of practice, regardless of the structure of that practice, leads to maximal performance. This is in contrast to what has been quantitatively demonstrated about advance skill performance. In the nineteenth century, Bryan and Harter (1899) studied the skill acquisition of Morse Code operators. They found that learners reached a plateau in their skills level for long periods, were unable to obtain further improvements. With extended efforts, trainees could restructure the skill to overcome these plateaus. Keller (1958) showed that these plateaus in Morse Code reception were not an inevitable characteristic of skill acquisition. He found that even very experienced Morse Code operators could dramatically increase their performance through deliberate efforts, e.g., when further improvements were required for promotions and external rewards (Bryan and Harter 1897). More generally, Thorndike (Thorndike and Woodworth 1901) suggested that adults perform at a level far from their maximal level, even for tasks they frequently carry out. Dvorak, Merrick, Dealey, and Ford (1936) reported substantial improvements (i.e., >50%) in experienced typists performance as a result of deliberate efforts. Probably the best monitored and measured performance characteristics of any group of elite performers are athletes. Performance in sport is usually measured under standardized conditions for the purposes of establishing local, national and world records. A review of performance data by Schulz and Curnow (1988) concluded that throughout the history of the Olympic Games, the best performance for all events has improved (in some cases by as much as 50%). It is generally recognized that some of these improvements are due to developments in equipment and rule changes. However, great improvements have also been observed in events such as running and swimming which have seen only minor changes in equipment and rules. For example, the marathon is one of the longest and most challenging tests of the human body. It is a centerpiece of athletic events throughout the world. In order for a performance to be ratified as a world record by the International Association Athletics Federations, the marathon course on which the performance occurred must be 42,195 km. There are a number of other stringent criteria that are applied when deciding whether an event is a recognized marathon. The methodology has been in place for the best part of a century. Robert Fowler (USA) set the world record for the marathon in 1908 in Yonkers, New York at 2 h 52 min and 45 s. Haile Gebrselassie (Ethiopia) set the world record in Berlin in 2008 with a time of 2 h 3 min and 59 s, which is an improvement of approximately 28% on the time set by Fowler. In virtually all domains, insights and knowledge are steadily accumulating and the criteria for eminent as well as expert performance undergo continuous change. To reach the status of an expert in any domain, it is sufficient to master the existing knowledge and techniques. To achieve eminent status means that the individual must first achieve the level of an expert and then in addition, they must surpass the achievements of already recognized eminent people and make innovative contributions to the domain.

In an extensive review and analysis of the performance attributes and characteristics of expert and exceptional performance, Ericsson and Lehmann (1996) argued that the highest levels of human performance in different domains can only be attained after around 10 years of extended, daily amounts of deliberate practice activities. They reported that laboratory analyses of expert performance in many domains such as chess, medicine, auditing, computer programming, bridge, physics, sports, typing, juggling, dance, and music revealed maximal adaptations of experts to domain-specific constraints. For example, performance characteristics of experts included acquired anticipatory skills which circumvented general limits on reaction time, distinctive memory skills which allowed a domain-specific expansion of working memory capacity to support planning, reasoning, and evaluation. It is the cumulative effect of deliberate practice on a range of human factors that defines expert performance. Furthermore, studies indicate a remarkable aging trend in North America. An accurate profile of the decline in physical and cognitive capabilities over time is essential to our understanding of the aging process. Baker, Deakin, Horton, and Pearce (2007) examined the maintenance of skilled performance across the careers of 96 professional golfers. Professional golfers are renowned for their detailed attention to deliberate practice. The data from Baker et al., (Baker et al. 2007) showed that performance of the golfers was maintained to a greater extent when compared with activities relying on biologically constrained abilities. Although the generalizability of these results to normal aging populations is not known, they suggest that acquired skills can be maintained to a large extent in the face of advancing age.

Gary Player probably did not craft the aphorism that links practice and luck, but he did tell the following story:

> "I was practicing in a bunker down in Texas and this good old boy with a big hat stopped to watch. The first shot he saw me hit went in the hole. He said, "You got 50 bucks if you knock the next one in." I holed the next one. Then he says, "You got $100 if you hole the next one." In it went for three in a row. As he peeled off the bills he said, "Boy, I've never seen anyone so lucky in my life." And I shot back, "Well, the harder I practice, the luckier I get." That's where the quote originated (Player 1962).

Whether this story is true or not and whether it originated from Gary Player is somewhat irrelevant. However, it does capture the quintessential nature and outcome of deliberate practice.

Deliberate Practice Characterized

Practice means to learn by repetition or systematic training by multiple repetitions. Deliberate practice is more than repetitive practice (or repeated experience) and is not just about working harder or deliberately engaging in more practice. Deliberate practice is designed specifically to improve performance and the operative word is "designed." Deliberate Practice is a system that anyone of any ability level (theoretically at least) can use as the backbone of their practice routine. People who engage in deliberate practice will look at areas of improvement and then set about creating a specific action plan which will take them just beyond their current abilities. They also invest both time and resources to ensure that they achieve the goals that they set or are set for them. It requires effort and attention to detail particularly when progress has been slowed or halted. It involves many of the factors that we have already discussed in this book as these principles and practices are what the "deliberate practice" is built on. Ericsson and his colleagues did not invent deliberate practice (Ericsson et al. 1993). Their contribution was to document the elements of deliberate practice and to show that, when rigorously applied by motivated individuals, this method is an efficient and effective process for gaining expertise in many domains and instructional settings. Interestingly, the elements themselves can be derived from commonly and long understood psychological principles and so in this sense, they are not new. However, what was new when Ericsson et al. (1993) first reported on their data was that the application of deliberate practice lay at the heart of the development of expertise across so many domains. In Chap. 9, we argued that in the preparation and delivery of didactic material, online content was *not* king; rather, it was the way that the content was configured that determined the effectiveness of didactic learning. The same is true for "practice" to be effective.

Deliberate Practice *not* Repetitive Practice

One of the main findings from the Ericsson et al. (1993) studies was the sheer amount of practice that experts engaged in. Deliberate practice for the violinists that they studied started with about 2–3 h/week when they were quite young (4–8 years of age) rising steadily throughout the teenage years with professional violinists and good students engaging in more than 24 h/week. All of the violinists studied by Ericsson et al. (1993) were either violin teachers, professional violinists, good and best student violinists. All of the students practiced more than the teachers had when they were teenagers and only the professional violinists practiced more than the good students. The same pattern emerged from their data on expert and amateur pianists. The other finding to emerge from this study was that deliberate practice extended over a considerable period of time, i.e., >10 years. The authors give three examples (work, play, and deliberate practice) which they suggest typifies the differences between "normal" activities and deliberate practice. Work includes public performance and services rendered for pay. Play includes activities that have no explicit goal and that are inherently enjoyable. Deliberate practice includes activities that have been specially designed to improve the current level of performance. The goals, costs and rewards of these three types of activities differ, as does the frequency with which individuals pursue them. Deliberate practice is also more than simple repetition of the same performance characteristics. After all, an individual can repeat the same sequence of performance characteristics during the same context, and be able to produce these performance characteristics reliably, but entirely inappropriately, i.e., they can make the same mistake repeatedly and not learn from it. Deliberate practice involves more structured activities which do not allow this situation to persist. The skills or performance characteristics that need to be developed are clearly identified at the outset. A strategy is then set out as to how these performance characteristics or skills are to be acquired. Traditionally, in surgery, these skills were acquired by the repeated practice of surgical procedures on patients throughout training, hence the persistent emphasis on procedure numbers completed by the trainee surgeon. Even more problematic with simple repetition is that it gives little or no indication of the quality of performance by the trainee and if in reality they were the first operator or even completed the procedure. Ericsson et al. (1993) found that elite performers had overcome a number of constraints that could have impinged negatively on their goals. They had obtained early access to instructors, maintained high levels of deliberate practice throughout the skills development process, and received continued personal and environmental support. The commitment to deliberate practice by expert performers distinguishes them from the vast majority of children and adults who have difficulty in meeting the much lower demands of practice in schools, adult education, and in physical exercise programs.

Another problem for training surgeons using the apprenticeship model is that unfortunately, during training, the time devoted to aspects such as technical skills is limited. The trainee surgeon has duties to attend on the ward, outpatient clinic, clinical audit, their own educational activities; hence, only a minority of their week is spent in the operating room. Even when they are allowed and present in the operating room, they may simply be there as an observer rather than operating or assisting. Furthermore, their exposure to patient cases is dictated by their work hours, whether a relevant case comes in on their day off or under another consultant with whom they are not working. In contrast, the ethos of deliberate practice takes the performance characteristics that are to be acquired, e.g., psychomotor skills for minimally invasive surgery and requires the trainee to deliberately practice them. Furthermore, the new development in training surgical and procedural-based medical skills is that these periods of deliberate practice should take place outside the operating room. One of the elegant aspects of simulation and particularly virtual reality simulation is that it allows for deliberate practice on the exact same model repeatedly. In the operating room (other than in exceptional circumstances), trainee surgeons cannot be guaranteed to get two consecutive cases that are remotely similar, never mind identical. While this represents the real world, it presents a situation that is not optimal for training, particularly during the early stages of learning. Virtual reality simulation, while not ideal, offers a training platform which can be optimally configured for skill acquisition and is not simply repetition.

Deliberate Practice Configured

Trainee Motivation

One of the most important aspects of deliberate practice is clearly identifying which skills or performance characteristics need to be developed. Just like the development of metrics that we described in Chap. 5, these goals need to be very specific and concrete if they are to be realized. The reason for this is that if very general or woolly goals are identified, they may be very difficult to measure. The ability to measure subtle aspects of performance is crucial for the effectiveness of a deliberate practice training program. (We shall return to this issue later) However, one performance characteristic that is crucial for the success of a deliberate practice program is the motivation of the trainee. In surgical training, motivation can come from at least two potential sources, i.e., requirement of the training program and/or from the trainee themselves. As trainers ourselves, we have no problems relying on training requirements as the motivating factor for trainees. While it is acceptable to rely on this foundation intermittently throughout training, it is worrying if it has to be relied on constantly. We prefer to observe motivation emanating from the trainee themselves. One of the reasons that we find the idea of delivering didactic material online very attractive is that it readily provides information on the motivation of the trainee, i.e., did they complete their online assignments, did they complete them in a timely fashion, and how well did they complete them? Also, we find proficiency-based progression training attractive for the same reasons. It removes ambiguity from a training scenario. If a trainee does not demonstrate proficiency on the didactic material delivered online, they may not attend requisite courses which are a pre-requisite for them making satisfactory career progression. Furthermore, the onus on demonstrating proficiency is solely on the trainee. The onus on the trainer is to provide adequate online material and educational support for the trainee to reach proficiency. That is not the current situation in surgical training, and in our view encourages considerable inefficiency in the learning process.

Trainees that present themselves for a course in the skills laboratory have to some extent demonstrated their motivation (by passing the online didactic portion). Also, they have quantitatively demonstrated that they have at the least a certain level of basic knowledge to help them get the most from the course. Trainees should be reminded throughout training that acquiring the performance characteristics to a sufficient level to practice as an independent surgeon, i.e., a consultant or an attending, should not necessarily be a painful process, but there is absolutely no guarantee that it will be painless. We do not hold with the philosophy of "no pain no gain" but we are aware of research on performance training emanating from sports science laboratories. For example, deliberate practice aimed at improving strength and endurance in sports clearly shows the importance of maximal effort during practice and the resulting fatigue. Untrained adults must obtain a minimum heart rate of around 140 beats per minute or 70% of their maximal heart rate for an extended time at least three times a week to see improvements (Lamb 1984). It is not clear how this proportion translates to cognitive or psychomotor training; however, it has been well documented that superior recall is associated with effortful learning. Furthermore, the best effects of effortful learning that have been demonstrated in minimally invasive surgery using a deliberate practice regime had used practice sessions of no more than 1 h duration (Seymour et al. 2002; Van Sickle et al. 2008). Optimal deliberate practice maintains an equilibrium between effort and recovery and through regular increases in amounts of practice (e.g., >20 min at a time) allows for adaptation and for memory consolidation (see Chaps. 3 and 9). Virtual reality simulation and online learning are ideally suited to this type of learning configuration.

Content Sequencing

The impact of deliberate practice on skill acquisition will be affected by the quality of the student's preparation for practical exercises, whether they be in the skills laboratory or in the operating room. Training in the latter is less likely to be effective, if the trainees do not understand the approach and context. This means that trainees need to know the anatomy and physiology, disease process, and treatments before learning the operative procedure. The benefits from deliberate practice do not accrue if the trainee simply goes through the motions of the task. As outlined in Chap. 9, recall and performance is optimized when the trainee understands why they are performing the procedure in a particular way. This also necessitates the thoughtful configuration and organization of learning materials. For example, there is little point in a trainee completing highly successfully the online didactic component for colorectal surgery if they are currently on an orthopedic rotation and their next skills lab session is emergency medicine! An optimal configuration would ensure that prior to the orthopedic rotation, the trainee had an introductory online didactic module on orthopedic surgery, which on demonstrating proficiency, they were then required to complete in an orthopedic basic skills laboratory. This would then be built on by requiring them to complete more advanced online modules in orthopedic surgery consolidated with orthopedic training sessions in the skills laboratory. Furthermore, in an ideal world, the optimal learning configurations would ensure that the skills lab training was followed by operating room experience directly related to the academic material they had covered online and in the laboratory. Again, didactic material delivered online and simulation training lends themselves readily to optimal configuration for maximum training impact. We have observed first-rate surgical training programs, with appropriate online modules, very good skills laboratory training programs, and outstanding support from very experienced consultant surgeons who were also good and enthusiastic teachers. However, the program fell down because these already available resources were not optimally aligned. This is surely wasteful.

Performance Feedback

Well-configured content sequencing affords the optimal opportunity for information to be learned and remembered (Chaps. 3 and 8) by trainees. However, one of the most powerful aids to learning and remembering is feedback from performance; it is immaterial whether learning is from online modules, the skills laboratory, or the operating room. The most important point is that the metrics should characterize important aspects of performance. Metrics should also be easy to use, be reliable, and valid. The task analysis of the procedure to be taught and the metrics that derive from this analysis are crucial to the deliberate practice method. In the absence of adequate feedback, efficient learning is considerably weakened and improvement reduced to minimal, even for highly motivated trainees (Anderson

1982). That is why repetition alone does not reliably predict improved performance (Chaps. 4, 9, and 10). Traditionally, in surgical practice (and opportunities where deliberate practice does exist), individuals develop advanced levels of skills under a process of supervision and direction from good teachers, tutors, and mentors. This teaching was mostly delivered on a one-to-one basis or in a small group instruction environment where trainees enjoy almost continuous feedback from their teacher about their progress. To ensure effective learning, trainees should ideally be given explicit instructions and contiguous feedback. As discussed in Chap. 10, this method of training is certainly very effective at producing trainees with advanced surgical skills such as intracorporeal suturing and knot tying; however, it is also a very expensive and a time-consuming way to conduct training. Simulation models for skills training are effective because they provide a context, organizational structure and focus to apply information retrieved from long-term memory and permit a practice of the sequencing of psychomotor skills to complete the task. However, the trainees also learn whether they performed the task well or not from the assessment of their performance. As pointed out in previous chapters (4 and 10) formative feedback (particularly feedback on errors) should be given proximate to performance so that the trainee can learn which aspect of their performance was erroneous and correct it. Summative feedback is valuable, but less effective at driving the learning process. For the trainee, summative feedback may provide motivation, but formative feedback tells them what they have to fix, and at what stage of the procedure.

Metric Fidelity

In the medical simulation literature, readers will find frequent reference to simulation fidelity. The general assumption being that the higher the fidelity the simulation achieves the more the trainees will learn. This is an incorrect assumption. The "potential" for vast amounts of learning are usually present with high-fidelity simulations but they are not always capitalized on. For example, until relatively recently, surgeons trained on the highest fidelity training model possible, i.e., real, live, (frequently sick) human patients, but some failed to learn. Why was this if training fidelity correlated with skill acquisition? The reasons are fairly straightforward, Chaps. 5 and 6 are directly relevant to the effectiveness of deliberate practice. It is widely assumed the "prettier" or more realistic a simulation looks, the greater the simulation fidelity. There is a relationship between how a simulation looks and its fidelity, but unfortunately, they are not as well correlated as we would like. Even more unfortunate is that most surgeons and physicians do not seem to know what to look for in the assessment of simulation fidelity. A high definition video recording of a surgical procedure may be very high fidelity, but it is not of much use as a technical training device other than showing trainees what they should do during a procedure, the order in which they should do it and with which surgical instruments. Unfortunately, this is about the level of fidelity of some "virtual reality simulators" that have been sold to surgical training programs as "high-fidelity simulations." These simulation platforms look like the real operating room, catheterization laboratory, or internal anatomy of the patient; they may even have a manikin with monitoring equipment bleeping in the background. However, this level of "eye candy" represents a very superficial aspect of what the fidelity of medical simulation should be about.

Under ideal circumstances, a medical simulator would have all of the above. However, more important than these aspects of the simulation is precisely what it is that you can measure about trainees' performance. A really good simulator provides all the "eye candy" and additionally provides a full physics–simulated operating environment where gross and subtle aspects of intraoperative performance can be assessed. Here we are talking about the ability of the simulation to deliver high-fidelity metric-based performance assessment. Take the example we have given in Chap. 6 (Fig. 6.7). The hypothetical performance graph that we have shown demonstrates improvement in performance or increasing skill against experience and learning. As can be seen, the greater the increase in performance and skill, the more subtle the information that is required to accurately and reliably assess performance. At the start of training, the metric "time" tells us how long they took but not whether they performed it right or wrong. As the trainees' skills improve, we will want more detail on performance such as whether the procedure was performed right or wrong. This means that the metric of time will not give us this information (although quite frequently, surgical trainers draw this inference). To capture this information, we need to be more precise about the questions we are asking. Then we may wish to know whether the procedure was done following the correct steps as laid out in the curriculum. Answering this question also answers whether the procedure was done right or wrong. What we are suggesting is that higher fidelity metric assessments can effectively act as surrogates for other useful pieces of information about performance. In Fig. 10.1 (Chap. 10) the metric information on subtle detail about intraoperative performance (level 5) subsumes information on all the previous metrics, i.e., it tells whether devices were used in the correct order, during the correct procedural step, using the correct instrument and whether or not the procedure was completed accurately. In addition, we can have information on time to perform the procedure, but this is only useful when combined with information on the quality of performance.

We are not suggesting that performance measures such as time are not useful. However, what we are suggesting is that, on their own, they provided inadequate information on which to assess performance. In Chap. 10 we discussed the development and application of performance metrics for assessing suturing and knot tying for Nissen fundoplication (Van Sickle et al. 2008). Previous studies have shown that time shows a learning curve for intracorporeal suturing and knot tying (Rosser et al. 1998). However, knowing that a trainee was able to suture and knot tie quickly gives little information on how efficiently they tied the knots (i.e., they could have omitted important steps and therefore recorded a fast time), how safe their performance was (they could have been stabbing other tissues with the needle or ripping through tissue with suture material that had been pulled too tight). Time also gives no information on the quality of the knot. In contrast, the KQS metric gives information on

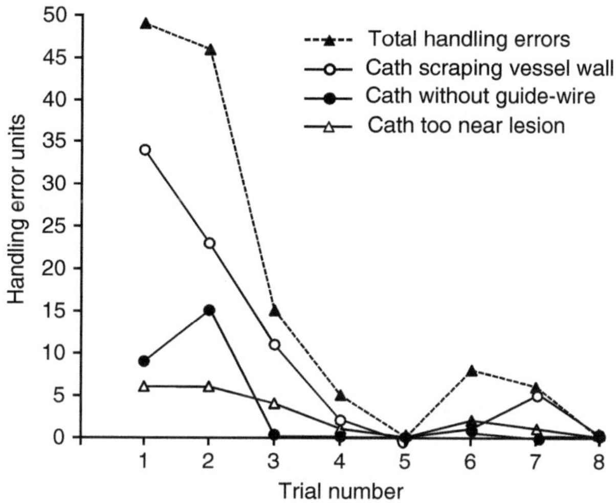

Fig. 11.1 VR metrics during carotid angiography training gives a more granularized picture of learning and skill acquisition across training trials and allows feedback about errors close to when they were performed

time to tie the knot and the quality of the knot (i.e., did it slip or not and if so at what tension).

The solid triangle and dashed line in Fig. 11.1 shows the frequency of the total number of handling errors enacted by a trainee for each of their eight training trials on the VIST simulator while training to perform carotid angiography. The data for this metric are the same as presented in Fig. 10.11 (Chap. 10). It shows a clear learning curve for the trainee. However, total handling errors is the sum of a number of other performance measures. These include moving the catheter with its tip scraping along the vessel wall (this runs the risk of breaking off debris from the vessel wall, which may advance into the brain and block off a small artery causing a stroke), advancing the catheter without a guidewire in front of it (means that the operator cannot fully control the movements at the tip of the catheter), and advancing the catheter too close to the lesion (thus running the risk of breaking off plaque which may advance into the brain). Although the overall metric is very sensitive to learning, the more detailed metric information allows the trainer and the trainee to be more precise on which aspects of performance need to be focused on for improvement. This performance information allows the trainer to give very precise feedback to the trainee about their performance. Furthermore, deliberate practice as a methodology requires the trainee to engage in evaluation of their own performance in order to identify suboptimal characteristics and then identify ways to correct these problems in subsequent practice sessions.

Metric Errors

Early intensive investigations of the skill acquisition process carefully monitored improvements in performance by subjects (Dvorak et al. 1936). They also collected as much self-report information from subjects as possible. The reason for this was that they wanted to identify what types of strategies subjects used to improve their performance. They found that subjects actively searched for methods to improve and that a change in performance methods were often strongly related to improvements. Chase and Ericsson (1982) have also shown that trainees actively try out different methods and refinements are a response to the errors they have made. Thus, the ability to investigate different performance strategies with accurate and timely feedback is an important facility in the development of optimal performance. One of the major advantages of a metric-based simulation training strategy is that trainees can make performance errors on the simulator without exposing patients to risk. Furthermore, they can get precise feedback on what it was that they did wrong. Despite elaborate metric feedback, sometimes trainees fail to discover precisely what they were doing wrong on the simulation, even after repeated attempts to resolve the problem themselves. It is at this point that the trainer should intervene and guide the trainee through this stage of performance refinement. Instructions to the trainee which helps them generate new methods or approaches to successfully performing the procedure or task can help them re-establish their learning curve performance trajectory which has temporarily arrested. As the complexity of the procedural skills increases, the logically possible methods to correctly and incorrectly perform the procedure increase as well. To ensure efficient learning and selection of the best method to perform the procedure, explicit instructions should be given to trainees. Furthermore, during these training sessions which are likely to occur during advanced courses, individualized supervision should be given. This in turn will facilitate early identification of performance errors which need to be dealt with. The best way to deal with them is to give informed feedback and where necessary remedial training. To ensure efficient use of the trainer's time, in the past, we have tended to supervise in pairs as we have found observational learning a very useful and efficient approach to learning during advanced or complex procedures.

Reinforcement of Proficiency Approximations

One of the major reasons that deliberate practice works is that it takes into account very powerful learning strategies such as shaping and reinforcement (Kazdin 1994). The performance characteristics that we wish to train are frequently so complex that their constituent elements are not in the behavioral repertoire of the individual we are trying to train. For example, at no point in their young life has a junior surgeon had to perform the behaviors remotely approximating the psychomotor coordination which are required for intracorporeal suturing and knot tying. In shaping, a training goal is achieved by reinforcing small steps or approximations toward the final goal rather than simply reinforcing the final response itself. Performance characteristics are reinforced when they resemble the final call (e.g., intracorporeal suturing and knot tying) or include components of the desired performance characteristics. By reinforcing successful approximations of the final goal, it is gradually achieved. Performance characteristics, increasingly similar to the final goal, are reinforced and they increase; performance characteristics dissimilar to the final goal are not reinforced and as a result, they extinguish. The chain of novel behaviors that are required from a trainee learning intracorporeal suturing and knot tying are almost impossible to learn all at once. If the trainee practices the skill of intracorporeal suturing and knot tying without some type of positive feedback they get frustrated with their efforts (usually failures) and give up before learning the skill or worse still, frequently believe that they can *never* learn these skills. Unfortunately, we have seen this reaction to learning these complex skills all too often. An alternative strategy, which is the one embraced by deliberate practice is to have numerous solvable sub-goals that approximate the final goal. These approximations are measured (by the simulator or the trainer) which the trainee finds reinforcing, because at least they are making some progress toward the final goal. These metric-based performance characteristics are what constitute the learning curve. It is immaterial whether the feedback is on correct performance or on performance errors as both provide reinforcement. When designing a training program, we have usually identified a sequence or cluster of performance characteristics that we wish to see when training is complete, so the trainee has a clear idea about what they must do that is correct. However, we also have error and efficiency goals. Errors are particularly useful for learning. One of the goals of training for the trainer and the trainee is to reduce intraoperative errors on the simulator to a performance criterion level (e.g., a level of proficiency). However, in the enactment of an error during training, which is unambiguously identified to the trainee, they learn, (1) they did "it" wrong; (2) they know to look for another strategy; and (3) they have been exposed to an error that could occur intraoperatively and so the experience will not be novel to them when they do experience it, thus helping them to avoid it in the future or better still, preparing them for how to deal with it. The distinction between work and training (or deliberate practice) is generally recognized. Individuals given a new job are often given some time period of transition or supervised activity during which they are supervised to acquire an acceptable level of reliable performance. Thereafter, individuals are expected to give of their best performance in work activities, and hence, individuals rely on previously well-established methods rather than exploring alternative methods with unknown reliability.

By using this approach to training, deliberate practice uses a less aversive learning strategy. Trainees get positive feedback on approximations to the final goal rather than simply the final goal itself. That is why intraoperative formative feedback is a much more powerful approach to learning than summative feedback. The ideal approach to shaping performance is where performance and feedback metrics are actual constituent units of the end goal such as in Fig. 11.1 where total handling error was the sum of a number of other technical errors. Indeed, that is the approach that we would take to the establishment of proficiency. By using this strategy, the trainee is forced to pay particular attention to the detailed technique of the skills that they are learning rather than aiming for the outcome goal. What distinguishes a master surgeon from a good surgeon is their attention to detail. These details on their own are probably inconsequential; however, the sum of their effects across the entire procedure means that the procedure is performed very well.

Rolling Proficiency Demonstration

Setting the goal of becoming a "good" or "competent" surgeon sets the bar very high for junior trainee surgeons. This means that their long training apprenticeship has minimal, positive reinforcement deliberately built into it. In contrast, a deliberate practice approach to training specifically programs in short-term goals which are achievable. They have the primary goal, which might be a level of proficiency while more immediate and reinforcing aspects of training are getting their scores and performance characteristics closer to the level of proficiency. Even if they are not reaching the proficiency level, they at least are improving their scores which they can see and on which they get feedback. In Chap. 8 we discussed in detail how we established our level of proficiency and how it was quantitatively defined. The current training paradigm in surgery is less concrete than a proficiency-based progression training paradigm. Furthermore, proficiency is achieved and demonstrated by performing well metric units of performance characteristics that actually constitute proficiency. The level of proficiency is quantitatively defined on the basis of performance characteristics of experienced operators. This assumes that the metric units which are used to assess performance characteristics of the experienced operators are actually valid and reliable. That is why we placed great emphasis on the development of metrics that were objective, transparent, fair, reliable, and valid (Chap. 8). These metric-based performance units can be applied to any aspect of knowledge and skill acquisition in the process of training a doctor, never mind a surgeon. Furthermore, a level of proficiency can be established for knowledge (e.g., an online didactic module), operative procedure in the skills laboratory, and/or in the operating room. Proficiency levels can also be established for specific modules, for specific years of training and for more advanced training. Indeed, this was the approach that the FDA recommended for the introduction of carotid artery stenting with embolic protection, i.e., attending vascular surgeons, interventional cardiologists; interventional radiologists and interventional neuroradiologist were required to demonstrate proficiency on a metric-based simulation before performing the procedure on a real patient (Gallagher and Cates 2004).

Figure 11.2 shows two hypothetical learning curves as a function of time in training. The steep solid curve with the different numbers along it shows the levels of performance that a trainee can reach with the different types of education/simulation training. It is the exact same learning curve as is shown in Fig. 10.1 (Chap. 10). The point we made previously is that the higher the level of training, the greater the fidelity of the simulation and metric-based feedback has to be to ensure optimal progression. The implicit assumption we made was that training was conducted on a proficiency-based progression training paradigm and proficiency was quantitatively defined on its constituent metric-based performance units. The other hypothetical learning curve shown in Fig. 11.2 is that from a more traditional approach to learning. The two learning curves show the same improvement in performance

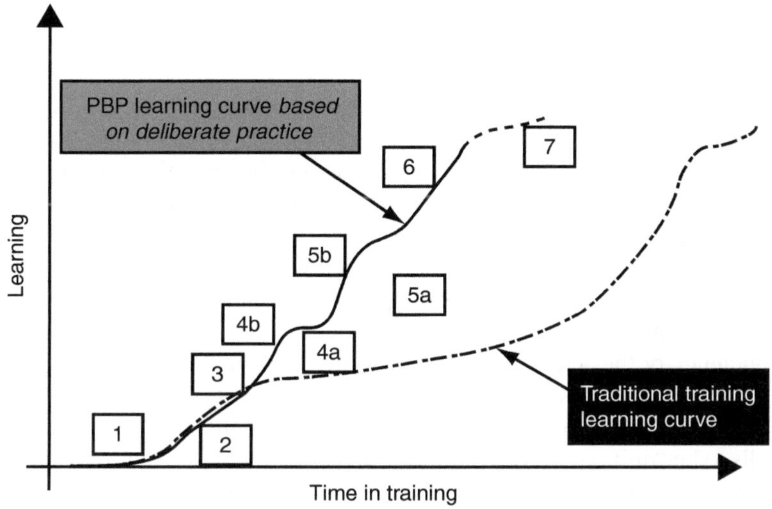

1. Simple explanation
2. Lecture
3. Formative assessed explanation (online)
4. Emulation models
   a. Silicon, animal tissue (no formative feedback)
   b. Silicon, animal tissue MIST VR (formative feedback)
5. VR Procedural simulation
   a. Full procedural VR simulation with summative metrics
   b. Full physics VR simulation with proximate formative & summative metrics
6. Real patients with good mentoring and feedback
7. Wisdom acquisition

Fig. 11.2 Diagrammatic representation of the "estimated" speed of learning with proficiency-based progression (PBP) training and traditional surgical training as a function of time in training

characteristics as a function of simple explanations and lectures. They start to diverge after proficiency-based progression on the online education that has been followed up with metric-based emulation or simulation-based training. It is assumed that the traditional trained group continues with a traditional training curriculum which involves random exposure to patient cases and intraoperative experience. The more traditional approach leads to a slower rate of learning (Anderson 1982). In contrast, deliberate practice training will lead to a faster rate of learning because the entire approach and ethos of the process concentrates on efficiency and effectiveness of the learning process. Trainees are given relevant and timely information to help them improve their performance. They are also given positive reinforcement as their performance characteristics approximate the desired level, i.e., reach proficiency, while the traditional trained surgeons rely on a summative assessment process which has vague endpoints and only intermittent and unpredictable positive reinforcement.

Proficiency Consolidation

Once proficient performance has been established in one domain, it needs consolidation. It is probably best if preliminary consolidation occurs in the skills laboratory. The worst possible outcome following proficiency demonstration is the complete absence of any practice of the skills. This leads to a process of extinction which happens quickly. Extinction is a decrease in the probability that an event will occur; for example, being less able to practice the skills that had been learned to a level of proficiency because of a lack of opportunity. In our skills laboratory studies, we observed some considerable skills decrement within 1–2 weeks of demonstrating proficiency or the acquiring the skills. Other evidence comes from friends (surgeons, interventional cardiologists, and interventional radiologists) who have returned to clinical practice after being on a 2–3-week break and found their operative skills to be "quite rusty." This was surprising to us but the frequency with which this phenomenon has been reported to us leads us to suspect that it is a reliable phenomenon, even with very experienced clinical practitioners whom we know to be good operators.

To consolidate their skills, the trainee should continue practicing on their particular training model and should start introducing unpredictable "events" to the scenario. If they are working on animal tissue or silicon models, the event might be as simple as one of the instruments or suture material that they wished to use not being available to them. How do they cope with this minor event? It is tempting to think that this type of scenario would have little impact on the performance of a trainee who had already demonstrated proficiency. Personal experience suggests otherwise. In the Nissen fundoplication study that we described in detail in Chap. 10 (Van Sickle et al. 2008) we described some of the difficulties that the researchers had in implementing the proficiency-based progression training paradigm and in collecting data on the intraoperative performance. However, an interesting example occurred during the study and involved one of the proficiency trainees. This subject had demonstrated proficiency in the skills laboratory and (informally) was considered one of the better trainees. Although his intraoperative performance was better than the control subjects, it was not as good as the researchers might have expected (nor as reported by the subject immediately after completing their assessed surgical procedure). Subsequent to performing the procedure in vivo and having it assessed, he was asked why he thought his performance in the operating room was not as good as he thought it should have been he explained that in the training lab, he would get ready to perform the intracorporeal sutures and knot tying and one of the researchers would hand him the needle (while holding the thread) oriented in the ideal position for him to grasp it with the needle holder when it had been inserted into the box trainer. In the operating room, he was operating with the chief of surgery which he found stressful. Furthermore, the nurse who was handing him the needle and thread never presented them to him in the ideal position. Thus when he grasped the thread and inserted it down through the port, the needle was invariably in an awkward position. This minor deviation from the training procedure on which he had demonstrated proficiency was enough to disrupt his performance. In light of this information, the researchers made an addition to the proficiency-based progression training program in the study. All subjects were trained to proficiency, but in addition to this, the needle and thread were no longer handed to trainees in the optimal position, toward the end of training. This problem did not occur again. It seemed the extra variability at the end of training prepared the trainee to cope with the detrimental effects of environment variability. How far this preparation should go is a question that is amenable to quantitative investigation.

Deliberate Exposure to "Events"

The situation we describe above occurred during the Nissen fundoplication clinical trial and could probably be best categorized as an event with no significant adverse consequences. The trainees did not perform the procedure as well as expected but did perform better than in the standard training group. Also, the event had no adverse consequences for the patient. However, events of this type and probably of greater magnitude occur often. This type of event is a significant occurrence or happening with no adverse outcome. Possibly, a less trained junior surgeon may not have coped with the situation as well as the trainee we describe and the same situation might have led to a poor outcome. Bad outcomes can occur for several reasons and it is increasingly recognized that some result directly from the performance of the surgeon (Regenbogen et al. 2007). These errors can occur because of unsafe acts committed by surgeons who are in direct contact with the patient or the care system. Reason (2000) has referred to these types of errors as "active failures" and they take a variety of forms which include, slips, lapses, fumbles, mistakes, and procedural violations. Errors are also caused by "latent conditions" which are the inevitable resident pathogens within the system. They are frequently described as the "accident" waiting to happen (but accident may not be the appropriate word to describe them). They arise from decisions made by someone in the system or organization, usually but not always at the level of management or design. Latent conditions have two kinds of adverse event; they can translate into error-provoking conditions within the local workplace (e.g., time pressure, understaffing, fatigue and inexperience) and they can create long-lasting predispositions to errors (e.g., untrustworthy alarms and indicators, unworkable procedures, design and construction deficiencies, etc.). These predisposing conglomerations may lie dormant within the system for years before they combine with active failures and local conditions to create an accident opportunity. Unlike active failures whose specific forms are often difficult to foresee, Reason (2000) suggests that they can be identified and remedied before the adverse event occurs. Understanding this process leads to proactive rather than reactive management.

One of the ways that we try to deal with the potential for latent errors is to stress-test the trainee who recently has consistently demonstrated proficiency. The example we have outlined above (i.e., the Nissen fundoplication) was a salutary lesson that taught us that very little can be taken for granted in the execution of well-practiced skills in what we perceive to be a relatively straightforward situation. We were once again reminded that in the operating room and catheterization laboratory, it is unwise to take anything for granted. That is why we introduce "events" into familiar and well-practiced clinical operating scenarios. These types of experiences help to ensure the trainees' procedural skills are less likely to be disrupted by unexpected events. However, they also ensure that the procedural skills of the trainee do not become too automated. This can happen when the trainee performs the skills they have learned unthinkingly in routine situations which, to some extent, is a desired state of affairs but not when they completely disintegrate with deviations from routine practice. Requiring the trainees to deal with unfamiliar and unpredictable events ensures that they are capable of the effortful recall of procedural information to the extent that they can consciously deal with procedural deviations with minimal effort and disruption to their effectiveness. Most of the virtual reality simulations currently available on the market have a variety of operative cases of increasing complexity on which the trainee can practice. However, few if any of the virtual reality simulations have the capacity for the trainer to control the introduction of an adverse event to the training scenario, although this is a common occurrence in anesthesia training (Gaba and DeAnda 1988).

The ideal situation would be to expose the trainees to a variety of clinical situations which were known to have happened in real operating rooms, with real strategies to deal with them and real outcomes. In surgery and medicine, there are well-documented and reported situations that went disastrously wrong, albeit infrequently. What would probably be of more use is an archive of "near-miss" cases. These are widely used in the aviation industry where they have a situation of no consequence reporting of near misses. Indeed, if the pilot has a near miss and fails to report it and this event subsequently becomes an issue, then he/she is not immune from the naturally occurring consequences. This is a very persuasive incentive for reporting near misses! There is no doubt that they would be invaluable in surgery and interventional medicine. However, until a culture can be created within medicine that is similar to the no-blame culture associated with reporting near misses in the aviation industry, many valuable potentially life-saving lessons will go unlearned.

Consolidated Cases and Mission Rehearsal

There is no doubt that procedural-based medical disciplines such as surgery could learn a lot from archived cases which did or did not go wrong. However, there is also an enormous amount that can be learned from operative cases which go entirely according to plan. Training in the Halstedian apprenticeship model means that if a trainee is off-duty when a particularly interesting case or even when a very straightforward case is operated on, they may never get the opportunity to learn from it. If they are fortunate, a considerate peer or consultant mentor may actually video-record the procedure for later viewing. One of the problems is that the majority of operating rooms are not equipped for video recording of live cases at short notice. This is a considerable failing in the link between the education system and clinical training which would be relatively easily rectified and would most certainly be a building block of an effective and efficient deliberate practice and proficiency-based progression training paradigm.

Indeed, the ideal approach would be to videotape the procedure and also to document an extensive patient background, clinical history, presenting symptoms, diagnosis, and treatment. This information could then be used for an online education unit with appropriate contextual information (e.g., anatomy and physiology) with formative and summative assessments. After successfully navigating through the online didactic unit, the trainee could then watch the intraoperative procedure which would have been edited by the consultant and/or their support staff. The edited version of the operative procedure would also include a running commentary of what was being done and why it was being done, as well as what went well, what did not go well and unanticipated events. At morbidity and mortality meetings or a seminar, trainees could question the operating surgeon so as to elicit further information and to clarify any ambiguities they had. This would be a very powerful learning resource which may not necessarily replicate being in the operating room while the procedure was being performed but would certainly come a very good second best. Indeed, as an educational resource, it is probably more effective at imparting information and technique than simply observing in the operating room because the operating surgeon may not have the attentional resources to hear, never mind answer the questions of inquisitive trainees.

The ultimate learning opportunity for the trainee would be the possible performance of the case themselves, i.e., perform the exact same case, using the exact same surgical devices, operating in the same sequence of operative steps as the original operating surgeon and then compare their operative performance against that of the original operating surgeon. Even better, if they could repeat the procedure as many times as possible until their performance was equivalent to that of the operating surgeon This situation is currently possible for certain endovascular procedures. In Paris 2005, magnetic resonance angiogram images of a real patient's vessels and anatomy were converted into a standard Digital Imaging and Communications in Medicine (DICOM) format and loaded on a virtual reality simulator and used to recreate the patient's vascular anatomy. The first time this was completed was for an interventional cardiology procedure (Gallagher et al. 2006). In the first part of this study patient-specific data was used to rehearse a case of multivessel coronary disease which required stenting. This case was then used to establish that very experienced interventional cardiologists performed the case significantly better than junior colleagues. The second case involved mission rehearsal for carotid artery stenting with embolic protection (Cates et al. 2007). The angiographic data from the patient was prepared in the same way and downloaded to the simulator for the operator to practice the procedure before operating on the patient. The researchers reported that the virtual reality–simulated and live-patient cases showed a high degree of similarity of the angiographic anatomy. All catheter movement and handling dynamics, catheter–catheter interaction, wire movement and dynamics, and embolic protective device deployment and retrieval demonstrated a one-to-one correlation of device movement in virtual reality compared with the live-patient case. Decisions about catheter selection (correct sizing of balloon, embolic protective device and stent) and catheter technique (catheter- and wire-handling dynamics) transferred directly and correlated with the live-patient procedure. The potential of this type of technology for deliberate practice and case rehearsal for training purposes is enormous. Unfortunately, only endovascular simulators (and possibly ophthalmic simulators) have the capability of handling patient-specific data. This is a direction that trainers of procedural-based medicine disciplines must pursue aggressively. Trainee surgeons and other interventionists will continue to receive less of their training in the operating room because of constraints on training time due to work hour limitations and pressures on consultant and attending surgeons to perform more cases. It has been consistently reported that surgical cases that are also used for training take significantly longer to complete (Bridges and Diamond 1999). The combination of these factors means that trainees will have limited exposure to different types of procedures and indeed case volume. It is not clear whether the latter will impact on performance as much as the former. More intense and deliberate practice with augmented feedback for the cases that trainee surgeons do operate on will probably mitigate much of the learning that correlated with case volume. However, it is more difficult to supplant experience and training on a wide variety of clinical cases.

Open Surgical Simulation

The appearance of problems in life should usually be viewed as an opportunity and not just a threat. In surgery, the development of less invasive ways of performing complex surgery caused many problems when it was first introduced. The end result of the MIS revolution was that surgery and medicine were forced to examine in detail why "smart" "well-educated" and apparently "well-trained" individuals had difficulty learning to use these approaches. Consequently surgery has had to reconsider the validity of what it considers as "well-trained." Furthermore, the process has provided significant insights into how junior and senior doctors can be trained and assessed. Other disciplines within medicine, such as interventional cardiology, interventional radiology, emergency medicine, and any discipline that uses procedural-based medicine, have been quick to learn from surgery's successes and failures. It is also fair to point out that the majority of these insights stem directly from developments in laparoscopic and endovascular training. To us this appears somewhat ironic as the majority of surgical procedures are still performed with a traditional open incision approach. For many years, one of us (AGG) was naive enough to think that the types of skills and problems that occurred with efforts to train a minimally invasive surgical skills base simply did not happen in open surgery. The rationalization was simple: open surgery simply did not have the information loss that minimally invasive and endovascular interventions had, i.e., degraded visual information, degraded, tactile information, degraded haptic information, counterintuitive movement of surgical instruments due to the fulcrum effect of the body wall, etc. Therefore, how could open surgery have a problem? While visiting a good friend in the USA, there was some cognitive restructuring of these beliefs. It was pointed out that open surgery had the same spread of skills as MIS (from the outstanding surgeon to the surgeon who can barely tie their own shoelaces). However, (mostly) it just did not seem to generate the same news headlines as the problems associated with the introduction of the relatively new technology. This friend also pointed out that there were certain operating surgeons who were persuaded to operate on nothing more complicated than lumps and bumps. However, even in this situation, things go wrong. On September 5, 2007, a patient was admitted to Fairfield General Hospital in greater Manchester to have a cyst removed from one of his testicles. Instead of removing the cyst, the operating surgeon mistakenly removed the whole testicle! The General Medical Council was told that the mistake was made as one nurse helping the surgeon turned her back to get a suture and when she turned around, the testicle had been removed.

Open surgical skills training, no matter how simple, requires efficient and effective training. Traditionally, high-fidelity training models, e.g., patients, have been how most surgeons have acquired their skills. As with other approaches to acquiring procedure skills (but not basic skills training), some part of training must take place on real patients. Cadavers, animal models and wet tissue, all serve useful functions in the training of basic surgical skills. The problem with these training models is that they require intense supervision to ensure that the trainee receives enough feedback for effective and efficient learning. Despite being a minority approach to the performance of surgical procedures, MIS (and endovascular) has the best developed virtual reality simulations in medicine. This situation is unacceptable. What is urgently required is a relatively inexpensive virtual reality simulator for the training and assessment of open surgical skills.

The development of a virtual reality simulator for open surgical skills will almost certainly benefit from the advances in MIS simulation development such as curriculum development, metric development, task analysis and validation studies. There may even be some insights from engineering developments. In a personal communication with Dr. Dwight Meglan, he informed us that the difficulties in developing an open surgical virtual reality simulation should not be underestimated. Dwight is probably one of the best engineers in this field, anywhere in the world. He, along with Drs. Steve Dawson and Stephane Cotin, developed the Interventional Cardiology Training System at CIMIT in Harvard which morphed into VIST (Mentice AB, Gothenburg, Sweden) which we believe is probably the best virtual reality simulator in medicine at this time. Dwight has also worked on a number of

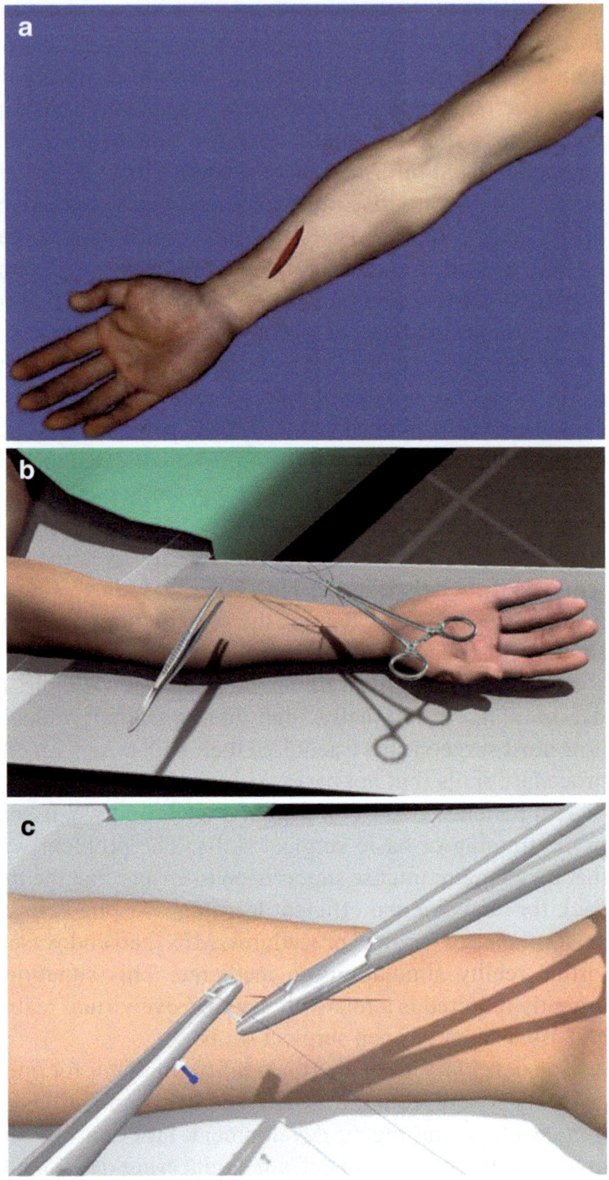

Fig. 11.3 (**a**–**c**) Showing (**a**) virtual wound on the right forearm; (**b**) needle holder, forceps, needle holder, suturing needle, and thread; and (**c**) more detailed view of view (**b**)

other advanced medical device projects and all of his contributions have been impressive. He along with Prof. Howard Champion (an internationally known trauma surgeon) is currently in the final stages of completing a full physics virtual reality wound simulator shown in Fig. 11.3a–c. This simulates, in a full physics environment, the suturing of a forearm wound with accurate and real-time detailed tool-tissue interaction, uniquely capable of suture simulation (developed from the engineering properties of the suture material itself), and hybrid tissue physics with integrated simulation of bleeding. If this simulator proves to be as good as other devices produced by Meglan, this will be one of the most capable (and expandable) simulation platforms in surgery. However, it is just a start to the enterprise of developing a range of full physics simulations for training and assessment of open surgery.

In relation to the development of an open surgical simulator, the level of engineering is more difficult because the user can see much higher levels of visual detail and feel much more complex and detailed forces/torques than you can in endovascular procedures. It is much more challenging to get the physics right in an open VR surgical simulator. The simulations are also potentially more diverse than with endovascular simulations. People are much more sensitive to wrongness with an open surgery simulator than they are with endovascular simulation. For endovascular simulation, the user has only the manipulation of the catheters/wires and the grainy fluoroscopy to guide them. Open surgery provides orders of magnitude more sensory, hence perceptual information, and so affords greater opportunity to see and feel that things are not "right." Also, the interactions of the tools with the tissue are more complex than with endovascular: grasping, cutting, needle insertion, thread pulling/looping/knotting, and so on. The fact that the user looks at the surgical field which is in the same direction as their hands makes for a more complex user interface than for laparoscopic and endovascular procedures. This would dictate the use of an augmented reality type display which adds complexity to the situation because of the need to align the images produced with the simulator with users' hands holding the actual tool handles. Endovascular simulation is much simpler since the operator does not (or at least should not) look at their hands. Finally, in endovascular simulation, the tools are largely flexible cylinders with some variations. With open surgery, there will be all manner of tool handles and tool tips with many variations in the potential actions of those tools (even for the same one) e.g., grasp and hold, grasp and slip out of jaws, grasp and crush, grasp and transect, etc. This will involve considerably more diverse simulation physics than for endovascular procedures. We will discuss this issue further in Chap. 12, but for now, suffice it to say that no open surgical simulation exists that is even approaching the sophistication of low-fidelity simulators that are available for simulation in laparoscopic and endovascular interventions. This is a very worrying state of affairs. In the interim, surgery would do well to heed the lessons from minimally invasive surgery and apply rigorous training and assessment methodologies such as proficiency-based progression in a deliberate practice training program.

Development of Wisdom

Medicine across the world has engaged in an extensive self-evaluation about who or what a doctor is. We have little doubt that these questions have in part been precipitated by high-profile medical error cases. However, it would be misleading to say that these questions stemmed from these developments alone. Medicine is fortunate to attract bright students who enter the profession for very noble reasons. The vast majority develop into first-rate doctors who are mindful of their multifaceted role and responsibilities within society. Many of the questions that have been raised have originated from doctors (many of them very senior) themselves who recognize that the way doctors have been trained and prepared for the practice of a lifetime in medicine is no longer fit for purpose. They also recognize that the way some doctors have behaved in the past was unacceptable. Across the world, groups of doctors have outlined as best they can the characteristics that they believe constitute a "good" doctor. The ACGME has identified the core competencies of Patient Care, Medical Knowledge, Interpersonal and communication skills, Professionalism, Practice-based Learning and improvement, and Systems-based practice. In the CanMEDS system, the roles of the doctor have been defined as: Medical Expert, Communicator, Collaborator, Manager, Health Advocate, Scholar, and Professional. As discussed in Chap. 8, what has been offered as definitions of these characteristics are probably no more than descriptions. Unfortunately, it is almost impossible to reliably measure descriptions and adding further detail to the description makes matters worse rather than better. Throughout this book, we have advocated a practice of objectivity, transparency, and fairness in the development and measurement of performance characteristics that are ascribed to a good medical trainee or practitioner.

While accepting the propositions put forward by the ACGME and CanMEDS, many of our colleagues in surgery argue that the essence of a "good surgeon" is their ability to make decisions. One of the difficulties that we have with this proposition is that on the one hand, we agree with the performance characteristics of a good doctor described by the Core Competencies and the CanMED system, but on the other hand, we are not entirely convinced that the sum of the parts contained within these descriptions captures the essence of the whole. We are certain that our colleagues' protestations that the "essence of a good surgeon is their ability to make decisions" is wide of the mark. We have thought on this issue and discussed it among ourselves for some time. One of the attributes that has impressed us about individuals whom we consider to be good practitioners is their apparent sense of balance. The description that probably best characterizes these individuals is that they seem to possess wisdom. There are a number of definitions but the one that we like characterizes wisdom as the power of judging rightly and following the soundest course of action, based on knowledge, experience and understanding. Unlike our colleagues, we do not think that decision making is the most important attribute of a practicing surgeon; we do however think it is important, but so also are the other attributes described by the Core Competencies and the CanMED system. We also think that "sound" technical ability is a fundamental building block of a "good" surgeon. The difficulty we have is that neither the Core Competencies nor the CanMEDs deal explicitly with this attribute of a surgeon or indeed for other procedural interventionalists. Our concern about this stems from the fact that a good surgeon can provide excellent patient care, have first class medical knowledge, be very socially skilled and always adhere to the highest professional standards with good awareness of practice-based learning and systems-based practice but these attributes are not substitutes for safe technical performance. All of these attributes enable them to make the correct formulation, make the right diagnosis in a timely fashion, and decide to do the correct surgical procedure; however, of what use are they if the surgeon cannot perform the procedure safely? This issue is not explicitly addressed in any of the characterizations of the modern doctor. Although we are discussing this problem in the context of surgical education and training, this problem exists in other areas of interventional medicine.

In our experience, the balanced surgeon is always a technically proficient surgeon, not necessarily outstanding, but definitely safe. This must be the bedrock that other physician attributes are built on. This attribute of the interventionist can now be reliably and validly assessed. What about the other attributes such as decision making? All too often, it is assumed that the ability to make decisions is acquired through mentoring, modeling, mimicry, experience, and sometimes by osmosis. Unfortunately, a bit like the current skill acquisition process, it is somewhat random how skilled individuals become good at making decisions. Individual supervision, formative assessment events, case conferences, and morbidity and mortality meetings are good opportunities in which to develop decision making during training. However, there appears to be no systematic way of training these skills. Somewhat more worrying, it is assumed that once the trainee becomes a consultant or attending surgeon, they have reached the pinnacle of their decision-making ability.

The process of wisdom development is almost certainly lifelong and it is also certainly a function of clinical experience. This is not just of patient cases but the experience and knowledge gained from discussions with colleagues. There is almost no discussion in the literature about the impact of reduced work hours and increased specialization on the acquisition of wisdom for surgeons currently in training. This problem is most likely to show itself in the near future when older surgeons who trained under the traditional Halstedian apprenticeship model have retired. The wisdom that they possess will largely be unavailable to newer consultant surgeons who have trained under a different training paradigm. The problem is that we are not entirely sure what this wisdom is or how we measure it, or acquire it efficiently; however, we recognize it when we see it. We believe that the foundation of wisdom in clinical practice is that the physician must first of all be proficient in practice of their chosen specialty whether that be surgery, anesthetics, internal medicine, or pathology. Very specifically, we do not mean they are proficient at talking about their chosen specialty but are proficient in their actual *practice* on patients. We believe this attribute is crucial, because it colours almost every other aspect of the doctor's attributes. In surgery, the attribute that seems to be most valued is the ability to make decisions effectively and efficiently. However, the decision making about whether or not to operate or when to operate will be different for a surgeon who is technically proficient than for a surgeon who is considerably less experienced or skilled. A surgeon who is technically proficient will have the cognitive resources (i.e., attentional capacity) and technical ability to deal with unexpected intraoperative events. A less experienced or skilled surgeon will not have these resources available and this almost certainly will influence the decisions they make about whether or not to operate. Decision-making ability is not simply about making decisions. If a decision is made and acted upon, it reduces uncertainty by at least 50%, i.e., the decision was right or wrong. This means that good decision-making ability must be underpinned with the ability to recover from error as in medical specialties such as surgery, the operator cannot be expected to get it right all of the time. However, what they can be expected to do is to recover from these events to reinstate a situation of safety. Just like the process of technical skill acquisition and assessment, decision-making performance is understandable and quantifiable before the surgeon reaches the stage of being a consultant. Furthermore, the wise consultant will realize that he or she is never too old, too experienced, or skilled to learn. The same effort that has been invested in understanding the process of skill acquisition now needs to be invested in understanding medical wisdom in procedural-based medical disciplines such as surgery.

Summary

Proficiency-based progression simulation training is effective and efficient at helping trainees acquire the skills for the practice of surgery because it affords the opportunity for deliberate practice. Traditional training provides the opportunity for repetitive practice. Deliberate practice differs from this traditional training methodology because performance feedback is more detailed and configured in such a way as to motivate trainees the more their performance approximates the proficiency goal. Trainees should be well prepared for training both in terms of knowledge and motivation. Metric fidelity of the simulation training program is crucial. Summative metrics are useful but formative metrics are the real drivers of performance improvement. Virtual reality simulators are more effective and efficient at delivering detailed performance feedback proximate to performance but effective performance feedback can also be delivered by trainers who closely supervise and monitor training. Although equally as effective, trainer-delivered performance feedback is inefficient and expensive. Once proficiency has been acquired, the trainee's skills should be inoculated against the disruptive effect that environmental events such as intraoperative complications can have on newly acquired skills by exposing the trainee to unanticipated events during the latter stages of their training process. Skills can be consolidated further with training on patient-specific data on a full physics virtual reality simulator as part of a well-configured and sequenced training program. These types of simulators currently only exist in endovascular medicine but there is an urgent need to develop them for training traditional open surgical skills. The development of virtual reality simulators for training open surgical skills will present some very difficult engineering and software problems that need to be confronted sooner rather than later. Traditional surgical skills are the foundation on which important medical skills such as decision making, professionalism, interpersonal and communication skills, and the other attributes of being a good doctor are built upon. Although we have descriptions of these characteristics, we have minimal quantitative and philosophical understanding of how they cluster together.

References

Anderson JR. Acquisition of cognitive skill. *Psychol Rev*. 1982;89(4):369-406.

Baker J, Deakin J, Horton S, Pearce GW. Maintenance of skilled performance with age: a descriptive examination of professional golfers. *J Aging Phys Act*. 2007;15(3):300.

Bridges M, Diamond DL. The financial impact of teaching surgical residents in the operating room. *Am J Surg*. 1999;177(1):28-32.

Bryan WL, Harter N. Studies in the physiology and psychology of the telegraphic language. *Psychol Rev*. 1897;4(1):27-53.

Bryan W, Harter N. Studies on the telegraphic language: the acquisition of a hierarchy of habits. *Psychol Rev*. 1899;6:345-375.

Cates CU, Patel AD, Nicholson WJ. Use of virtual reality simulation for mission rehearsal for carotid stenting. *J Am Med Assoc*. 2007;297(3):265.

Chase WG, Ericsson KA. Skill and working memory. In: Bower GH, ed. *The Psychology of Learning and Motivation: Advances in Research and Theory*, vol. 16. New York: Academic Press; 1982:1-58.

Dvorak A, Merrick NL, Dealey WL, Ford GC. *Typewriting Behavior*. New York: American Book Company; 1936.

Ericsson KA, Lehmann AC. Expert and exceptional performance: evidence of maximal adaptation to task constraints. *Annu Rev Psychol*. 1996;47(1):273-305.

Ericsson KA, Krampe RT, Tesch-Römer C. The role of deliberate practice in the acquisition of expert performance. *Psychol Rev*. 1993;100(3):363-406.

Gaba DM, DeAnda A. A comprehensive anesthesia simulation environment: re-creating the operating room for research and training. *Anesthesiology*. 1988;69(3):387-394.

Gallagher AG, Cates CU. Approval of virtual reality training for carotid stenting: what this means for procedural-based medicine. *J Am Med Assoc*. 2004;292(24):3024-3026.

Gallagher AG, Renkin J, Buyl H, Lambert H, Marco J. Development and construct validation of performance metrics for multivessel coronary interventions on the VIST virtual reality simulator at PCR2005. *EuroIntervention*. 2006;2(1):101-106.

Kazdin AE. *Behavior Modification in Applied Settings*. Pacific Grove: Brooks/Cole Publishing Co.; 1994.

Keller FS. The phantom plateau. *J Exp Anal Behav*. 1958;1(1):1.

Kohn LT, Corrigan JM, Donaldson MS. *To Err Is Human: Building a Safer Health System*. Washington: National Academy Press; 2000:196-197.

Lamb DR. *Physiology of Exercise: Responses and Adaptations*. New York: Macmillan; 1984.

Player G. *Gary Player's Golf Secrets*. USA: Prentice-Hall; 1962.

Reason J. Human error: models and management. *Br Med J*. 2000;320(7237):768.

Regenbogen SE, Greenberg CC, Studdert DM, Lipsitz SR, Zinner MJ, Gawande AA. Patterns of technical error among surgical malpractice claims: an analysis of strategies to prevent injury to surgical patients. *Ann Surg*. 2007;246(5):705.

Rosser JC Jr, Rosser LE, Savalgi RS. Objective evaluation of a laparoscopic surgical skill program for residents and senior surgeons. *Arch Surg*. 1998;133(6):657.

Schulz R, Curnow C. Peak performance and age among superathletes: track and field, swimming, baseball, tennis, and golf. *J Gerontol*. 1988;43(5):P113.

Senate of Surgery. *Response to the General Medical Council Determination on the Bristol Case: Senate Paper 5*. London: The Senate of Surgery of Great Britain and Ireland; 1998.

Seymour NE, Gallagher AG, Roman SA, et al. Virtual reality training improves operating room performance: results of a randomized, double-blinded study. *Ann Surg*. 2002;236(4):458-463; discussion 463-454.

Thorndike EL, Woodworth RS. The influence of improvement in one mental function upon the efficiency of other functions. *Psychol Rev*. 1901;8(3):247-261.

Van Sickle K, Baghai M, Huang IP, Goldenberg A, Smith CD, Ritter EM. Construct validity of an objective assessment method for laparoscopic intracorporeal suturing and knot tying. *Am J Surg*. 2008;196(1):74-80.

Chapter 12
Proficiency-Based Progression Simulation Training: A To-Do List for Medicine

There is no excuse for the surgeon to learn on the patient
William H. Mayo M.D. (pp. 1378, 1927)

Change has been the order of the day in medicine, but particularly in disciplines such as surgery. Surgery has changed the way it treats patients with interventions becoming less invasive but also becoming more difficult to learn and to practice. Sometimes these changes were patient driven. One of these changes, minimally invasive surgery (MIS) was introduced on a wave of enthusiasm in the early 1990s (Centres 1991). It was a disruptive technology and had unforeseen and wide-reaching implications and ramifications for the entire practice of medicine. In the original description of this phenomenon, the authors argued that "disruptive innovations can hurt successful, well managed companies that are responsive to their customers and have excellent research and development. These companies tend to ignore the markets most susceptible to disruptive innovations (Bower and Christensen 1995)." That is how MIS took hold of the field of surgery, i.e., patient demand. The complications that were associated with the practice of this new type of surgery became very public and pointed to a skills deficit in the operating surgeon. It is unfortunate for surgery that these developments occurred around about the same time as high-profile medical errors cases were being investigated (e.g., The Bristol Case (Senate of Surgery 1998)) in the UK and the "To Err is Human" Report (Kohn et al. 2000) in the USA. We believe that both of these developments had a profound influence on medicine for the better. The introduction of MIS forced the surgical community to investigate why this type of surgery was more difficult to learn than the traditional open approach, and as a result surgery in particular and medicine in general had to closely examine how they prepared doctors to treat patients. The high-profile error cases forced the medical community to confront an uncomfortable truth which is that some patients are made sicker or die as a direct result of the care they are given by their doctor. While this was not a new phenomenon the patients were being told about it on the media. Worse still was that in some cases, the public were told that the medical community knew about "it" and did nothing until the issue had been made public. The hemorrhage of public confidence from medicine as a result of these incidents cannot be underestimated.

A.G. Gallagher and G.C. O'Sullivan, *Fundamentals of Surgical Simulation*, Improving Medical Outcome - Zero Tolerance,
DOI 10.1007/978-0-85729-763-1_12, © Springer-Verlag London Limited 2012

As a result of the investigations into medical errors, it became clear that a high proportion of them occurred in surgery. Regenbogen et al. (2007) have suggested that between one half and two thirds of hospital adverse events are attributable to surgery and surgical care. Also, the sorts of errors that occur in surgical care tend to be different from those that occur on medical services, making many of the studies of medication errors in hospital not easily generalizable to surgical care. The big difference is that most surgical errors occur in the operating room and most are technical in nature. Technical errors are errors in which some aspect of the surgery is not done properly and concern manual skills and errors of surgical judgment or knowledge. Surgery is unique among medical specialties in that while doing operations, surgeons are constantly making decisions in real time and acting on them. These sorts of errors can occur at any phase of surgical care and have been attributed to low hospital volume, breakdown in communications, systems failures, fatigue, lack of experience in trainees and many other causes. The results from the Regenbogen et al. (2007) study are not unique. Similar results have been reported in Belgium using a similar type of research methodology. Somville et al. (2010) retrospectively reviewed surgical malpractice claims from 3,202 malpractice liability cases, in which patients alleged error, between 1996 and 2006. They identified surgical errors that resulted in patient injury in 427 study claims. The results showed that 63% of these cases involved a significant or major error injury and 6% involved death. In most cases (48%), errors occurred in intraoperative care, 15% in preoperative care and 37% in postoperative care. The leading factors which were associated with errors were inexperience/lack of technical competence (57%) and communication breakdown (42%). Furthermore, cases involving technical errors were more likely to occur during elective surgery. These findings were not available at the time surgery and medicine were conducting root and branch analysis of how they practice medicine; however, they serve as reinforcement that the analyses was appropriate.

Training Efficiently

Whether as a result of these medical errors or as an evolution of common sense in medical training, the number of hours which junior doctors are required to work have been reduced dramatically. This did not happen in one country, but in almost every country with a well-developed medical training system. Neither of us can recall going to a conference during the last decade and NOT hearing a senior surgeon bemoaning the reduction in training hours for junior surgeons. The same is true in other disciplines in medicine. No amount of complaining will change the situation regarding training hours. What is rarely discussed by leaders in medicine is the inefficiency of the current training system. In the USA, it takes 5–7 years to train a surgeon, assuming they undertake a Fellowship in their specialty. In the UK and Ireland, it takes between 11 and 13 years to train. The question should be asked: is the performance of surgeons in the USA who finish after 5 or 7 years so much inferior to the performance of surgeons who finish in the UK and Ireland after 11–13 years? This may not be a politically polite question.

The simple fact of the matter is that surgery and medicine are training doctors for twenty-first century medicine using a nineteenth century training paradigm. Halsted developed and implemented his apprenticeship model in the late nineteenth century because there was nothing else available in the USA that was as systematic and presumably effective. He did what he could with the resources he had available to him. At the start of the twenty-first century, we are duty bound to build on Halsted's legacy. We know considerably more about how human beings learn, how they acquire knowledge and skills, the limits of their sensory and perceptual system, and how all of these human factors can be facilitated and augmented to better achieve "education and training." By constructing an apprenticeship-based curriculum for surgical training, Halsted was configuring and organizing the information that the trainee acquired which in turn facilitated them in becoming a safe surgeon. What we have proposed here in this book simply builds on that methodology. In the past, medicine was learned from books, lectures, tutorials, and practicals. It was also learned from repeated practice on real patients. The methodology that we are proposing here really does not differ significantly from what has been done in the past in terms of content. However, where it does significantly depart from what has been done in the past is how that content is delivered. We have argued that content alone does not make an education and training program effective. What makes education and training effective and efficient is how the content is delivered and how the delivery is configured. Human beings are not simply passive information processors; they are not simply vessels that we can pour knowledge and skills into (mores the pity). This means that when we teach trainees, we cannot assume that they have learned the material or understand it, nor can we assume that they can do something that we trained them to do (never mind do it to a certain standard).

Human beings are more likely to remember information that has been organized for them and has been sequenced in a logical and meaningful order. Furthermore, we cannot assume that they have learned the material; we must check. Likewise, skill acquisition should be organized in a sequential and sensible fashion where basic skills are acquired before more complex skills and performance must be assessed. The trainee must know how they are performing and the trainer must know how a trainee is progressing. The trainee will learn fastest and most efficiently if they have formative feedback during their training. Furthermore, for training to be effective, trainees cannot simply engage in repeated practice; they must engage in deliberate practice. Deliberate practice differs from repeated practice in terms of how training is configured but more importantly or the formative and summative feedback that the trainee is given.

Proficiency-Based Progression

This information is not new but what is new is how it is applied to the acquisition and practice of procedural skills such as surgery and to those that would suggest that we are just spoon-feeding the trainees, we would point out that what we are advocating is simply good educational and training practices that are well grounded in quantitative research. If anything, our proposals place a greater emphasis on the effort made by the trainee. Ericsson et al. (1993) have shown that performance excellence is not something that individuals are born with rather it is something that has been acquired over 10 years of deliberate practice. Many surgical trainees will find this an uncomfortable truth. What we have proposed here is that deliberate practice should be used for the effective and efficient acquisition of skills and knowledge. However, this process cannot be continued ad *infinitum* by educational and training institutions. That is more the responsibility of the trainee, and the regulatory agencies have been particularly good at ensuring continuing professional development as an integral and non-negotiable part of medicine. We have suggested that training should continue until the trainee has reached a performance criterion level. Furthermore, that performance criterion level should be quantified on the basis of real-world surgical/medical skills. Unfortunately, there continues to be too much ambiguity and debate about precisely what constitutes "competency." To circumvent these issues, we have objectively defined and quantitatively assessed proficiency. Dreyfus et al. (1986) have proposed that proficient skills are those that have been developed to a stage beyond competent skills. This means that if skills are demonstrated to be proficient, by default, they must be competent. To quantify the performance level of proficiency, we have used the performance of experienced practicing surgeons. There can be little doubt that the vast majority of these individuals' performance is at least competent. Using this approach, we have been able to establish a quantitative goal for the trainee based on the real skills of real practicing surgeons. It also means that the benchmark that has been established is fair, objective and transparent. Furthermore, it is a sufficiently flexible approach to training to allow the gifted trainee to progress through the training cycle quicker than those trainees who take longer to reach the level of proficiency. Moreover, it does not discriminate against the trainees who acquire their skills at a slower rate. The ethos of training is that once the proficiency level has been demonstrated (consistently), that part of training is completed. The other advantage with proficiency-based progression training is that it ensures that ALL individuals in the training program have successfully demonstrated the required skill level. This is not the case with the traditional training approach. Unfortunately, in the traditional training approach, the same amount of time in training is presumed to fit all when it is obvious that this is not the case.

A proficiency-based progression training paradigm places the onus on the trainers to provide the facilities and the learning resources for the trainee to acquire the skills and knowledge to learn their craft. However, it places the onus on the trainee to unambiguously demonstrate that they have reached the prescribed level of performance. This approach to training is far removed from the "spoon-feeding" approach that some individuals might so caricature. This is a relatively new approach to training, and few assumptions are made about the knowledge and skill level of the graduating trainee. Rather, they must demonstrate that they have the knowledge and skills before graduating; otherwise they do not progress. The development of metrics for the assessment process on which proficiency is established will be new to most of medicine. However, it is a well-established and validated protocol in the behavioral sciences (Kazdin 1994; Martin et al. 1993). Furthermore, it is relatively straightforward, and once users have experienced the entire process a couple of times, they will develop a comfortable familiarity with it. It is a process that Halsted would probably have been comfortable with because it pays attention to detail. In fact, the effectiveness of the training and assessment system relies on reliably capturing performance detail. The thesis behind the system is that proficient surgeons are good at what they do because of their attention to small but apparently inconsequential details of task performance which they probably perform automatically and unthinkingly. However, it is the attention of the surgeon to these details that makes their performance proficient or better. For example, it probably does not make that much difference when suturing a wound closed whether or not all of the knots are aligned on one side of the wound, whether or not they are spaced equally apartnd and the suture tails are approximately equal (not too short, not too long), etc. However, it is attention to these types of detail that probably typify the approach of the operator to other and less inconsequential aspects of the procedure.

What was demonstrated in the past is that if a trainee has been trained to the level of proficiency which has been based on the performance scores of experienced and practicing surgeons (in that particular task or procedure), those trainees outperform their peers who have gone through a traditional curricular training program (Ahlberg et al. 2007; Seymour et al. 2002; Van Sickle et al. 2008b). These studies have been prospective randomized and blinded in their assessment of the proficiency-based progression training paradigm. Although the subject numbers in each of the studies were small, the differences between the traditionally and the proficiency-based progression trained surgeons were large. Some surgeons may claim that the number of subjects in the studies were too small from which to generalize the results. In response to this, we would point out that science is about the unambiguous establishment of cause-and-effect relationships. These studies have unambiguously demonstrated in a prospective, randomized, and blinded fashion that proficiency-based progression trainees perform better.

Metric Validation

We have no illusions that there will be critics of this approach to training, and in the best traditions of the scientific enterprise we will be the first to celebrate the verification of an alternative strategy with the same scientific rigor that has been applied to proficiency-based progression. One of the cornerstones of proficiency-based progression training is the performance metrics. These will be developed from rigorous task analyses by experienced groups of surgeons proficient at performing the surgical task or operation in question. The performance characteristics that they identify during the task analysis will be explicitly operationally defined in a way that they are refutable. This is a crucial aspect of an objective, transparent and fair assessment system. We have been critical of assessment strategies which are less explicit, e.g., OSATS (Martin et al. 1997). Although we are sympathetic to their goals, attempting to score the performance characteristics of procedural medicine such as surgery on a Likert scale is more difficult than it should be, using OSATS. Trying to establish high inter-rater reliability using a Likert scale scoring system is almost impossible or, at least, will take more time to accomplish than most consultant surgeon assessors are prepared to give. It is much easier to establish high levels of inter-rater reliability with a checklist scoring system. However, the checklist that has been constructed for the assessment of performance on any task or procedure must be comprehensive and incisive. Furthermore, it needs to be valid. The metrics that have been identified as part of the task analysis should be shown to distinguish between the performance of experts and novices or at least experienced practitioners and novices. If metric-based performance does not distinguish between these groups, the metrics are flawed, and probably important aspects of the performance of the procedure have not been well characterized. However, we have not encountered a set of metrics that have been developed using the methodology that we have described that did not distinguish between experts and novices (with one exception). If a surgical task is so simple that a brief explanation and one demonstration is sufficient to transfer the skills and knowledge to a trainee, construct validity (i.e., being able to show a difference between the performance of experts and novices) will be difficult to demonstrate (indeed, we would suggest pointless).

Surgery and other procedural-based disciplines in medicine must move away from ambiguous definitions of performance characteristics. They are difficult to measure and have the tendency to allow bias and possibly even unfair practices to creep into the assessment system. There is some evidence that the new assessment systems that are being introduced into the training programs in the UK are becoming more explicit about what they assess. The DOPS system uses a Likert-type scale for the assessment of performance; however, it is only used for formative assessments (Chap. 7). For high stakes assessment, such as PBAs, a checklist scoring system is used (Chap. 8). However, attempting to reliably assess performance characteristics that have been defined as, "optimum" (without definition), "adequate," "sound," and "purposeful" leaves too much room for individual interpretation and will almost certainly impact on inter-rater reliability levels.

In Chap. 7 we examined the issue of inter-rater reliability levels in great detail. That was because these are the metric units of performance on which trainees within a training program will be passed or failed. In our opinion, the least that the person being assessed can expect is that the examiners agreed on at least 80% of their assessment scores (as the performance characteristics have been defined). It does not mean that the assessors agree 80% of the time for the entire class that is being assessed; it does not mean that the correlation between the two examiners scores is $r \geq 0.8$, nor does it mean that the alpha coefficient between the two raters is ≥ 0.8. However, that is what some researchers are reporting in validation studies (Bann et al. 2003; Khan et al. 2007; Larsen et al. 2006) in some of the highest impact journals in surgery and medicine. Inter-rater reliability means the percentage of agreement between the two examiners on the individual who is being assessed. Anything less rigorous than this approach to validation may lead to successful litigation claims by trainees whose training progress has been halted because they failed to demonstrate proficiency using metrics that had been validated using a validation process other than 80% agreement between assessors. Proficiency-based progression training ensures the quality of performance of the trainee. However, it also makes the system that they are being assessed by much more transparent than it has been in the past. Furthermore, these assessments are not called high stakes by coincidence; these assessments determine whether the trainee progresses in their training. Some trainees who fail to progress will almost certainly seek legal redress as they will have already invested many years in education and training. Anything less than transparently rigorous validation of all levels of proficiency-based progression training programs, and in particular the metric-based assessment units, will lead to successful legal challenges. Ironically, it is easier to get the process right than it is to do it wrong!

Proficiency Refined

The skill acquisition framework that we have proposed here derives from the model proposed by Dreyfus and Dreyfus (Dreyfus et al. 1986). Although the Dreyfus and Dreyfus model proposes a conceptual framework, it does not offer nor advocate a measurement strategy. The quantification strategy that we dovetailed with this model comes from the behavioral sciences and has been used for more than half a century. We are satisfied that they complement each other well; however, we do have some philosophical questions that have practical implications about the characterization and implementation of proficiency-based training. Proficiency as characterized by us is the performance of experienced surgeons; these individuals are experienced in performing the task or the surgical procedure which we wish to set a level of proficiency. They, preferably are, not the leading surgeons in the world at performing the task or procedure and likewise they are not at the opposite end of that scale. Rather, their performance lies somewhere around the middle of that performance spectrum. Metrics that are developed from the analysis of the task or procedure should be capable of characterizing the performance of these individuals to the extent that it can reliably distinguish between their performance and that of novices or less experienced operators. This may seem imprecise and that is because it is. We developed this strategy to avoid the alternative which is the development and application of standardized operating procedures. The methodology is robust enough to ensure that it is fairly representative of the vast majority of operating surgeons who perform the procedure or task; however, it also sets a high enough standard so that trainees who reach that level perform significantly better intraoperatively than trainees who go through the traditional training program. Furthermore, benchmarks established on the performance of these experienced surgeons appear to be reachable by the vast majority of surgical trainees who persist in deliberate practice training sessions.

The first time a proficiency-based progression training strategy (based on the methodology that we have described here) was used was in the original VR to OR study conducted at Yale University in the USA (Seymour et al. 2002). In that study, virtual reality training subjects trained on the simulator in a 1-h session until they reached the performance criteria level (or level of proficiency) with both hands, on two consecutive trials. The reasoning was:

1. That the surgical task that they were to perform (i.e., dissection of the gallbladder from the liver bed using electrocautery) was a bimanual task and therefore they had to be equally skilled with both hands.
2. They had to reach the level of proficiency on two consecutive trials, because they could demonstrate proficiency once potentially by accident, but not twice in a row.
3. Proficiency was quantitatively defined on the basis of five attending surgeons' performance on the training task.
4. Furthermore, it was the mean performance of the surgeons that constituted the performance criteria levels for errors and economy of diathermy.

One of the problems that we have with the characterization of proficiency as described here is that for the trainees to demonstrate proficiency, must, on average, perform better than 50% of the surgeons on whom proficiency was quantified. Furthermore, why does proficiency have to be the mean of the performance of the experienced operators? why could it not be the mean plus one standard deviation, or indeed the median? Also, why has proficiency to be demonstrated on two consecutive trials; why not more than two? These are questions that need to be quantitatively addressed probably sooner than later. An alternative strategy would be to investigate the receiver operating characteristic (ROC) of proficiency development and the clinical implications of adopting different training strategies. ROC analysis provides tools to select possible optimal models and to discard suboptimal ones independently from (and prior to specifying) the cost context or the class distribution. ROC analysis is related in a direct and natural way to cost/benefit analysis of diagnostic decision making. The ROC curve was first developed by electrical engineers and radar engineers during World War II for detecting enemy objects in battle fields, also known as the signal detection theory and was soon introduced in psychology to account for perceptual detection of signals (Swets 1996). Whatever strategy is eventually decided upon, it will be a difficult balancing act to fulfill. The level of proficiency must be conservative enough to ensure that it confers a uniform and high standard of intraoperative performance that optimizes patient safety. The standard must not be set so high that trainees find it very difficult, if not impossible to reach. The way that proficiency is currently construed appears to work fairly well, but we believe that it can be improved further.

Proficient Experts?

One of the problems that relates to the quantitative definition of proficiency is the much wider issue of objective assessment of technical performance in surgery. Much of the methodology that we have discussed in this book is about the objective and fair assessment of performance and how this might be approached.

This approach was then validated and the validated metric units were used to establish performance benchmarks. These benchmarks were based on the performance of experienced operators. The assumption being that these experienced operators were "good" at what they did. What do we do if they are not? This is not a hypothetical situation. One of the first studies to report the performance of some surgeons who are performing significantly worse than their peers was by Gallagher et al. (2003c). They found that some other surgeons who participated in the study could not complete any part of the relatively simple box trainer and virtual reality laparoscopic tasks. Furthermore, some of those who were able to complete the tasks were performing more than 20 standard deviations from the mean. The data were checked and rechecked; the relationship between the operative experience of the surgeon and their performance was checked, as was the reliability of the simulator. All of these potential explanations were rejected as reasonable explanations for the performance of this small group of surgeons. These surgeons' performances were always *more* than two standard deviations worse than their peers and frequently worse than the trainees to whom we were comparing them for the establishment of construct validity! The alternative explanation was that they simply performed badly on the tasks on the day that they were assessed and that this probably bore no resemblance to their intraoperative clinical performance.

As the years have passed and more experience in the objective assessment of the surgical skills has been accrued, this explanation also seems unlikely. For a small minority of surgeons that we have encountered, there appears to be no correlation between their objectively assessed performance and their self-reports of their own intraoperative performance. We have not systematically nor aggressively pursued a scientific answer to this question even though we suspect we know the answers. However, from personal experience, we believe that a strong correlation does exist between objectively assessed performance and intraoperative performance. Informally acquired information on some operators (e.g., surgeons, interventional cardiologists, etc.) seems to corroborate the suspicion that individuals who do not perform well in the skills laboratory also perform poorly intraoperatively. If these were trainees, there really would not be a problem. The problem arises from the fact that these individuals are consultant or attending surgeons. These are the very individuals whom we wish to benchmark so that we can use their performance as a training goal for their juniors. Take for example, a consultant surgeon who when objectively assessed is performing five standard deviations worse than their peers. The ethos of the proficiency-based progression training program is that proficiency should be established on the basis of experienced operators' performance, and therefore, their performance measures should be included in the proficiency definition. After all, these individuals are experienced operators. How should these individuals be dealt with?

We are not sure how to deal with them. In general, the surgical community are aware that these individuals exist, but in the past it was extremely difficult to quantify their performance other than in terms of bad outcomes and their outcomes were not "significantly" worse than some of their peers. That situation has changed and we can now reliably and validly assess intraoperative performance which simple logic dictates has to be related to intraoperative performance. Some in the surgical community might argue that our intraoperative performance characterization (e.g., metric-based assessment) does not really capture the performance of a surgeon and the hypothesized relationship between objectively assessed intraoperative performance and outcomes has never been established. However, the intraoperative performance metrics that we use to assess performance have been identified by a group of experienced operators who have identified characteristics that they believe distinguish between optimal and suboptimal performance. Van Sickle et al. (2008a) found that when they compared the objectively assessed intraoperative performance of attending surgeons to surgical residents on an intracorporeal suturing task, the intraoperative metrics reliably distinguished between the groups of surgeons. Furthermore, these types of detailed task performance metrics constitute the same types of parameters that the aviation industry uses in their analysis of near misses. The logic that the aviation industry uses is that each near miss is an accident waiting to happen. As pointed out previously, the performance units that we use in the objective assessment of performance may be better construed as "events" which are best defined by their outcomes but that each event set the occasion for a potential bad outcome to occur. These are what Reason (2000) refers to as the latent conditions in the chain of error causation. It should also be recalled that Reason was very clear that latent conditions are much easier to deal with than active failures. In essence, the technically poor performing surgeon is the latent condition that sets the occasion for active failures. Also, as discussed in Chaps. 4, 8, and 10, surgeons who struggle with relatively straightforward skills–based scenarios will not be able to cope with intraoperative clinical situations that are more demanding. In one sense, it is not their fault as they simply do not have the cognitive attentional resources to deal with the situation. However, who should recognize and act appropriately with this as a potential latent error situation: the surgeon? the hospital? their profession? A previous head of department once said that if he ignored some problems long enough, they just went away. We strongly suspect that this one would not and will in fact probably get worse as more and more evidence accrues linking bad outcome to the intraoperative performance of the operator. Also, this is not just a problem for surgery but for all of procedural-based medicine. Surgery just happens to be grasping the nettle first. We are fully aware that bad things happen to good surgeons and are very sympathetic to this view. Surgeons and other interventionalists have a very difficult and complex job to do. Unlike many other medical disciplines, they have to perform well technically while at the same time having to make difficult intraoperative decisions 'on-the-fly'. When many surgeons see a bad outcome happening to one of their peers, they think "there but for the grace of god go I." The surgeons with whom these infrequent events occur are not the surgeons we are alluding to.

Our approach to individuals who perform badly on the objective assessment is simply to exclude them from the proficiency definition process and take the matter no further. After all, their performance does not accurately reflect the vast majority of their peers' performance. Furthermore, the rule of thumb that we use in the exclusion is performance that is more than 1.96 standard deviations away from the mean (in a negative direction). It could be argued that performance in a positive direction creates as much of a problem; but to date, we have not found this to the case. Not everyone is happy with this approach, least of all the person who has been excluded from the proficiency definition. However, there is little else that can be done at this stage. This is not simply a matter for the surgical community to resolve. We have made the same observations in other procedural-based disciplines in medicine. The scientific issue that begs to be resolved is the unambiguous establishment of a relationship and the strength of that relationship between objectively assessed intraoperative performance and clinical outcomes. This question is answerable. The study would need to be very large and conducted independently in the countries around the world who carry major responsibilities for training large numbers of procedural-based specialists. It should also be noted that the vast majority of operating surgeon's have absolutely nothing to fear from this process. It will quantitatively confirm what we already know and that is that the majority of operating surgeons perform similar to their peers. A small number will be outstanding performers and a very small minority will demonstrate considerable skills deficits.

Regional, National, and International Levels of Proficiency

In the USA, the American Boards of Surgery and Internal Medicine, etc., are responsible for the examination and licensure of surgeons and physicians across the entire country. Currently their examination system consists mainly of knowledge and decision-making assessments. However, with wider acceptance of the validity of technical skills assessment, it offers the opportunity to standardize assessment of this aspect of surgical performance across the USA. Furthermore, these assessment and credentialing boards are well known for the rigor with which they apply to the assessment process. This assessment process could be used as a liberal inclusion process rather than a conservative exclusion process. However, the outcome would almost certainly mean that individuals whose technical performance may best be characterized as "outliers" would almost disappear. In the USA, re-credentialing is a non-negotiable part of practicing as a doctor. This process would also ensure less performance variability across the country. The data could also be used to establish where on the performance distribution surgical graduates from other countries lay. The process could even facilitate the credentialing of international surgical graduates who wished to work in the USA. Although no equivalent credentialing system exists in the UK and Ireland, there are urgent plans to implement a similar system. One of the problems that the UK and Irish system have is that surgical graduates from outside the jurisdiction are entitled to apply for training positions and jobs. However, there is little or no way of objectively establishing how good, bad, or indifferent is the applicant's performance. A valid and reliable system for the assessment of technical skills would considerably simplify answering that question. This would ensure a much fairer approach to the applicant and an even fairer treatment of the patient.

This approach to credentialing has other, possibly less attractive ramifications for procedural specialties like surgery. We have possibly seen a glimpse of the future in the FDA decision on carotid artery stenting with an embolic protection device. In the rollout of this relatively new approach to treatment for carotid artery disease, vascular surgeons who normally treated this condition found themselves in competition with interventional cardiologists, interventional radiologists, interventional neuroradiologists, and neurosurgeons. The decision of the FDA and The Centers for Medicare and Medicaid Services (or CMS) was that all interested medical specialties who could demonstrate proficiency in performing the procedure could claim reimbursement (Gallagher and Cates 2004a). This was made possible because part of the FDA decision included an acceptance that proficiency could be achieved in part by training on a high-fidelity virtual reality simulation. Furthermore, rather than simply relying on procedural numbers, proficiency demonstration on the simulator could be underpinned with metric-based performance characterization. Although the FDA decision related to the marketing and sale of the device, the impact radiates outward to medical practice as no physician of any procedure specialty could use the device in the absence of other skills associated with making appropriate interventional judgments about the patient's care. The physician may be proficient in the use of the device, capable of deploying the device in the correct fashion, but the physician may still not be allowed to perform the procedure. To ensure safe care of patients, an operating physician requires patient-specific knowledge of the anatomy, pathophysiology, treatment effects, and robust knowledge of the overall clinical status of the patient. Simulator training may be necessary for proficiency to be demonstrated, but simulator training alone is not sufficient for a physician to be certified as competent to perform interventional care (Dawson 2006).

Dawson (2006) also argues that simulator-based training is not a replacement for clinical experience. We tend to disagree with him on this point. We agree with him that simulation will not entirely replace clinical experience. However, it will supplant a large part of it particularly in the early stage of the learning curve where it is very difficult to justify basic procedural training on a sick patient. The full impact and ramifications of the FDA decision have not been fully realized yet. However, the FDA decision has levelled the playing field in terms of which medical specialty can perform interventional procedures. We believe that this decision will impact on who can be credentialed to perform other procedures such as colonoscopy, natural orifice total endoscopic surgery and a wide range of new percutaneous endovascular procedures. The FDA decision means that large governmental organizations now know that they do not have to take an individual physician's or medical specialties' word about their capability to perform a given procedure safely. They can now insist on quantitative evidence to demonstrate this fact. We are not entirely sure where this development is going to lead but we feel certain that it will have profound implications for the practice of safe interventional medicine. The FDA decision may have no legal implications outside the USA but precedents are difficult to ignore when grappling with similar issues in similar circumstances.

What is the Relationship Between Proficiency and Competency?

In the Dreyfus et al. (1986) model of skill acquisition, they describe proficiency as a more advanced stage of skill acquisition than competency. Their proposal is a useful heuristic in trying to conceptualize the process of learning skills. However, their proposal contributes very little to the operational definition and measurement of the different levels of skills development that they outline. What they propose for the different levels of skills development are nothing more than descriptive indicators which are really not much better than the descriptions of competency outlined by the Accreditation Council for Medical Education (Beall 1999) in the USA and the General Medical Council (1993) in the UK. The clinical trials conducted on proficiency-based progression training have avoided the term "competency"-based progression because of the lack of an unambiguous and agreed-upon definition of what is competence. Ironically, the operational definition of competence is purely a matter of words and agreement within the medical profession itself. The difference between the concept of proficiency that we propose here and that has been operationalized in previous clinical trials (Ahlberg et al. 2007; Seymour et al. 2002; Van Sickle et al. 2008b) is that there is a general consensus among physicians and surgeons that doctors currently in practice are at least competent, probably proficient, and some are expert. The other difference is that proficiency has been quantitatively defined based on the performance of doctors whom most people agree are competent and/or proficient. Hence, the definition is parsimonious, i.e., proficiency is what proficient doctors do. This means that by default, proficiency has already been quantified for some tasks and surgical procedures. Furthermore, this methodology has been validated both in terms of metric validation and clinical validation. Would this approach solve the impasse on the issue of competence? We suspect not.

The issues that medicine has about competency are not to do with measurement they are more to do with agreeing on a definition. Once a benchmark has been set for the measurement of competence, the logical conclusion of this process means that some individuals will be measured as "not competent." There is considerable trepidation among physicians and surgeons about this eventuality even though as stated earlier that the majority of practitioners have absolutely nothing to fear. Our concern is that at some point, medicine may be forced to quantitatively define competence at a time and over an issue that is not of medicines choosing. At some point, someone, possibly a legislator, possibly a failed trainee, possibly the very wealthy parents of a failed trainee, is going to ask, "When exactly is someone deemed competent or conversely when are they deemed incompetent?" An individual who failed to progress in the competency-based training system in the USA or in the UK must have failed to demonstrate one or more specific competencies. The concept of competency, if it is to be at all meaningful, must be verifiable and falsifiable (Popper 1979). That is probably one of the first questions that the lawyer will ask of a training organization that stopped the training of the litigant. Using the word "competency" and "competence" numerous times during their answer will not be an adequate defense. The lawyer will want to know the specific criteria that are objective, measurable, transparent and fair, and which clearly demarcates the difference between competent and incompetent performance. As things currently stand, medicine would be in considerable difficulties. This is a very difficult issue to resolve.

Compounding this problem is our suspicion that the profession of medicine and the general public (and remember politicians and senior civil servants make up the general public as well) have contradictory notions about precisely what competence means. Medicine probably construes competency as something closer to the dictionary definition. In contrast, we believe that the general public's views of medical competence is something more akin to the dictionary definition of proficiency.

- *Competence*: describes those behaviors required for satisfactory ("threshold competence") performance in a job
- *Proficiency*: describes the ability to perform a specific behavior (e.g., task) to the established performance standard in order to demonstrate mastery of the behavior; skillfulness in the command of fundamentals deriving from practice and familiarity

This is a relatively straightforward question to answer but the response may pose even more difficulties for medicine. It is our belief that the general public does not construe "medical competence" or just passing and no more. Medical competence appears to be construed as performing at a higher level. However, it would be useful if medicine could quantitatively answer this question and so avoid potentially awkward questions and possibly even more awkward answers. Damaging public confidence in medicine further is probably not a good idea at the present time!

Dreyfus et al. (1986) suggested that in the process of skill progression, there is never a clear demarcation between one level and the next (Chap. 8). This means, for example, that the performance characteristics of the novice will at certain times be more similar to the advanced beginner than they are to the novice level. This does not mean that at these times, the novice is a fully fledged advanced beginner. They may demonstrate some of the performance characteristics, but this is likely to be in superficial aspects such as technical skill and not in characteristics such as wisdom. This is most likely to be the case in surgical skill progression. For example, in the proficiency-based progression clinical trials that have already been conducted, the researchers would not argue that the proficiency-trained surgical trainees had the same procedural wisdom as the attending and consultant surgeons on whom their technical skill benchmark was based. All that the trainees did was demonstrate the proficiency benchmark of the more experienced surgeons on two consecutive training trials and having done this, they also demonstrated superior objectively assessed intraoperative performance than a traditional trained group. This means that the trainees demonstrated performance characteristics of proficient surgeons but this does not mean that the trainees themselves are proficient. Only one specific aspect of the performance was trained and tested during the clinical trial. We find the simplicity of this approach very appealing because it avoids convoluted discussions which have been ongoing for some period of time but at the same time does not compromise the quality of trainee performance.

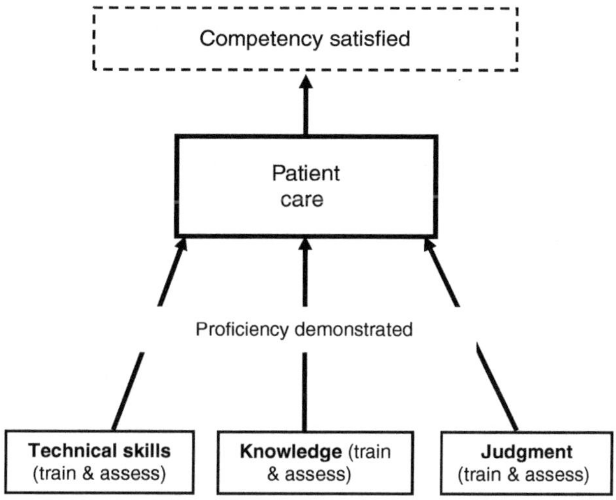

Fig. 12.1 A core competency satisfied, built on real-world defined attributes that are objectively assessable and based on empirically demonstrable characteristics which are defendable!

Figure 12.1 shows how this approach might be implemented in a manner similar to proficiency-based progression clinical trials that have already been conducted. It shows a hypothetical process of meeting the ACGME “Patient Care” core competency. Metric-based assessment for the constituent components for the patient care competency, i.e., technical skills, knowledge, and judgment could be developed very much in the manner we described in Chap. 5. These could then be used to characterize how experienced surgeons perform against these metrics, thus establishing a proficiency level. Trainees would then be required to demonstrate proficiency on the performance characteristics. Once demonstrated on all three performance characteristics, by default, the trainee has just demonstrated competency in this core competency. The precise number of times that the trainees should demonstrate proficiency or the methodology used for a trainee to demonstrate proficiency will still need some discussion but this is a relatively straightforward question that can be answered quantitatively. In its simplest form, the question asks: how many times must proficiency be demonstrated so that the trainee is assessed as safe as can be hoped for without significantly compromising the amount of time it takes to fully train a surgeon. Figure 12.2 shows how this approach might be applied to trainee surgeons demonstrating all six ACGME core competencies. After demonstrating proficiency in the different performance characteristics that constitute the core competency, the trainee is, by default, competent.

This approach to competency-based training avoids some of the difficulties of trying to operationally define competence in a way that the vast majority medical of practitioners will agree. It also ensures that there is no compromise in the quality of the skills the surgeon brings to patient treatment and care. It does however deal with the question of “What is the demarcation between competence and failure to reach competence”? Furthermore, it has answered the question of how to actually define what is competence. This approach is also flexible enough to allow the progression to be optimally paced for the trainee while still not compromising on the quality of

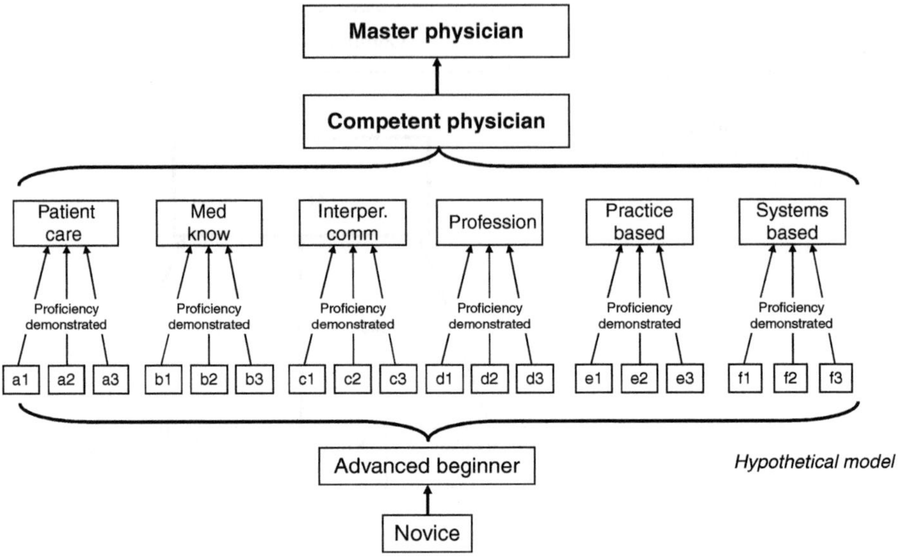

Fig. 12.2 The ACGME six core competencies: An alternative hypothetical model for acquiring and demonstrating "medical competence"

training. Furthermore, it provides a very clear quantitative benchmark which has been unambiguously defined for trainees and potential litigants. The GMC in the UK has the assessment infrastructure already in place to implement such a strategy. They have formative assessments in the form of the DOPS and they have summative assessments in the form of PBAs (Chap. 8). The PBAs may need some development work so as to eliminate assessment items such as, "optimum" (without definition), "adequate," "sound," and "purposeful." This is a relatively simple matter. They could then be used to quantitatively define levels of proficiency for the index procedures already identified. This would make a very robust assessment system.

Whatever approach is taken to solve the verification or falsifiability issue, a less ambiguous training endpoint will have to be developed by the major surgical training bodies around the world. As we have clearly indicated throughout this book, time in training is not a good predictor of skill and if, as the training bodies state, they have a competency-based training program, why not have competency or proficiency as the indicator of training completion rather than the time in training. If the trainees are given end of training benchmarks such as levels of proficiency that have been quantitatively defined on the basis of experienced surgeons performance, they will probably find that acceptable or very difficult to disagree with. Of course, this assumption is based on the premise that the training facilities are made available to them in order to demonstrate the level of proficiency. That means that they must have access to training facilities where they can engage in deliberate practice. Defining an unambiguous training endpoint could possibly create its own problems. For example, assuming that the issues pertaining to proficiency and competency are satisfactorily resolved with an unambiguous outcome, resulting in a clearly defined quantitative end of training based on objectively assessed performance of the trainee, what are training bodies going to do with trainee surgeons who progress rapidly through the proficiency-based progression training cycle? It is assumed that proficiency will have been demonstrated in the process with something like their PBAs on real patients. Should the trainees who demonstrate proficiency first give up their operative cases so that their peers have more opportunities to demonstrate proficiency? or should they progress to the next training rotation? (Oh, but for such a problem)! This sort of scenario could play havoc with training rotations and the administration of a training program. However, it could also offer the opportunity to radically reduce the number of years in training without compromising the quality of the graduating surgeon.

Optimized Training Availability

There is a growing body of data from clinical studies that shows proficiency-based progression training on simulation models is a better way to train procedural-based surgical skills. It is also clear that these training models work because they afford the opportunity for the trainee to engage in deliberate practice. Deliberate practice differs from repeated practice (the ethos of the traditional approach to training) because of the way the curriculum content is configured, delivered, and assessed. Trainees on a proficiency-based progression training schedule engage in deliberate practice with formative feedback, which shapes and optimizes their performance. The optimal application of this type of training program assumes that the trainee engages in a didactic educational program (which is also proficiency-based progression) before being offered technical skills training. The evidence from clinical trials shows that proficiency-based progression training using this approach has resulted in superior objectively assessed intraoperative performance when compared to the traditionally trained surgeons. These results have been demonstrated for basic laparoscopic procedures such as cholecystectomy and for advanced procedures such as laparoscopic Nissen fundoplication. The training for laparoscopic cholecystectomy was conducted on virtual reality simulation (Ahlberg et al. 2007; Seymour et al. 2002) and Nissen fundoplication training was completed on improvised simulation models (Van Sickle et al. 2008b). Deliberate practice coupled with formative feedback on both types of simulations significantly improved objectively assessed intraoperative performance in comparison to traditionally trained surgeons. However, one of the most important lessons learned from these studies was the additional effort that had to be invested to implement a proficiency-based progression training program on a simulation that was not computer generated. The simulation models used in the Van Sickle et al. study were perfectly adequate for achieving the goals of the training program and did a good job at facilitating the acquisition of intracorporeal suturing skills that transferred to intracorporeal suturing in Nissen fundoplication. The problem with this training program was the implementation of the formative and summative assessments. In vivo training on these simulation models had to be supervised by a researcher who was very familiar with the application of the performance metrics. They also had to assess the quality on all of the knots tied during training. Possibly the process could have been made more efficient by training two subjects at a time rather than just one subject. However, even with this strategy, it is a very expensive approach to training; imagine a standard class size of 20–30 trainees. These are the sorts of numbers the Royal College of Surgeons in Ireland train daily in its skills laboratory.

One of the most important lessons learned from the Van Sickle et al. study was the value of computer-generated and scored virtual reality tasks. It makes the entire training process orders of magnitude more efficient. This is an important lesson because surgical training programs that opt to conduct this type of surgical training purely for training purposes and not for research purposes are very unlikely to have the personnel resources to invest. Although all of the researchers conducting the training in the Van Sickle et al. study were highly trained on the implementation of the formative metrics; the fact that they were delivered by a person rather than a computer can allow subjectivity to creep into the assessment process. Even if the researchers had implemented assessment of psychomotor performance using something like ICSAD for measuring hand movements, intra-operative task performance would still be required, during training, to comply with the formative assessment aspect of training. These findings and conclusions point to the urgent need for wider availability and use of computer-generated and scored virtual reality simulation tasks for training procedural-based skills such as surgery. Evidence clearly shows that they are effective and efficient at delivering deliberate practice training as part of a proficiency-based progression skill acquisition program. One of the problems that disciplines like surgery have is that most of the virtual reality simulations available commercially are for minimally invasive or endovascular procedures.

Open Surgical Simulation

The traditional open incision remains the most common approach to performing surgical procedures. In spite of this, practically all of the surgical simulations that are currently available on the market are for some type of minimally invasive intervention such as laparoscopic, endoscopic, or endovascular. A range of silicone-based and animal tissue models are currently used for the training and assessment of surgical skills for open surgery. However, one of the problems with these tasks is that the silicone models vary in the degree they approximate the actual surgical task/procedure on a real patient. For example, some of the silicone models for training suturing are inappropriate for training a subcuticular suturing technique as the suture material tends to rip through the foam material. The bowel and anastomosis models also have similar problems, and while they may look acceptable when the task has been completed, they are really not very good for assessments such as leakage of the anastomosis. The water tends to seep through the small holes through which the needle passed. The advantage of these types of models is that they can be used in almost any teaching space. Animal tissue can be used as an alternative to silicone with the advantage that in general, they have many of the properties of human tissue. However, the problem with these tasks is that they require specialist facilities for use and disposal, e.g., specialist tables, flooring, cleaning, etc. Both of these types of simulation training models have been used for training purposes for decades. However, with a better understanding of how to achieve effective and efficient training, e.g., deliberate practice, and pressures on the amount of time available for training, these models look increasingly unattractive. The greatest problem with using them is providing performance and summative feedback to the trainee in an efficient and cost-effective manner. Procedural-based medicine trainers and educationalists (undergraduate and postgraduate) should come to the realization that there is an urgent need to develop virtual reality simulations for the training of open surgical skills. There are some simulations that claim to train open surgical skills such as giving an intravenous injection or taking blood. There are also a number of fairly large projects which are underway around the world whose outputs look as though it would take relatively little effort to develop them into full-blown virtual reality simulations for open surgical skills. The Virtual Physiological Human project (http://www.vph-noe.eu) is an extension of the virtual human project that is trying to do a multi-scale model of the human body. There is also the 3D Anatomical Human (http://3dah.miralab.ch) which claims to be more aligned with real-time interactive simulations of humans for practical applications rather than the basic science focus of the VPH project. The Simulation Open Framework Architecture (SOFA) is an Open Source framework primarily targeted at real-time simulation, with an emphasis on medical simulation. It is mostly intended for the research community to help develop newer algorithms, but can also be used as an efficient prototyping tool (http://www.sofa-framework.org/home). These efforts are to be commended but the problem with these approaches is that they are mostly proof-of-concept systems or designed for research and development. Furthermore, showing high-quality anatomical images is all well and good for display purposes to show what is possible with virtual reality. The problems come when they are required to be used for interactive hands-on simulation training.

Open Surgical Simulation: What Would It Take?

One of the major problems for the development of an open simulator is producing generalized solutions that are physics-appropriate and yet can run in real time. The more complex the interactions between tools, tissues, etc., the more complex the computation of the interactions become. For example, in a simple suturing task, the interactions will include needle holder grasping the needle that punctures tissue while needing to stabilize the tissue with another tool and also looping the suture thread around tools to begin cinching down the two sides of the wound which must contact one another and produce appropriate contact stresses and result in the proper inversion/eversion of the wound sides. These highly complex interactions are currently being tackled by Dr. Dwight Meglan and Prof. Howard Champion's (Simquest, Silver Springs, USA) team in their construction of a simple open surgery wound closure task. One of the major problems in creating an open simulation that is physics based is that there are very few people in the world who are experienced at developing this technology for a real-world application.

To develop solutions for the problem of open surgical simulation will require a very focused effort and considerable developments in existing knowledge, including physics-based simulation and engineering. To create a generalize able model of an open surgical procedure interacting with the anatomy of a human, it should probably start with putting together measurement tools that can define exactly what is physically happening in surgery, e.g., movements of tools, forces/torques/pressures at the interface of tool-tissue, etc. Then catalogs need to be developed for all of the tissues that need to be simulated in terms of their mechanics and construction (heterogeneous materials like muscles, nerves, blood vessels, lymph ducts, etc.), and the like. Also included in this catalog would be how the tissues are interconnected. In addition, a catalog of all tool-tissue interactions, both in type as well as in mechanics – details like how grasp really happens (friction, mechanical interference, etc.), the process of tissue failure in cutting, ablation mechanics, etc. From these units of information, an engineering approach would need to be developed to construct various entities at a foundational level and form more complex tissues from these. As a lot of this information will be novel, quantitative engineering tests would need to be conducted at each level of construction to prove how well the simulations match reality, both in terms of mechanics as well as in terms of speed of computation. Simultaneous with the tissue buildup, detailed tool–tissue interaction physics would need to be developed and managed with the same approach for doing deconstructed simulations at the lowest level first and building up from those with the same engineering property and simulation assessments being conducted at each level.

To ensure optimal functionality, this project would require focus around one deliverable simulation project; large enough that it answers a lot of simulation, physics and, engineering questions about building an open surgical simulator, but is also something that was manageable. This would minimize the development of disparate entities with their own research and development agendas. To undertake this challenging project would require people who are good at computational numerics and who also appreciate the need for real-time results. It would also need people familiar with computed interactions because we have been informed that this turns out to be much harder than doing the physics of the objects (like finite elements) especially when you want to do it in real time. Obviously, an open surgical simulator would require haptics and graphics developers. Development would also require individuals who are comfortable at undertaking task deconstruction of the surgeries and defining an approach/architecture to build up a general solution. Finally, the simulation development would require high-level developers who would concentrate on the construction of the learning scenarios (tools and data), defining the learning focus of the scenarios, assembling some form of automated instruction/

mentoring as well as formative and summative metric aspects as well as verification and validation studies.

Who Is Going to Pay?

A textbook on fundamental principles of surgical simulation would be incomplete if we did not attempt to address how the principles and practices that we have described and discussed are going to be implemented and paid for. If the decision is taken by a surgical training program to implement even part of a simulation-based deliberate practice regime for proficiency-based progression training, they are going to require more resources. The least that they will require is experienced assessors to ensure that trainees get sufficient formative feedback on their performance during training. This assumes of course that the program leaders have already conducted the task analysis, developed the intraoperative or task performance metrics, and validated them, including the development of proficiency levels. These developments will significantly improve the effectiveness of current training, particularly if they were coupled with an online didactic education program linked to the skills laboratory training and schedule in the appropriate order. The use of staff to provide performance assessment during training is not a particularly efficient approach. In the short term, we really do not see that medicine will have an alternative but to make the training of procedural skills more effective. Doing nothing is not a sensible option.

A more efficient approach would use computer-generated virtual reality tasks for training. Unfortunately, a virtual reality simulator for training open surgical skills does not currently exist. We have some idea of what it would take to develop an open surgical simulation platform (which we described above). The development of one simulation platform for a specific open surgical procedure would cost between £50 and £100 million and probably take 3–5 years to complete assuming that the appropriate expertise could be found and employed to build it. The development of virtual reality simulations which can be used as actual training devices is orders of magnitude more difficult than producing virtual reality images, no matter how sophisticated those images are. At the moment, it is not clear who will pay for the development of such a device. We shall come back to this issue after we had discussed funding for the simulators that currently do exist.

As we have pointed out on a number of occasions, virtual reality simulations currently exist for minimally invasive and endovascular procedure. Although these approaches still represent a minority of approaches to interventional procedural-based medicine, these types of procedures still constitute a substantial number of operations per year. Furthermore, these procedures are significantly more difficult to learn than the traditional open approach to surgery. Some of these simulators have been developed since the mid-1990s (e.g., MIST VR) and clinical data showing their effectiveness as training tools has been available since the start of the twenty-first century. There remains no consensus about who should pay for these devices. In the USA, the ACGME has insisted that surgical training programs should provide access to simulations and simulators. Despite a relatively standardized training program in the USA, there appears to be no coherent approach to the purchase and implementation of surgical simulation. The American College of Surgeons launched a program to accredit institutions which aimed to enhance access to educational opportunities in surgical training (Haluck et al. 2007). No extra monies were available to fund accredited institutions even though it was acknowledged that the financial and logistical considerations of establishing an institution were considerable. One of the good things about this effort was that it was National with implicit agreement to share experiences (both good and bad) in relation to training and simulation. This approach at least ensures that institutions do not replicate the same mistakes.

Ironically, simulations for minimally invasive approaches to performing procedures are probably the easiest to fund. Medical device companies continue to refine and develop new instruments for performing surgical and other interventional procedures. Currently, most of the training that these companies conduct to ensure that the surgeon or physician are familiar with the instruments is conducted in animal laboratories. This is a very expensive way to train to use relatively straightforward devices. The medical device manufacturers who produce endovascular devices such as catheters, stents, and wires probably have the greatest incentive to use virtual reality simulations for training as the animal models that currently exist bare little similarity to operating on patients. Furthermore, training using full physics virtual reality simulations means that the doctor can be trained to use the exact same device, in the exact same order, on more or less the same anatomy as they would in a real patient. Although these companies have invested heavily in these devices, their attitude toward virtual reality simulations indicates that they are not really sure what a huge business opportunity full physics virtual reality simulation represents for them. This is probably because they do not fully understand the capabilities of full physics virtual reality simulation. Some of them may even believe that it does not look or feel like operating on a real patient. As we have explained in Chaps. 3 and 10, the sensations that individuals detect from operating on real patient human anatomy and surgical instruments are perceived differently by each individual and the function of virtual reality simulation is not to simulate each individual's perceptual experience, rather it is to provide a reference case that is anatomically correct which can facilitate completion of a full procedure using the exact same devices as on a real patient.

Virtual reality training is a less expensive way for device manufacturers to train their sales staff who in turn can provide training for doctors to use the device. We are surprised that more multinational medical device companies have not made greater use of full physics virtual reality simulation in the design and marketing of their product. Engine design, automobile manufacturers, and Formula 1 racing teams currently make extensive use of virtual reality simulation in the design and preparation of their products. We are not entirely sure of the budget ratio between marketing and manufacturing of a new medical device but we do know that it is substantial. It would seem to us that more aggressive use of virtual reality simulation would give considerable manufacturing and marketing advantage which proportionately would almost certainly convert into increased sales. Furthermore, we would have thought that the FDA decision on including virtual reality training as part of the roll out of carotid artery stenting with embolic protection would have given a very clear lead on this issue (Gallagher and Cates 2004a).

Although medical device companies may not have used virtual reality simulation to its full potential in their research and development of a product, they certainly have been keen to sponsor training events that utilize simulation. At most of the major medical conferences for procedural-based disciplines such as surgery, interventional cardiology and interventional radiology, etc., virtual reality simulations are now a common sight in the booths of the large medical device manufacturers. There has been some discussion within the professional societies about approaching the large multinational medical device manufacturers and requesting that they pay (fairly large sums of money) for simulators for surgical training centers. However, even if the manufacturers paid for or "sponsored" the simulators, they would have no say on how the simulators would be used, nor of the curriculum content which from the manufacturers' perspective may not seem a very good deal. As it currently stands, the medical device industry is relatively generous with its arm's-length sponsorship of courses and events. However, the medical device industry continues to appear bemused by the potential of this very powerful technology. Paying for further original development of simulations does not appear to be imminent from this source.

The Royal College of Surgeons in Ireland has a well-developed surgical training center and pursues a training and assessment strategy using a wide range of simulations and simulators. They have also adopted one of the most innovative approaches to the implementation of a training and assessment strategy using simulation. Surgical trainees in Ireland *must* attend the national surgical training center for a minimum of 6 days per year for training. To pay for this facility, each trainee is charged €3,000 per year (which is tax deductible). However, this does not even cover 50% of what it costs to train trainee surgeons for the 6-days training provided. Irish surgical trainees would probably be considerably more disgruntled if they were charged in excess of €7,000 per year for their simulation-based training. The unwritten and unspoken understanding in postgraduate medical training in the USA seems to be that the trainee will work long hours, accept relatively poor pay and help to look after the attending surgeons' patients in return for being trained as a surgeon. However, with reduced work hours and consequently reduced opportunities for training, especially in the operating room, this unwritten "arrangement" seems to be under increasing pressure. Furthermore, surgical trainees in the USA and mainland Europe simply can not afford the full costs of skills laboratory training.

One possibility that could be used to subsidize training within institutions is for attending/consultant surgeons to develop procedure-specific teaching modules that are accompanied with a fully developed didactic module and an edited video recording of a specific procedure with running commentary. For some operations such as endovascular procedures, the surgeon could also make available the patient-specific data that could be downloaded into a virtual reality simulator for the trainee to practice the procedure that they had just studied. This for fee service could then be used by trainees (as well as much more experienced interventionists) to consolidate and expand their procedure experience. Indeed, whether or not this service develops commercially, we fully envisage it developing over the next decade to supplement the experience of experienced surgeons whose practice will probably be forced to become more and more specialized.

The possibility of professional societies and medical device manufacturers coming together to run and finance simulation-based training is currently a reality. Almost all of the procedural-based medical disciplines around the world rely heavily on the sponsorship of industry to help finance courses that they organize. This financial support reduces the cost of the courses but does not cover them completely. In general, this sponsorship is usually only available for trainees who are fairly advanced in their training or for consultant/attending courses. Furthermore, it seems highly likely that industry sponsorship for these types of courses in the future will become more and more restrictive as national governmental organizations and audit offices monitor ever closer the relationship between medical device companies and physicians. It is difficult to see what this relationship will morph into but we find it hard to believe that medical device manufacturers will not have a significant role in financing courses in the future. It may be that they sponsor or own the simulators on which the courses are run. The fact remains that interventional attending specialist courses must have hands-on experience with the devices they are going to use on real patients. Full physics virtual reality simulation certainly seems to us to be the best model on which to train and we do not see how training can be conducted without using the actual physical devices. Furthermore, it is probably best if an expert from the manufacturing company explains to the trainees how best to use the devices rather than have a surgeon or other interventionist explain how they use it. In our experience, these two accounts do not always correlate, and for safety and insurance purposes, it is probably best that the surgeon or interventionist hears directly from the manufacturers of the device how it should be used. Then, if the surgeon or interventionist decides not to use it the way suggested by the manufacturer, there can be little ambiguity where the fault lies if anything goes wrong.

An interesting development has been ongoing in Massachusetts at the Harvard Risk Management Foundation which provides malpractice insurance for doctors working in their health-care system. Anesthetists as well as obstetricians and gynecologists who have undergone a rigorous simulation and training program are eligible for up to 10% discount if they successfully complete the risk reduction course which involves team training simulation. Malpractice insurance for physicians in the USA is very expensive and a 10% reduction represents a substantial amount of money. We believe that the system could be optimized even further if the insurers insisted that course participants demonstrated a level of proficiency and that proficiency was based on the performance of a large group of interventionalists, e.g., surgeons, interventional cardiologists, and interventional radiologists. We believe that this would considerably reduce the risk of something untoward happening for the majority of physicians. We are very surprised that malpractice insurers have not made greater use of this facility particularly given the validation evidence that currently exists and the very clear relationship between proficiency-based progression and improved intraoperative performance.

In the UK and Ireland, it is not uncommon for institutional changes of the magnitude that we have outlined here to be financed by central government. If we return to the issue of paying for the development of an open surgical simulator, none of the organizations that we have discussed thus far either have the resources or the inclination to invest in such a development. Instruments that are used to perform open surgery are (in general) not disposable and do not really change that much over the years; the simulation companies who could potentially develop an open simulator do not have £50–£100 million to invest; it is probable that the professional societies do not have that amount of spare cash lying around and even if they did, getting agreement from them as to which open surgical procedure should be simulated first would be an interesting exercise; anyway, surgical training has been conducted perfectly satisfactorily for centuries on real patients. None of these answers leads to a satisfactory state of affairs. The fact is that an open surgical simulator is urgently required. Even starting today, it would take 3–5 years to build a working prototype that could be copied. It would probably take another 5 years of concerted effort to get an open surgical simulator to the same level of fidelity that we have for endovascular interventions. Furthermore, there is a latent landmine waiting to explode. As interventional medicine becomes less and less invasive for more and more procedures, how are the surgical community expected to retain their expertise and skill level for open surgical procedures that are common today but will almost certainly become infrequent in the near future? Avoiding these difficult questions will not make them go away.

We believe that a number of fairly straightforward developments would clarify matters pertaining to the financing of training and simulation developments. Training systems in the USA, UK, and Ireland seem to agree that competency-based training programs are the way forward. However, the problem is that they cannot or would not agree on a quantitative definition of competency that is verifiable or falsifiable. Whether the training system is based on competency or proficiency may be considered a matter of semantics. An agreed-upon quantitative measure such as those that have been used in a number of studies and proposed here adds considerable clarity to the issue of how training should be conducted in the future. If a level of proficiency was mandated and training progression was dependent upon it, then organizations that run training courses would have a much clearer idea of the market they had to deal with. Proficiency-based progression training on a deliberate practice regime leads to superior intraoperative performance in comparison to traditional training; there can be little doubt about the data. It would be a very foolish pundit who would bet against these results translating into improved operative outcomes. This means that a number of national or regional training centers would be responsible for deliberate practice training regimes in skills laboratories. There would also be a National Curriculum with a coherent e-learning program which would also be proficiency-based and implemented as a pre-requisite for attending skills linked courses at the regional or national training center. Establishment of these centers would almost certainly have to be funded from governmental sources and where possible subsidized or co-sponsored by industry. It should be remembered that the industry will want to use these facilities as well to train interventionists on their devices. This type of setup, with regional training centers possibly linked with an overarching informal organizational group such as the one set up by the American College of Surgeons would almost certainly ensure more efficient and effective training with national benchmarks.

In the financial year 2008/2009, Germany invested/spent €144 million, France €111 million, and the UK €107 million in The European Organization for Nuclear Research (Organisation Européenne pour la Recherche Nucléaire or originally *Conseil Européen pour la Recherche Nucléaire*) known as CERN. It is the largest particle physics laboratory in the world situated in the northwest suburbs of Geneva on the Franco–Swiss border (established in 1954). Each of these governments would argue that this money was invested/spent for the national and international good of mankind. In the USA, the Centers for Medicare and Medicaid Services (CMS) which is the equivalent of the NHS in the UK has an annual budget of approximately $780 billion per year. In the UK, the Department of Health spent £100 billion in 2008/9. It is difficult to envisage why the finance necessary to fund the *proper* establishment of simulation and training centers cannot be found. The same is true about the development of an open surgical simulator.

As the development of new minimally invasive technologies are implemented into healthcare, it is very easy to forget that if something goes wrong, it is probably a surgeon performing an open surgical procedure who will have to pick up the pieces. The changes in work practices, the opportunities to acquire procedural expertise and wisdom are contracting dramatically. Furthermore, acquiring the basic surgical skills on real patients is no longer acceptable. Professionals in disciplines like surgery are now aware that the process of acquiring proficient skills can be made more effective and efficient with a regime of deliberate practice. However, the current curriculum needs to be reconfigured and new tools are required for the delivery of a newly configured curriculum. Simulation-based regional and national training centers that can deliver the curriculum are required urgently. These centers will not be cheap to establish and maintain. Furthermore, they need to be appropriately staffed as the absence of high-fidelity simulation that can provide formative feedback on performance must be substituted with experienced supervision and the application of the same metrics. The development of a full physics virtual reality simulator for training open surgical skills is extremely urgent and we would propose that it should be considered as a national or indeed international priority development in healthcare.

Summary

Proficiency-based progression training on a simulator is a new approach to training doctors. Much of the ethos that is fundamental to proficiency-based progression training is not new. "Competency-based curriculum in any setting assumes that the many roles and functions involved in the doctor's work can be defined and clearly expressed. It does not imply that the things defined are the only elements of competence, but rather that those that can be defined represent a critical point of departure in curriculum development. Careful delineation of these components of medical practice is the first and most critical step in designing a competency-based curriculum" (McGaghie et al. 1978). Whether a training program is called competency-based progression or proficiency-based progression is a matter of semantics. However, as clearly stated by McGaghie et al., a training goal must be defined before it is established. No training program that currently claims to train competency-based progression has unambiguously defined competency endpoints that are falsifiable. In contrast, proficiency-based progression training studies have defined endpoints based on experienced surgeons' performance and established clear endpoints that are verifiable and falsifiable.

Proficiency-based progression training works because of well-proven principles and practices of learning. To ensure the optimal effectiveness of a proficiency-based progression training program does not require a radical change in the current curriculum content. However, what does require radical change is how that curriculum is delivered and implemented. Virtual reality simulation is a very powerful training tool for the delivery of deliberate practice coupled to formative and summative metrics on performance. In the absence of computer-generated simulation, formative metrics on training performance needs to be delivered by a trainer who is very experienced at performance assessment. Some virtual reality simulators currently exist in minimally invasive surgery and endovascular procedures. There are none for the training of open surgical procedures despite the fact that open surgery remains the most common type of procedural intervention and is also associated with the highest rate of errors. This situation needs to be addressed urgently.

A training program that has a clear end point must provide the facilities and opportunities for learning to meet the level of proficiency. A deliberate practice training regime affords the opportunity for independent pacing of skill acquisition; a coherent curriculum with appropriately sequenced learning material; and a variety of learning experiences (lecturers, seminars, small group teaching, e-learning, silicon models, virtual reality emulators, high-fidelity virtual reality simulators and real patients) optimize learning availability; and formative and summative metric–based assessments maximize the probability of learning. Although this approach to medical education and training may be conceptually and intellectually appealing, it represents a paradigm shift in how doctors are educated and trained.

References

Ahlberg G, Enochsson L, Gallagher AG, et al. Proficiency-based virtual reality training significantly reduces the error rate for residents during their first 10 laparoscopic cholecystectomies. *Am J Surg*. 2007;193(6):797-804.

Bann S, Kwok KF, Lo CY, Darzi A, Wong J. Objective assessment of technical skills of surgical trainees in Hong Kong. *Br J Surg*. 2003;90(10):1294-1299.

Beall DP. The ACGME institutional requirements: what residents need to know. *J Am Med Assoc*. 1999;281(24):2352.

Bower JL, Christensen CM. Disruptive technologies: catching the wave. *Harv Bus Rev*. 1995;73: 43-53.

Centres R. Cholecystectomy practice transformed. *Lancet*. 1991;338(8770):789-790.

Dawson S. Procedural simulation: a primer1. *Radiology*. 2006;241(1):17.

Dreyfus HL, Dreyfus SE, Athanasiou T. *Mind Over Machine*. New York: Free Press; 1986.

Ericsson KA, Krampe RT, Tesch-Römer C. The role of deliberate practice in the acquisition of expert performance. *Psychol Rev*. 1993;100(3):363-406.

Gallagher AG, Cates CU. Approval of virtual reality training for carotid stenting: what this means for procedural-based medicine. *J Am Med Assoc*. 2004a;292(24):3024-3026.

Gallagher AG, Cates CU. Virtual reality training for the operating room and cardiac catheterisation laboratory. *Lancet*. 2004b;364(9444):1538-1540.

Gallagher AG, Cowie R, Crothers I, Jordan-Black JA, Satava RM. PicSOr: an objective test of perceptual skill that predicts laparoscopic technical skill in three initial studies of laparoscopic performance. *Surg Endosc*. 2003a;17(9):1468-1471.

Gallagher AG, Ritter EM, Satava RM. Fundamental principles of validation, and reliability: rigorous science for the assessment of surgical education and training. *Surg Endosc*. 2003b;17(10): 1525-1529.

Gallagher AG, Smith CD, Bowers SP, et al. Psychomotor skills assessment in practicing surgeons experienced in performing advanced laparoscopic procedures. *J Am Coll Surg*. 2003c;197(3): 479-488.

General Medical Council. *Tomorrow's Doctors: Recommendations on Undergraduate Medical Education*. London: GMC; 1993.

Haluck RS, Satava RM, Fried G, et al. Establishing a simulation center for surgical skills: what to do and how to do it. *Surg Endosc*. 2007;21(7):1223-1232.

Kazdin AE. *Behavior Modification in Applied Settings*. Pacific Grove: Brooks/Cole Publishing Co.; 1994.

Khan M, Bann S, Darzi A, Butler P. Assessing surgical skill using bench station models. *Plast Reconstr Surg*. 2007;120(3):793-800.

Kohn LT, Corrigan JM, Donaldson MS. *To Err Is Human: Building a Safer Health System*. Washington DC: National Academy Press; 2000:196-197.

Larsen CR, Grantcharov T, Aggarwal R, et al. Objective assessment of gynecologic laparoscopic skills using the LapSimGyn virtual reality simulator. *Surg Endosc*. 2006;20(9): 1460-1466.

Martin P, Martin PR, Bateson P. *Measuring Behaviour: An Introductory Guide*. Cambridge: Cambridge University Press; 1993.

Martin JA, Regehr G, Reznick R, et al. Objective structured assessment of technical skill (OSATS) for surgical residents. *Br J Surg*. 1997;84(2):273-278.

Mayo WJ. Medical education for the general practitioner. *Journal of the American Medical Association*, 1927;88(18):1377-1378.

McGaghie WC, Sajid AW, Miller GE, Telder TV, Lipson L. *Competency-based curriculum development in medical education: an introduction; Competency-based curriculum development in medical education: an introduction*: Geneva: World Health Organization 1978.

Popper KR. *Objective Knowledge: An Evolutionary Approach*. Oxford: Clarendon Press; 1979.

Reason J. Human error: models and management. *Br Med J*. 2000;320(7237):768.

Regenbogen SE, Greenberg CC, Studdert DM, Lipsitz SR, Zinner MJ, Gawande AA. Patterns of technical error among surgical malpractice claims: an analysis of strategies to prevent injury to surgical patients. *Ann Surg*. 2007;246(5):705.

Senate of Surgery. *Response to the General Medical Council Determination on the Bristol Case: Senate Paper 5*. London: The Senate of Surgery of Great Britain and Ireland; 1998.

Seymour NE, Gallagher AG, Roman SA, et al. Virtual reality training improves operating room performance: results of a randomized, double-blinded study. *Ann Surg*. 2002;236(4):458-463; discussion 463-454.

Somville F, van Sprundel M, Somville J. Analysis of surgical errors in malpractice claims in Belgium. *Acta Chir Belg*. 2010;110(1):11-18.

Swets JA. *Signal Detection Theory and ROC Analysis in Psychology and Diagnostics: Collected Papers*. Mahwah: Lawrence Erlbaum Associates; 1996.

Van Sickle K, Baghai M, Huang IP, Goldenberg A, Smith CD, Ritter EM. Construct validity of an objective assessment method for laparoscopic intracorporeal suturing and knot tying. *Am J Surg*. 2008a;196(1):74-80.

Van Sickle K, Ritter EM, Baghai M, et al. Prospective, randomized, double-blind trial of curriculum-based training for intracorporeal suturing and knot tying. *J Am Coll Surg*. 2008b;207(4): 560-568.

Author Index

A.G. Gallagher and G.C. O'Sullivan, *Fundamentals of Surgical Simulation*, Improving Medical Outcome - Zero Tolerance,
DOI 10.1007/978-0-85729-763-1, © Springer-Verlag London Limited 2012

Subject Index

MIX
Papier aus verantwortungsvollen Quellen
Paper from responsible sources
FSC® C105338

If you have any concerns about our products,
you can contact us on
ProductSafety@springernature.com

In case Publisher is established outside the EU,
the EU authorized representative is:
Springer Nature Customer Service Center GmbH
Europaplatz 3, 69115 Heidelberg, Germany

Printed by Libri Plureos GmbH
in Hamburg, Germany